Pumping INSULIN

Everything You Need to Succeed on an Insulin Pump

Edition 5.1

by John Walsh, P.A., C.D.T.C., and Ruth Roberts, M.A.

Torrey Pines Press
San Diego

Torrey Pines Press
1030 West Upas Street
San Diego, California 92103-3821
1-619-497-0900

Library of Congress Cataloging in Publication Data

Walsh, John and Roberts, Ruth

Pumping Insulin:

> Everything you need to succeed on an insulin pump, edition 5.1
> by John Walsh, PA, CDTC, and Ruth Roberts, MA

p. cm.
Includes bibliographical references.
Includes index.
1. Diabetes Popular Books
2. Diabetes Insulin
3. Diabetes Insulin-dependent diabetes
4. Diabetes Research
5. Insulin Therapeutic use
I. Title

Library of Congress Control Number: 2012935075
ISBN 1-884804-12-8 $27.95 Paperback

Printed in the United States of America

10 9 8 7 6 5 4 3 2

More Praise...

The deeper I read into **Pumping Insulin 5**, the clearer everything became. The word that kept popping into mind was "clarity." Every subject is covered in several ways until it becomes crystal clear to the reader – chapter previews, text, short summaries sidebars, and graphs. It is jam-packed with the most up-to-the-minute technical information on insulin pumps along with how to apply the information to one's everyday pump use.

> — Judith Jones Ambrosini
> Journalist, Author of **The Sisterhood of Diabetes**
> Type 1 and pumper
> Sea Girt, NJ

When I first started on an insulin pump 6 years ago, I was confused, afraid, and un-comfortable. My doctor at the time was little help and I wasn't familiar with the diabetes online community. I hated my pump because I didn't understand it. If I had been handed **Pumping Insulin** then, my transition from MDI to a pump would have been seamless. This book has all the tools to benefit people with diabetes. I feel so much more empowered because I finally know what is happening.

If you have diabetes and are even considering an insulin pump – READ THIS BOOK. It makes all the difference in the world!

> — Elizabeth Zabell Edelman
> Co-Founder and CEO, DiabetesDaily.com

Pumping Insulin is the quintessential guide to using an insulin pump. Each and every insulin pump manufacturer calculates suggested amounts of insulin differently and this book explains how to fully understand your insulin pump, when to follow its suggestions, and when to override them.

Kudos to John Walsh and Ruth Roberts for writing another outstanding edition of the "bible" of insulin pumping with a great guide for using a continuous glucose monitor (CGM).

> — Ellen H. Ullman, MSW
> Advocate for persons with diabetes

The 5th edition of **Pumping Insulin** is the most comprehensive, up-to-date resource for every piece of information related to starting, using or teaching insulin pumps. Whether you are a person with diabetes or a healthcare provider, I am certain the information in this book will benefit you.

> — Joe Largay, PAC, CDE
> Clinical Instructor, School of Medicine
> University of North Carolina Diabetes Care Center
> Durham, NC

This book provides an amazing wealth of information at your fingertips! It is an outstanding reference for patients and professionals alike who want to know about optimal management and diabetes care.

— Judy Gates, RN, MPH, CDE
Yucaipa, CA

This fantastic book keeps getting better and more comprehensive with each edition. I refer patients to it regularly, both type 1 and type 2, and MDI as well as pumpers or wannabe pumpers. The basic information on the important aspects of diabetes control with regard to carbohydrates, insulin, activity, exercise, menses, stress, illness, and growth are all addressed in a relatively easy and straightforward way. John and Ruth make this complex disease more comprehensible to physicians and people with diabetes alike. Kudos to them once again!

— Nancy JV Bohannon MD, FACP, FACE
1580 Valencia St. Suite #109
San Francisco, CA 94110-4415

I recommend **Pumping Insulin** to all my patients using insulin pumps and I frequently refer them back to the sections on testing bolus and basal rate doses, as well as the section on adjustments for exercise.

— Diane Krieger, MD
Medical Director Nutrition/Endocrinology, Miami Research Associates
Miami, FL

A great format allows you to quickly identify key information. This is the single "must have" book for pumpers and those considering pumping! **Pumping Insulin** benefits those on pumps from the improved control and increased flexibility that pumping can provide.

— Melany Hellstern
www.insulinpumps.ca
Mother of a successful pumper
Oakville, ON, Canada

The authors of **Pumping Insulin** lead us through the diabetes wilderness to safety with precision and wisdom. I thank them for sharing their knowledge and insights in this comprehensive guide to successful pumping. They truly show us that the most important thing we have to give people with diabetes is hope.

— Virginia Valentine CNS, BC-ADM, CDE
Clinical Nurse Specialist and person living well with diabetes, Diabetes Network®, Inc.
Albuquerque, New Mexico

Sometimes, a book can change your life. My A1c had never hit target before -- not in 16 years of type 1 diabetes, or doing 10-12 blood tests a day. **Pumping Insulin** gave me the techniques I needed to manage my diabetes with confidence. My A1c hit target just three weeks later, and I felt an energy that I didn't know I was missing.

Imagine swimming for 10 hours straight and having every single blood test come up exactly where you want it? Thanks to John and Ruth, I've done it! Diabetes feels like a different disease for me now, thanks to **Pumping Insulin**.

— Jen Alexander
Marathon swimmer
Recognized by the International Marathon Swimming Hall of Fame
Diabetes Exercise and Sports Assocation "Athlete of the Year" in 2008
Halifax, Nova Scotia

The new version of the classic **Pumping Insulin**, by Walsh and Roberts, is even better than before. It is packed with useful information on how to achieve and maintain control of type 1 diabetes using an insulin pump. This edition has lots of new information, including recommendations on the use of continuous glucose monitors and on how to use dietary information such as the effect of glycemic index and the effect of protein and fat. Most importantly, there is a multitude of practical, well thought-out bits of advice that will help the person with diabetes live a better, healthier life.

I give this book my highest recommendation for both patients and health professionals.

— W. Kenneth Ward, MD
Associate Professor of Endocrinology & Diabetes
Oregon Health and Science University
Senior Scientist, Legacy Health System
Portland, OR

It not often that you find a book that can be used equally by patients, educators, pump trainers, care givers and industry. This up-to-date version is well organized and approachable for all to use to optimize insulin delivery and diabetes care. I learn something new every time I pick it up.

— Howard Zisser, MD
Director of Clinical Research and Diabetes Technology
Sansum Diabetes Research Institute
Adjunct Professor/ Dept Chemical Engineering
University of California Santa Barbara
Santa Barbara, CA

I always recommend **Pumping Insulin** to my patients and their families who want to go into depth about using an insulin pump. It is also great reading for physicians, diabetes nurses and dietitians who care for children and adolescents on pumps. I wish it was available in Swedish to get a wider audience.

> — Ragnar Hanas, MD, PhD
> Author of **Type 1 Diabetes**
> Uddevalla Hospital, NU Hospital Group
> Uddevalla, Sweden

If you are already on an insulin pump or thinking about going on one – John and Ruth's book is one of the most comprehensive insulin pump books that you will want to keep as a reference guide.

> — Nadia Al-Samarrie
> Publisher/Editor in Chief, *Diabetes Health Magazine*
> Novato, CA

This book is a wonderful and sophisticated compendium of key aspects of insulin pump use. It is appropriate for anyone who is serious about pumping - both patients and their providers can benefit from it. The tables, worksheets, and examples are extremely helpful.

> — Robert A. Vigersky, MD
> Colonel, Medical Corps
> Director, Diabetes Institute
> Walter Reed National Military Medical Center
> Past-President of The Endocrine Society
> Professor of Medicine
> Uniformed Services University of the Health Science

The 5th edition of **Pumping Insulin** remains the Gold Standard on insulin pump therapy for both patients and health care providers. It provides nearly all of the information a person needs from considering whether to use a pump to solving most self-management problems. I recommend this book as the primary source of information about pumping to all of our patients, allied health care providers involved in diabetes care, as well as our medical students, medical residents, and diabetes fellows.

> — Frank Schwartz, MD, FACE
> Director, ARHI Diabetes Center
> Professor of Endocrinology
> Ohio University, Athens, OH

As an insulin pump and CGM user, and author of the German standard work to this topic, I thank John Walsh and Ruth Roberts for this brilliant American point of view. Very pragmatic outline, clear and direct language, many many text boxes, tables and figures – thank you!

> — Bernhard T. Gehr, Dr. med.
> Author of **CGM und Insulinpumpenfibel** and **Diabetes und Sportfibel**
> Centre for Diabetes and Metabolism
> Fachklinik Bad Heilbrunn, Germany

Pumping Insulin is an extremely informative and comprehensive resource on using an insulin pump, and in this new version, a CGM - so valuable! From data analysis to pregnancy, John Walsh and Ruth Roberts do an excellent job covering the specifics of how to use the best technology to achieve glucose control.

Although I've had diabetes for 25 years, been using an insulin pump for 15 years, and writing a free monthly newsletter on diabetes research and products for five-plus years, I've still learned plenty reading - and re-reading! - this book.

A must-have for anyone who wants to optimize their diabetes control.

> — Kelly L. Close
> Principal, Close Concerns (www.closeconcerns.com), and pumper
> Editor-in-Chief, diaTribe (www.diaTribe.us)
> San Francisco, CA

I first read **Pumping Insulin** before putting my own diabetes on the pump almost 15 years ago. Today, I use **Pumping Insulin** to help me teach my patients to make the most of pump therapy. Thank you for teaching us all how to use an insulin pump to its full potential and live better with diabetes.

> — Jen Block, RN, CDE
> Department of Pediatric Endocrinology, Stanford University
> Palo Alto, CA

This definitive guide helps us understand and utilize all the tools currently at our disposal for the informed management of diabetes. John and Ruth's narrative, charts, graphs, tables, and work sheets enable us to problem solve and become more self-assured about caring for this always challenging, often complex condition. We owe them a debt of gratitude for their comprehensive and practical 'how-to' manual.

> — Sydney Christensen Bush, BSN, RN, CDE, CPT
> Diabetes Nurse Educator, Cottage Health System
> Living successfully with Type 1 for 60 years
> Santa Barbara, CA

This book is a perfect resource for anyone who uses an insulin pump or would like to learn to use an insulin pump. I heartily endorse this book for all patients that want to improve their knowledge of insulin pumps.

— Ken Cathcart, DO, FACE
Northside Internal Medicine
Spokane, WA

Those who can read can be helped - a CGM and insulin pump provide the best technologie in diabetes you can get, but technologie itself does not make for good diabetes control. Like a computer, the machine is as smart as the user behind it. So get as much knowledge as you can regarding your own diabetes therapy when you exercise, travel, and make adjustments for every day life. **Pumping Insulin** is the best source you can get for diabetes technologie. Learn to use these brilliant tools to get the best diabetes control possible by knowing how to use them - so start reading and start being your own best diabetologist, every day of your life. Learn to think like a pancreas and have fun doing it.

— Ulrike Thurm, RN, CDE,
On an insulin pump over 25 years and CGM over 5 years
Author of **CGM und Insulinpumpenfibel** and **Diabetes und Sportfibel**
Berlin, Germany

About the Authors

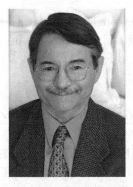

John Walsh, P.A., C.D.T.C., is a Physician Assistant and Diabetes Clinical Specialist who has provided clinical care to thousands of people with diabetes for more than 30 years in a wide variety of clinical settings, including private practice, HMO and university settings. He has pumped for 30 years and worn almost every insulin pump released during that time. He has also started hundreds of people on pumps and provided their clinical care.

Mr. Walsh is a popular presenter on a wide variety of diabetes topics to physicians, health professionals, diabetes educators, and people with diabetes, including the American Diabetes Association, Canadian Diabetes Association, Diabetic Sports and Exercise Association, Children With Diabetes, and pump support groups.

He serves as President of Diabetes Services, Inc. and is webmaster of www.diabetesnet. com, a highly trafficked source of diabetes information and online store. He has authored or coauthored numerous diabetes articles, abstracts. diabetes books and booklets. He is a consultant for medical corporations, and has developed many of the theories and assisted in the design of many of the dose-related features in today's and tomorrow's pumps and devices. He is considered an authority on pumps, devices, and intensive diabetes management, and sees patients at Advanced Metabolic Care and Research in Escondido, CA.

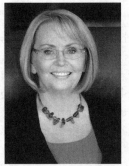

Ruth Roberts, M.A., is CEO of Diabetes Services, Inc, Diabetes Mall and Torrey Pines Press, and a widely-read medical writer and editor. She has served as a corporate training administrator, technical writer, and instructional designer for twenty years in San Diego. She has coauthored several books on diabetes, edited a weekly internet newsletter, "Diabetes This Week," and written numerous articles on diabetes.

She is a consultant for medical corporations and business start-ups specializing in diabetes products and services. She is a professional member of the American Diabetes Association and past board member of the International Diabetes Athletes Association, now DESA.

Other books by John Walsh, PA, CDTC, and Ruth Roberts, MA:

Using Insulin, Torrey Pines Press, 2003

Pumping Insulin, 1st, 2nd, 3rd, and 4th edition, Torrey Pines Press, 1989-2006

STOP the Rollercoaster, Torrey Pines Press, 1996

Pocket Pancreas, Torrey Pines Press, 1995, 1998, 2000

Smart Charts, My Other CheckBook record book, Torrey Pines Press, 1995, 2000

Insulin Pump Therapy Handbook, 1990

Diabetes Advanced Workbook, 1988

Acknowledgments

Pumping Insulin is the product of years of personal and professional experience with diabetes and insulin pumps. During this time, major contributions have been made by our mentors, colleagues, patients, friends, and fellow travelers. We owe all a great debt of gratitude,

Our heartfelt thanks go to these individuals who graciously and critically reviewed and improved upon this fifth edition of Pumping Insulin:

Ragnar Hanas, MD, PhD; William D. Zigrang, MD, FACE, CCC, CEC; David C. Klonoff, MD, FACP; W. Kenneth Ward, MD; Jen Alexander; Sydney Christensen Bush, BSN, RN, CDE, CPT; Jen Block, RN, CDE; Prof. Dr. Lutz Heinemann, PhD; Jacqueline Hosch, RD, CDE; Bernhard T. Gehr, Dr. med.; Judy Gates, RN, MPH, CDE; Robert A. Vigersky, MD; Ulrike Thurm, RN, CDE; Howard Zisser, MD; Ellen H. Ullman, MSW; Satish Garg, MD; Malinda Duke, MSN, CPNP, CDE; Sheri Colberg, PhD; Evelyne Fleury-Milfort, C-RNP, BC-ADM, CDE; Sue Amidon, RN, CDE; Elizabeth Zabell Edelman; Frank Schwartz, MD, FACE; Nancy JV Bohannon MD, FACP, FACE; Joe Largay, PAC, CDE; Melany Hellstern; Virginia Valentine CNS, BC-ADM, CDE; Timothy Bailey, MD, FACP; Daniel Einhorn, MD, FACP, FACE; Steve V. Edelman, MD; Judith Jones Ambrosini; Ken Cathcart, DO, FACE; Diane Krieger, MD; Jeff Hitchcock; Bruce Perkins, MD, MPH; and Kelly Close.

Special thanks to San Diego graphics artist Richard B. Morris, III for the cover design, chapter headings, and all the wonderful tables, figures, text boxes and workspaces that present complex information in a clear, crisp way. Richard's work can also be seen at our website www.diabetesnet.com where he supplies expertise in design and programming, as well as at his website at www.atingeofplatt.com.

We and everyone with diabetes are indebted to:

The American Diabetes Association, the Juvenile Diabetes Research Foundation, the National Institute of Health, and other national agencies that support diabetes education and research.

All the health professionals and the 1,441 volunteers with diabetes who participated in the Diabetes Control and Complications Trial which confirmed what early pumpers and pump proponents had already assumed—that controlling glucoses makes people healthier and reduces their risk for complications.

Table of Contents

Boxes

Tables

Workspaces

Clever Pump or CGM Tricks

Figures

Examples

Important Note

This 5th edition of **Pumping Insulin** is a guide to successful glucose control with an insulin pump. Many figures, charts, examples, tables, and tips provide basic and advanced pump information. The information included in this book should be used only as a guide. Insulin requirements and treatment protocols can differ significantly from one person to the next. **Pumping Insulin** can never substitute for the sound medical advice of your personal physician and health care team.

Specific treatment plans, insulin dosages, and other aspects of health care for a person with diabetes must be based on individualized treatment protocols under the guidance of your physician or health care team. The information in this book is provided to enhance your understanding of diabetes and your insulin pump so that you can manage the daily challenges you face. It can never be relied upon as a sole source for your personal diabetes regimen.

While every reasonable precaution has been taken in the preparation of this information, the authors and publishers assume no responsibility for errors or omissions, nor for the uses made of the materials contained herein and the decisions based on such use. No warranties are made, expressed, or implied, with regard to the contents of this work or to its applicability to specific individuals. The authors and publishers shall not be liable for direct, indirect, special, incidental, or consequential damages arising out of the use of or inability to use the contents of this book.

Read This!

We provide the best information and tools available to help you work with your health care professional to normalize your glucose. Never use this book on your own! Any suggestions made in this book for improving your glucose should have the approval and guidance of your personal physician and health care team.

This book by itself is not enough. We have worked with pumpers who have used this information together with the guidance of their physician and they have excelled. We have also seen pumpers who get themselves into trouble by a selective use of this or other material, and by ignoring or not seeking excellent medical advice.

No book can ever help you as much as your physician and health care team. They have the benefits of knowing you personally and the objectivity and experience gained from working with other pumpers. Your own participation in the process of good control is essential, but never minimize the importance of good professional advice and support. Teams win where individuals fail, and teamwork takes trust and communication from everyone.

We wish everyone who reads this book good health and great glucose management!

Foreword

Pumping Insulin by John Walsh and Ruth Roberts is the world's best book about how to use insulin pumps. It explains the basics as well as the most sophisticated concepts in a clear stepwise way so that a patient can understand how to use a pump and a health care professional can understand many features of the pump that allow for fine tuning of glucose control. The book covers pumps in a logical sequences, starting with getting ready to use a pump, training essentials, how to select doses of insulin, fine tuning and problem solving, and considerations for special types of patients.

When I read this book I feel like I am learning the most useful tips and explanations of everything that I need to know in order to teach my patients not only the basics, but the fine points of using insulin pump technology. The more that the health care professional and the patient both know about a complicated product, like an insulin pump, the safer the device will be for maintaining control and the more effective the device can be, as well.

The latest edition of **Pumping Insulin** contains a discussion of very recent material about bolus calculator software. This type of software accounts for insulin that has not yet been absorbed from a prior bolus dose and each pump manufacturer calculates the amount of leftover insulin differently. Walsh and Roberts carefully take the reader through a process to understand best practices in bolus dosing. They begin with how to calculate your own accurate carbohydrate boluses, then how to check how your own pump handles bolus insulin on board, how to set or adjust your duration of insulin action time.

The book discusses which types of prior boluses each of the five largest pump manufacturers consider as part of their bolus on board formulae and how bolus on board is applied to carbohydrate or correction boluses. This is a sophisticated discussion. They even include presentations on when to override your bolus calculator bolus dose recommendation, and when to watch out for a blind spot with your bolus calculator.

This edition of **Pumping Insulin** clearly presents important information about determining total daily doses, basal rates, carbohydrate factors, and correction factors, using clear tables and brief case studies. The latest edition of the book contains new material about continuous glucose monitors (CGM), including tips for calibration, site selection, alarm settings, verifying continuous data with self-monitoring of blood glucose (SMBG), and how to magnify the amplitude of a hypoglycemic alarm. The book discusses how to use CGM to prevent and correct lows and highs.

A chapter on pattern management with solutions is very helpful for patients who might be overwhelmed with data from SMBG or CGM. A chapter on troubleshooting is a must-read for every pump patient and it presents specific solutions to problems with clogs, blockages, leaks, detached sets, infections, and bad insulin. How to avoid episodes of hypoglycemia, hyperglycemic spikes, and ketoacidosis is fully discussed. A practical chapter on the effects of insulin is helpful for every type of athlete and a chapter on pumping during pregnancy presents detailed advice on adjusting calories, exercise and insulin dosing as the pregnancy progresses and then beyond through labor & delivery and the postpartum state. This book is chock full of practical tips for patients new to technology, experienced patients, and health care professionals.

Pumping Insulin is full of clearly designed figures, lists, tables, and graphs of data presentation from monitoring equipment. I highly recommend this book for anyone who wants to match sophisticated insulin delivery technology with fluctuating glucose levels to achieve successful control of their diabetes.

David C. Klonoff, M.D., F.A.C.P.

Clinical Professor of Medicine, U.C. San Francisco

Editor-in-Chief, Journal of Diabetes Science and Technology

Medical Director, Diabetes Research Institute, Mills-Peninsula Health Services

San Mateo, California 94401

For Clinicians

Since its introduction to diabetes clinical practice more than 30 years ago, insulin pump therapy has become widely accepted and continues to increase in popularity. Nonetheless, many clinicians leave their formal academic training with limited experience in pump therapy. Most prescribers of insulin pumps are self-taught or have acquired their knowledge from infrequent manufacturer-sponsored seminars and training classes. Thus the full potential of insulin pump therapy has often been unrecognized.

The game changer in this situation is **Pumping Insulin**. Introduced in 1989, this book has provided a systematic and thorough introduction to pumps, their promise and their pitfalls. Revised and expanded, the book now includes topics such as pregnancy, exercise and athletics, and continuous glucose monitoring.

Pumping Insulin, the fifth edition, is a detailed master course in advanced insulin therapy, with descriptions of the differences between various pumps, their Bolus Calculators and settings, and infusion sets. It's really a distillation of both academic and practical experience in insulin therapeutics as well as of the contributions over time of what I call the "pumping underground." The various charts, tables and worksheets guide the patient and clinician through the process of choosing and initiating the pump and of refining appropriate insulin delivery.

Although I have extensive experience over decades of pump therapy, with each new edition I find topics and wrinkles that I had not considered previously in depth.

William D. Zigrang, M.D., F.A.C.E., C.C.C., C.E.C.

Board-certified Endocrinologist

Burlingame, CA

Introduction

If you're considering an insulin pump, beginning to use a pump, or already on one but your glucose management is less than you desire, this book provides the in-depth detail you need for success on a pump.

Pumping Insulin is for:

- Everyone considering or beginning to use an insulin pump
- Existing pumpers who want to improve their glucose management
- Physicians, nurses, dietitians, physician assistants, nurse practitioners, family members and others who support people on pumps
- Everyone who wants to lower their glucose exposure and variability
- Everyone who wants to match insulin need with insulin delivery

Pumping Insulin tells you:

- What a pump is, how to set it up, and how to get the most from it
- How to manage basal rates and boluses for more stable readings
- How to use a CGM to normalize glucoses
- How to count carbs
- How to avoid and treat low and high glucoses
- How to minimize and solve pump problems
- How to feel better and live a healthier life
- When to seek help

This book guides you through new pump features, how to evaluate your glucose management, how to set and test basal and bolus doses, and how to determine and use your personal carb and correction factors.

Included are step-by-step instructions for starting on a pump, using a CGM, how to test your pump settings, checklists to improve glucoses, and specific examples of glucose management techniques, as well as charting methods, carbohydrate counting instructions, approaches to exercise and pregnancy, and specific directions for children and teens.

If you are preparing to start on a pump, read the first 13 chapters in **Pumping Insulin** before you start. These chapters explain how a pump works, how to switch from injected doses to a pump, and how to estimate and test your starting doses.

Consult specific chapters for issues as you continue on a pump. Keep it close at hand as a reference when glucose management is less than you desire.

Pump Terms and Acronyms

Basal Insulin or Basal Rate – An all day insulin delivery that matches background insulin need. Once correctly set, the glucose does not rise or fall in daily situations while the person is fasting.

Basal/Bolus Balance – Basal insulin usually makes up half (40-60%) of the total daily dose with the rest as boluses.

Bolus – A quick release of insulin from the pump to cover carbs or lower a high glucose.

Bolus Calculator (BC) – A part of the insulin pump software that uses settings and logic to make bolus recommendations to match carbs, bring down high readings and, by tracking BOB, minimize insulin stacking.

Bolus On Board (BOB) – A pump feature that tells how much insulin from a recent bolus insulin is left to lower the glucose. Also called insulin on board, unused insulin, or active insulin.

Bolus Stacking – Caused when frequent boluses overlap, resulting in a low glucose. Today's pumps help prevent stacking by tracking BOB and by having an appropriate DIA.

Carb Bolus – A bolus delivered to match carbohydrates in an upcoming meal or snack.

Carb Factor (CarbF) – How many grams of carbohydrate one unit of insulin will cover.

Continuous Glucose Monitor (CGM) – A computerized device that provides a constant stream of readings that helps the wearer know the glucose value and whether it is rising, falling or steady.

Correction Bolus – A bolus delivered to bring a high glucose back to your target.

Correction Factor (CorrF) – How many mg/dl (or mmol/L) one unit of insulin lowers the glucose. Used to correct highs.

Correction Target or Target Range – The glucose target or target range that the BC aims for with its correction bolus recommendation.

Duration of Insulin Action (DIA) – How long a bolus of insulin actively lowers glucose.

Infusion Set – Inserted through the skin to deliver insulin from a reservoir (cartridge) to the body. Includes a hub (connection), catheter (tubing), and insertion set. It may be a fine metal needle that remains under the skin, or a larger metal needle that is removed to leave a small Teflon catheter.

Insulin Pump – A computerized device about the size of a small cell phone that is programmed to deliver basal insulin and carb or correction boluses. Insulin is delivered from a reservoir through flexible tubing to a Teflon or small metal needle inserted through the skin. Delivers doses as small as 0.025 to 0.001 unit. Input from frequent glucose monitoring from a meter or CGM is required to manage dosing.

Total Daily Dose (TDD) – The total units of insulin a person uses in a day. Includes basal doses and bolus doses. It is used to determine the basal rate and carb and correction factors.

Why Use an Insulin Pump?

The use of insulin pumps has risen dramatically over the last 35 years to nearly a million people worldwide. The number of satisfied users continues to grow as pump technology and its benefits for control evolve.

Enthusiastic pump wearers of all ages propel this growth when they share their experiences with others. They see their pump as a turning point in diabetes care, saying "For the first time in years, I can eat when I want to," or "I can really control my blood sugars now and I feel better, too."

One enthusiastic pumper who started at age 70 says, "My insecurity is gone. My A1c said my control was good on injections, but I couldn't avoid overnight lows and that created stress day after day. On my pump, I feel positive and really in charge of my body." An 11 year-old was happy to "eat just like my friends if I count my carbs and cover them with boluses" and added, "Going on hikes this year at diabetes camp was easy."

This chapter reviews
- Why people choose insulin pumps
- Pump benefits
- How a pump works and how it delivers insulin
- Pump drawbacks

Pump benefits include fewer injections, the ability to give insulin easily for spontaneous events, with faster insulin adjustments for changes in eating, exercise, and activity. Unlike injections, a pump uses only rapid-acting insulin. The large depot of long-acting insulin under the skin that is absorbed differently from day to day as temperature or activity changes is no longer needed. The infusion site stays in place for about three days rather than being injected into different locations with different absorption characteristics several times a day. Insulin stacking from previous boluses can be avoided for more consistent insulin activity.

A pump offers convenience, more consistent insulin action from day to day, easier problem solving, easier tracking of insulin use, less hypoglycemia, less risk of hypoglycemia unawareness, and fewer morning highs. A built-in *bolus calculator (BC)* uses personalized settings to make bolus doses more accurate and glucoses more stable. In the background, important insulin dosing and glucose history gets recorded to solve control issues.

An insulin pump may seem complicated, but wearers quickly become advocates when they can finally match their needs with the right amount of insulin at the right time. Powered by AAA, AA, or rechargeable batteries, pumps benefit people of all ages, from infants to those in their 80s and 90s.

People on multiple injections who have to eat meals on a rigid schedule, require a snack every night before bed, wake up at 3 a.m. sweating profusely, return to consciousness in an emergency room, face high morning readings that ruin the rest of the day, or want to sleep late on the weekend, find that changing to a pump offers a new confidence and a freer lifestyle.

> ## 1.1 A Pump Really Helps Those Who:
> - Want better control and more stable readings
> - Need or desire a freer lifestyle
> - Have an A1c over 7%
> - Are very sensitive or very resistant to insulin
> - Use less than 35 units a day
> - Want to give insulin discreetly.
> - Have problems with lows
> - Keep their glucose high from fear of lows
> - Live alone
> - Want to prevent long-term complications
> - Want to stop insulin stacking
> - Participate in intensive exercise
> - Want an easy way to track their data
> - Travel or do shift work
> - Want peace of mind

Even the large pumps introduced as early as 1979[1] were well received. One study which reviewed 18 different research studies completed before 1991 found that 62.5% of the 520 participants who used both a pump and multiple daily injections (MDI) during crossover trials chose to remain on these early model pumps at the end of their study.[2]

Today's pumps offer many more useful features for convenience and safety as they perform the complicated math you need to calculate bolus doses.

Pump features include:

- A bolus calculator with settings for a carb factor, correction factor, target glucose, and duration of insulin action
- An integrated glucose meter and often the display of CGM readings
- Carb counting aids
- Tracking of bolus on board (BOB) to reduce insulin stacking
- History to track insulin usage (basal/bolus balance, correction bolus percentage, etc.) and glucose values
- Helpful reminders and alerts

The precise insulin delivery of a pump is especially helpful when combined with feedback from a *continuous glucose monitor (CGM)*. A CGM helps change behavior as alarms warn of highs and lows. The results of under-counting carbs, late bolusing, over-treating lows, and being on too little or too much insulin are quickly seen in CGM trend lines. The reliability and accuracy of CGMs continue to improve and will eventually allow glucose readings to be directly entered into a pump *bolus calculator (BC)* for bolus calculations. Although integrating pumps and CGMs will take time, early features needed for automatic control when the glucose goes low, such as stopping basal insulin delivery for a period of time, are beginning to appear.

1.2 Health Care Professionals Recommend Pumps For:

- Poor glycemic control
- Frequent or severe hypoglycemia
- Hypoglycemia unawareness
- Nighttime hypoglycemia
- "Brittle" diabetes or high glucose variability
- Post-meal hyperglycemia
- Dawn Phenomenon
- Frequent ketoacidosis
- Insulin requirement less than 35 units a day
- Frequent travel or a variable work schedule
- Help in tracking insulin doses, carbs, glucose levels, and other information critical to control
- Pregnancy and preparing for conception
- Improved control during growth and puberty
- Managing gastroparesis
- Less insulin resistance in Type 2 diabetes

Diabetes devices continue to improve with better CGM integration, smaller sizes, color screens, more infusion set choices, faster insulin analogs, and better trend analysis and pattern recognition. *A pump helps manage the complex interactions between insulin levels, blood glucose and carbs with less effort.* To get the most out of your pump and improve your glucose levels, you might want to learn and apply the principles in this book.

Pump Benefits

Better Control and More Stable Readings

Large research studies published in the last 10 years have shown that people on pumps have lower A1c values, less hypoglycemia, and more stable glucose readings compared to those on multiple daily injections.[3-7] Hypoglycemia generally becomes less frequent and less severe. In one study of 225 pumpers, severe hypoglycemia dropped from 138 events for every 100 years in the previous year on MDI to 22 per 100 years in the first year of pump use.[8] This lower rate persisted for pumpers during the four-year study.

1.3 Insulin Delivery on a Pump	
Basal Rates	An all-day insulin delivery that matches background insulin need to keep the glucose normal. Measured in units per hour, basal rates often range between 0.4 to 1.6 u/hr for most adults, and make up about half of the ***total daily insulin dose (TDD)***.
Carb Bolus	A spurt (bolus) of insulin used to counterbalance the glucose-increasing effect of carbs in a meal or snack. Adults and children often use 1 unit for every 5 to 22 grams of carb.
Correction Bolus	A bolus delivered to bring a high glucose back to your target. Adults often use one unit to lower the glucose between 20 and 120 mg/dl (1 to 6.7 mmol/L) per unit.

In 1998, the Disetronic (now Roche Accu-Chek) pump company surveyed 6,890 pump users in the U.S. and Europe. In this group, 62% reported that their hypoglycemia was less frequent, while 17% reported it was more frequent, and 21% said it was about the same compared to when they were on injections.

Insulin pumps and CGMs work together to avoid hypoglycemia (See Table 1.8). A pump can remind the user to measure their glucose after boluses, recommend doses based on a meal's carb count and the current blood sugar, and adjust dose recommendations to account for any remaining ***bolus on board (BOB)***. Tracking of active insulin allows it to determine about how many carbs are needed to prevent an upcoming low reading once a glucose test is done, as discussed in Box 10.4. Continuous monitors are able to track glucose trends and sound an alarm when the glucose falls or rises faster than expected.

Convenient Dosing

Work or school hours can vary, events pop up, and meals be delayed or missed from day to day. On weekends, you may want to rise early or sleep late, and be more or less active at different times of the day. Larger family or holiday meals and late dining are easier to manage. The use of rapid-acting insulin for basal and bolus doses allows insulin delivery to be more easily tailored to life's variety.

A pump wearer can quickly deliver insulin doses and no longer has to take long-acting insulin at the same time each day to avoid glucose fluctuations. A pump wearer does not need to have an insulin vial and syringe or an insulin pen to give insulin at home, at a restaurant, or in a public rest room.

More Precise Bolus Doses

Many people benefit from a pump's precise dosing, especially those who are sensitive to insulin and those who use less than 35 to 40 units a day. Even a small miscalculation can spell disaster for slender adults and children whose glucose may fall by 100 mg/dl (5.6 mmol/L) or more on each unit of insulin. The precision of a pump gives more stable glucose levels.

> **1.4 Why Injected Insulin Action Varies**
> * Size of the insulin dose
> * Where the injection is given
> * Depth of the injection into muscle or fat
> * Exercise length and intensity
> * Local heat or massage
> * Outside temperature
> * Mixing of different insulins
> * Smoking

A pump *bolus calculator (BC)* simplifies the division of grams of carb in a meal by your carb factor (grams of carb covered by one unit), the subtraction of your current reading from your target glucose and division of this result by your correction factor (how far your glucose drops on one unit). The resulting bolus dose is then adjusted for any remaining insulin activity from recent boluses. You simply enter how many carbs you'll eat and your glucose, and the bolus calculator recommends the bolus you need. You can then modify its recommendation as needed for factors like activity or illness.

More Flexible Basal Delivery

A pump usually provides more stable glucose readings than multiple daily injections.[9] Long-acting insulins like Lantus® (glargine) and Levemir® (detemir) were designed to have less peaking than older NPH insulin, which varied in activity as much as 25% from one day to the next.[10] But even these insulins can have variable peaks and valleys in insulin levels as gaps or stacking of insulin appear when injection timing changes, such as on weekends.

Lantus® and Levemir® have some peaking activity between 6 and 10 hours, and lower a person's glucose over 16 to 26 hours. Many diabetes clinics prefer to have Lantus® and Levemir® users take two injections a day to minimize spiking, avoid gaps in action, and better match lifestyle variations like sleeping in late on weekends.

Basal rates can be adjusted every 1 to 30 minutes in increments as small as 0.01 to 0.025 unit/hr, such as for an increase to offset a Dawn Phenomenon in the early morning hours or a decrease for longer periods of activity. A pump's basal delivery and the choice of multiple daily basal rates provides a better match to the variable background insulin needs of someone who experiences a Dawn Phenomenon, who changes their waking or work hours, or who periodically engages in strenuous exercise. Precise basal delivery helps those sensitive to insulin, such as infants, adults on low doses, and athletes. Over 90% of pumpers use more than one basal rate a day.

Easier Problem Solving

If your glucose goes high or low on injections, it is difficult to determine whether the long-acting insulin is peaking erratically, or a rapid-acting insulin dose was the wrong amount or given at the wrong time. On a pump, rapid insulin is used for basal and bolus doses with no long-acting insulin to cause confusion.

Basal delivery and carb and correction boluses are easier to determine on a pump. First, you test and adjust basal delivery until it keeps the glucose steady when you are not eating. Next, you adjust a carb factor to keep the glucose controlled after meals with a minimum of lows and highs. If the basal rate is correct, but the carb count for a meal is not accurate, the meal bolus will be the cause for the high or low reading that follows. This simplifies problem solving.

A pump history lets you and your doctor know exactly how much insulin you use per day. On injections, neither of you know your real insulin usage unless you never vary your doses or you record every dose you take. Knowing your average total insulin dose (TDD) let's your doctor and you select the settings you need in your pump for great control. **Pumping Insulin** shows how to do this.

> ### 1.5 Expect Better Control on a Pump
>
> Precise insulin delivery from a pump should allow you to achieve relatively normal glucose readings most of the time. If your glucose often goes high or low on a pump, then a basal rate, carb factor, correction factor, or duration of insulin action needs to change
>
> Never accept frequent highs, frequent lows, or erratic readings. If this happens, talk with your doctor about how to modify your lifestyle and adjust your doses until your control improves.

Fewer Lows and Less Hypoglycemia Unawareness

Hypoglycemia unawareness occurs when someone is no longer aware that they are going low. Their symptoms are so reduced by previous lows that thinking becomes severely impaired before symptoms occur. This is more common in those who have had diabetes for many years, especially when excessive insulin doses and frequent lows have depleted typical stress responses. This can be dangerous if no one is around to help.

More precise dosing from a pump gives the wearer fewer lows overall and less rapid declines in glucose. This gives more time to recognize symptoms and consume carbs.[11] Many undetected lows and most episodes of hypoglycemia unawareness occur during sleep. A pump can be programmed to deliver nighttime basal rates that better match a person's real need. Prevention of nighttime lows often allows a person to sense their daytime lows again.[12]

How a Pump Works

Similarities to and Differences from the Pancreas

An insulin pump mimics the pancreas in giving small doses of insulin around the clock to match ongoing insulin need, as well as being able to give bursts or boluses of insulin when food is eaten. *Although a pump is currently the best way to manage diabetes, it does not mimic the pancreas perfectly.* Normal beta cells release insulin in a system of very rapid checks and balances that keep the glucose within a narrow range. Figure 1.6 shows 24-hour glucose levels (top) and insulin levels (bottom) in people without diabetes. Glucose levels range between 72 and 143 mg/dl (4 to 8 mmol/L), with the white line showing the average glucose and the shaded area showing all glucose values.

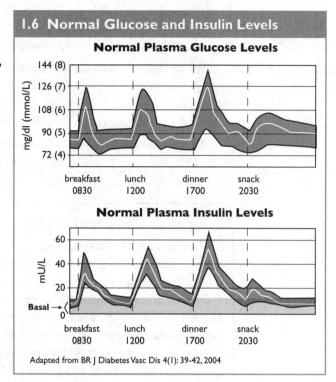

1.6 Normal Glucose and Insulin Levels

Normal Plasma Glucose Levels

mg/dl (mmol/L)

144 (8)
126 (7)
108 (6)
90 (5)
72 (4)

breakfast 0830 lunch 1200 dinner 1700 snack 2030

Normal Plasma Insulin Levels

mU/L

60
40
20
Basal → 0

breakfast 0830 lunch 1200 dinner 1700 snack 2030

Adapted from BR J Diabetes Vasc Dis 4(1): 39-42, 2004

The bottom graphic shows how insulin levels change over 24 hours. Basal insulin delivery is shown as the light grey in the bottom graphic. People without diabetes release about half of their total daily production of insulin as basal insulin.[13] Basal insulin requirements remain relatively constant for most people from day to day to balance glucose production by the liver, with some changes needed to balance activity, stress, and changes in other hormones. The spikes in the bottom graphic show insulin release at mealtimes to cover carbs. This release matches the number of carbs and the number of meals that are eaten.

The pancreas has two advantages over a pump or injections:

1. At mealtime, the pancreas quickly releases a spurt of stored insulin directly into the portal vein that goes to the liver. This *first phase insulin release* causes levels of insulin to rise dramatically in the liver to allow liver enzymes to quickly move glucose into liver glycogen. Blood insulin levels rise at the same time to move any remaining glucose into muscle and fat cells. More insulin is released shortly after this as insulin production begins.

2. Insulin is quickly released from the pancreas to prevent rises and falls in the blood glucose level.

If a pump were compared to a car, it would be slower than the cars most people drive because it can't deliver insulin into the portal vein (accelerate quickly), nor release a lot of insulin into the liver shortly after eating (fuel injection). Rather, it delivers insulin beneath the skin that gradually absorbs into the blood. This greatly delays insulin's arrival in the portal vein, never reaching the levels of a healthy pancreas. These factors make glucose levels more likely to spike after meals unless steps are taken to counteract them.

When you are climbing a hill (rising glucose), more gas (insulin) is needed, while when going down a hill (falling glucose) braking gets trickier. Without a pancreas' automatic brakes, you have to slam on the brakes (lower basal delivery) or put the car in reverse (eat carbs) to maintain control on downhill glucoses.

To compensate for these delivery limitations when a meal's carb content is known, boluses can be given 15 to 20 minutes before eating to improve post-meal control. A bolus calculator helps match each bolus dose to carb intake and the current glucose level.

1.7 Pumps Compared to MDI

Two research studies summarized data from smaller studies where people with Type 1 diabetes were randomly assigned to *multiple daily injections (MDI)* or a pump. The average A1c level was found to be 0.5% to 0.6% lower on pumps than on MDI. One summary with 600 people who participated in a dozen smaller studies found that pumps lowered the A1c by 0.51% compared to MDI. Those on pumps experienced less glucose variability and required 7.6 fewer units of insulin per day.[14]

The second study found that the A1c fell by 0.61% on pumps and daily insulin requirements fell by 11.9 units per day.[15] A later study of 24 people taking either Lantus® (glargine) or on a pump found no difference in the A1c, but glycemic variability (ups and downs in the glucose) and insulin requirements were both lower on a pump.[16]

Unfortunately, both those using MDI and classic pumps had an average A1c that was above 8.2% to 9% in these studies. This is much higher than the goal of 7% or less recommended by the American Diabetes Association and considerably higher than the 6.5% goal jointly recommended by the American Association of Clinical Endocrinologists and the International Diabetes Federation.[17,18]

A recent study reviewed how many teens had eye complications over time at the University of Wisconsin. A marked drop in retinopathy was seen from 53% of teens in the 1990 to 1994 group to 12% in those studied between 2005 to 2009. A1c levels fell by only 0.6% from 9.1% to 8.5% during this time, but a sharp increase from 17% to 88% was seen in the number using either a pump or multiple injections.

A nearly statistically significant advantage was found in glucose stability for pumps (CSII) over MDI. The authors concluded there was "evidence for reduced risk for retinopathy in those treated with CSII compared with MDI. Given there was no difference in A1C between groups, we hypothesize that reduced glycemic variability may have contributed to this difference." [19]

Less *glycemic variability* (fewer ups and downs) may lessen the risk of heart and organ damage.[20,21] Insulin pumps have been shown to help people with neuropathy,[22,23] early kidney disease,[24,25] and retinopathy.[26] Pumps also benefit those who have Dawn Phenomenon, erratic control,[27,28] or insulin resistance.[29] Improved control has even been shown to reverse some complications of diabetes in humans and animals.[30,31]

1.8 Ways That a Pump Helps Prevent Lows	
What Causes Lows	**How a Pump Helps**
Too much insulin	Protects against excess boluses once an appropriate carb factor and correction factor are programmed.
Insulin stacking	Bolus on board (BOB) that is still active from previous boluses is taken into account when a new bolus is given.
Increased exercise or activity	Bolus doses can be adjusted and temporary basal reductions can be used to lessen the risk of hypoglycemia during and after exercise.
Faster insulin absorption during hot weather	The pool of rapid insulin under the skin is much smaller than that of long-acting insulin. Less insulin gets released during hot weather or in a sauna.
A bolus is delivered but meal is delayed or missed	A temporary basal reduction can offset some of the bolus that was given, but the wearer has to consume the other carbs they need.

Without the advantage of a pancreas, even those in excellent control have readings that stray outside an ideal range. No health professional expects perfect control, but decades of clinical research show that the closer to normal and the more stable your glucose readings, the better. Many people find the pump a better way to manage their glucose.

How a Pump Delivers Insulin

Basal Insulin

A pump delivers rapid-acting insulin through the day as needed to provide the *basal* or *background* insulin need. Basal rates can be adjusted every 1 to 60 minutes, depending on the brand of pump, *to keep glucose levels flat through the night or during the day when a meal is skipped*. Accurate rates keep the glucose from rising or falling more than 30 mg/dl (1.7 mmol/L) during eight hours of sleep or during five to eight hours of daytime fasting.

"If I wake up high, my whole day is shot!" is a common complaint when basal rates are too low to match a person's need. Low night insulin levels let the liver release glucose and cause morning highs. These highs are harder to bring down because the liver is actively making glucose. Teens and younger adults often need higher basal rates in the predawn hours to counteract a *Dawn Phenomenon* caused by a natural increase in growth hormone in the early morning hours.[32,33] In the early morning hours, basal rates can be easily adjusted compared to long-acting insulin to balance the rise in growth hormone levels.

Adjustments in the nighttime basal rate are timed to prevent excess glucose production by the liver and excess fat release from fat cells, while increasing glucose uptake by muscle cells. This allows a person with Type 1 diabetes who has a strong Dawn Phenomenon or someone with Type 2 and insulin resistance to wake up with normal glucose readings.

Once the overnight basal rate is correctly set, you can:
- Go to bed with a glucose in your target range, eat little or no bedtime snack, and wake up in the morning with a reading close to the same number, assuming that no BOB remains at bedtime and the day was not unusually active.
- Correct a high glucose at bedtime and wake up with a reading in your target range the next morning
- Let yourself and your spouse, parents, children, and doctor rest peacefully during the night

Pumps also offer temporary basal rates and alternate basal profiles. A ***temporary basal rate*** is a temporary increase or decrease in basal delivery in 1% to 10% increments from 30 minutes to either 24 or 72 hours, depending on the pump. Temporary basal rates can be increased to handle occasional illnesses or decreased during and after longer periods of exercise or activity. An ***alternate basal rate*** allows a pumper to set up and switch between alternate basal profiles when basal requirements differ between weekdays and weekends, before menses for women, or on days when daily activity differs.

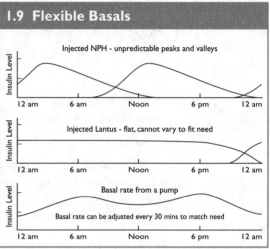

1.9 Flexible Basals

Injected NPH - unpredictable peaks and valleys

Injected Lantus - flat, cannot vary to fit need

Basal rate from a pump

Basal rate can be adjusted every 30 mins to match need

Bolus Insulin

Boluses are quick doses of insulin you can give with your pump as needed to cover carbs or to correct a high glucose reading.

Carb Boluses

Carb boluses are given for all carbs except when these carbs are used to compensate for a low glucose or extra activity. How many carbs a meal or snack contains largely determines the size of the carb bolus you need to cover it. The more carbohydrate, the larger the carb bolus that is needed. Accurate carb counting is critical for getting the most from your pump.

Boluses can be delivered in doses as small as 0.05 (five hundredths) of a unit, compared to 0.5 unit (five tenths) with a syringe. This precision, plus tracking of any bolus insulin still active, prevents the insulin stacking and hypoglycemia that can plague those using a syringe.

1.10 Will Starting on a Pump Harm My Eyes?

With the presence of moderate or advanced retinopathy, eye damage can temporarily worsen if glucose levels are rapidly improved on a pump or multiple injections because this raises VEGF levels.[34-36] A rise in VEGF or vascular endothelial growth factor levels appears to increase proliferative retinopathy (growth of new weak blood vessels into the clear fluid of the eye) and macular edema (swelling from leaky blood vessels).[37]

If your previous control has been poor, your physician may advise that you gradually lower your glucose over a few weeks to minimize VEGF release. If you have retinopathy, it is important to be followed by an experienced ophthalmologist to avoid making eye damage worse during early pump use. After 6 to 12 months of improved control, retinopathy usually stabilizes and may actually improve. Work with your ophthalmologist to ensure that this happens. Some success in reducing severe retinopathy has been shown by injecting VEGF-blockers into the clear vitreous of the eye.

Your personal *carb factor* (CarbF) or *insulin-to-carb ratio* is determined in Chapter 12. Your pump uses the carb count and your CarbF to calculate an accurate carb bolus for each meal and snack. Accurate carb counts put you well on your way to reliable control.

When carb counting and the CarbF are accurate and boluses well timed, the glucose usually rises no more than 40 to 80 mg/dl (2.2 to 4.4 mmol/L) 1 to 2 hours after a meal.

Correction Boluses

The person with a normal pancreas does not have high glucose levels. When a high reading occurs while using a pump, an accurate correction bolus can bring it down safely.

Similar to the number of grams of carb covered by one unit of insulin for the CarbF, *your correction factor (CorrF) is how much your glucose will fall per unit of insulin.* (See Chapter 13.) An accurate CorrF can be closely estimated. Once entered into your pump, your CorrF is used to determine the correction bolus needed to bring a high reading down to your target without going low.

A CorrF is accurately set when correction boluses consistently bring high glucose readings back to target 4 to 5 hours later.

Some Drawbacks to Pumping

A pump requires a willing and conscientious user to get the best results. It is not the answer for everyone. Consider the drawbacks below compared to MDI before you decide.

Being Attached

Although today's small pumps weigh only a few ounces, concern about being attached to a pump may exist. This concern almost always disappears after a day or two of wear, as the wearer experiences the pump's convenience and benefits.

Weight Gain

Weight gain may occur when a pump is first worn. If glucose levels were often over 200 mg/dl (11.1 mmol/L) prior to pumping, excess calories are often being eaten and excess glucose is being passed into the urine. Once insulin doses are appropriately adjusted and glucose levels improve on a pump, these excess calories are no longer lost. Eating habits have to change as control improves to avoid weight gain. Appropriate basal and bolus dose adjustments can also prevent hypoglycemia, so the wearer is less likely to eat excess calories when treating lows.

Site Infections

Skin is our most important defense against infection. Infections are rare with injections, but this risk rises slightly on a pump because the infusion set remains in place for two or more days. Site infections can be prevented with good site technique and appropriate hygiene. See page 86.

Ketoacidosis

On a pump, if delivery of rapid-acting insulin under the skin is interrupted by an infusion set problem, glucose levels can begin to rise within 90 minutes. If the set completely detaches, insulin levels can fall to half their original level in about three hours. Most cells then mobilize fat to replace glucose as fuel. When cells use fat instead of glucose, an acidic by-product called ketones is produced. Four to five hours after insulin delivery stops, *ketosis* (excess ketone levels) can start and be quickly followed by a dangerous acidic state called ***ketoacidosis***.[38] With MDI, a pool of long-acting insulin under the skin prevents this excessive glucose rise for up to 24 hours.

In the 1980s, ketoacidosis requiring an emergency room or hospital visit occurred once in every 6.5 years of pump use.[39] Advances in pump therapy have decreased this risk,[40] and in seven studies between 1985 and 1990, the occurrence of ketoacidosis dropped to once for every 10 to 25 years of use.[41] Even so, ketoacidosis is a serious risk that a pump wearer must keep in mind. See Chapter 16.

Cost

Insulin pump expenses include the cost of the pump and ongoing costs for supplies. Insurance covers most of this cost, but talk with your insurer to find out what your out-of-pocket expenses will be. Over time, research indicates that an insulin pump is often less expensive than MDI due to improved health and longevity.[42,43]

Summary

Managing your blood sugar in diabetes requires good decisions and lifestyle choices several times a day. An insulin pump makes it easier to skip meals, exercise when you want, work varied schedules, eat late, or alter how many carbs you eat with less chance of having high or low readings. When an elevated glucose, exercise, stress, or illness occurs, a pumper can push the buttons on their pump or press a touch screen to

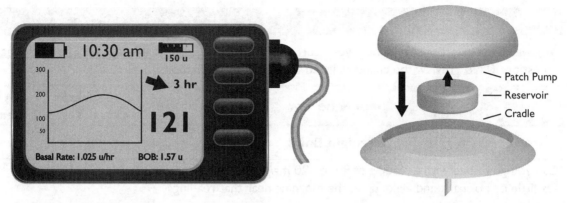

Line Pump - showing CGM information, current basal rate, Bolus on Board (BOB), battery life, and insulin left in reservoir

Patch Pump - low–profile delivery system attached to skin, has a separate controller

quickly adjust doses. The immediacy of giving insulin from a pump and the precise adjustment it offers brings freedom and lessens the risk of developing health problems related to diabetes. Many people on insulin find that a pump allows them to live a more normal life.

Having normal glucose levels is important to both physical and mental health. Confidence about good diabetes management enables a pump wearer to feel more in control of daily living. "My friends (family, coworkers) say that I look healthier and more alert" is a frequently heard comment. This book assists you in becoming a pro at using an insulin pump. It helps you set and achieve reasonable blood sugar goals, and it guides you in the use of all the tools that are available.

Even after your glucose is well controlled, ongoing basal and bolus adjustments will be needed as changes occur in weight, activity, or seasons. The time you spend now learning, adjusting, and analyzing will be more than offset by a greater sense of well-being and a more flexible lifestyle. With awareness and experience, you can reduce blood sugar swings, feel better, and prevent or reverse complications.

The Checklist on the next page shows a path toward optimal pump use.

Never be afraid to try something new. Remember that a lone amateur built the Ark.
A large group of professionals built the Titanic.

Dave Barry

1.11 Pump Tune-Up Checklist

Answer these questions to identify your current control issues. If you answer "Yes", go to the next question. If "No", review the chapters listed to the right for solutions.

Check & Review	Check if Yes	If No, read:
Overnight Basal Can you go to bed with a reading of 90 to 120 mg/dl (5.0 to 6.7 mmol/L), eat little or no snack and wake up in the morning near that reading?	☐	Chapter 11
Daytime Basal With a normal reading before a meal, can you skip eating, take no bolus and have your glucose rise or fall no more than 30 mg/dl (1.7 mmol/L)?	☐	Chapter 11
Carb Counting/Carb Bolus Can you accurately count the carbs you eat and, with a relatively normal reading before a meal, cover them with a carb bolus so your glucose returns to your target 4 to 5 hours later?	☐	Chapter 3 & 12
Correction Bolus Can you take correction boluses for high readings and have your glucose return to your target 4 to 5 hours after the bolus without going low?	☐	Chapter 13
Bolus On Board/Insulin Stacking When you give 2 or more boluses within 5 hours of each other, can you return to your target 4 to 5 hours later without going low?	☐	Chapter 8
Hypoglycemia Are you able to avoid frequent lows, severe lows, and rebound highs?	☐	Chapter 19 & 20
Handling Highs Can you avoid frequent highs and bring occasional highs down safely?	☐	Chapter 14 & 15
Exercise Can you exercise with good readings before, during, and afterward?	☐	Chapter 22

No problems? Terrific! Check again later!

Are You Ready to Pump?

This chapter is for those still considering an insulin pump. To evaluate your readiness, discuss any issues with family members, friends, and healthcare professionals. Ask questions and share your concerns with them and, if possible, with someone who wears a pump. Open, frank discussions will help determine whether you and a pump are a good match.

This chapter includes

- Questions to ask yourself
- Questions for parents of a child or teen considering a pump
- Examples of people who became successful pumpers
- Myths and truths about pumps

An insulin pump often seems complicated or overwhelming before you wear one. Fortunately, diabetes educators and pump companies provide excellent information and training materials.

Measure Your Readiness

The questions below will help you and your health care professional assess your readiness for pumping.

Motivation

1. On a 1 to 7 scale, how interested are you in using a pump?
   not interested 1 2 3 4 5 6 7 very interested

2. How motivated are you to control your glucose levels?
   not motivated 1 2 3 4 5 6 7 very motivated

3. Are you willing to check your glucose more often, and keep/download glucose records?
   ❑ yes ❑ no ❑ maybe

4. How likely do you believe you can control your glucoses day-to-day?
   not likely 1 2 3 4 5 6 7 very likely

5. How convenient will a pump be in your daily life?
   not convenient 1 2 3 4 5 6 7 convenient

6. Will better glucose control improve your health?

not likely 1 2 3 4 5 6 7 very likely

7. How comfortable are you about having diabetes – discussing it with friends, checking glucose in front of others, using an insulin pen or syringe in public?

not comfortable 1 2 3 4 5 6 7 very comfortable

8. Will others accept you if you wear a pump?

not likely 1 2 3 4 5 6 7 very likely

9. How excited are you about adapting new technology to control your diabetes?

not excited 1 2 3 4 5 6 7 very excited

10. Have you considered, or discussed with others, situations that might make wearing a pump inconvenient, such as athletics, work environment, etc.?

❑ yes ❑ no ❑ not yet   Which situations may present problems?

_____

11. Who can you rely on for support if pump problems arise?

_____

Need

1. How close is your most recent A1c or average glucose level to your goal?

not close 1 2 3 4 5 6 7 very close   ❑ Don't know

2. Are frequent highs or lows a problem?

❑ yes ❑ no ❑ sometimes

3. Have your lows been severe – ER visit, need other's help, hypoglycemia unawareness?

❑ yes ❑ no ❑ rarely

4. Do you have night lows or frequent morning highs?

❑ yes ❑ no

5. Do you use less than 40 units of insulin a day and need precise insulin doses?

❑ yes ❑ no

6. Do you travel frequently, have a varied school schedule, or work split shifts?

❑ yes ❑ no

7. Do you live alone and need safety features like BOB tracking, Auto-Off where the pump shuts off automatically, basal suspend for hypoglycemia with a CGM?

❑ yes ❑ no

Preparation

1. Number of insulin injections per day:
   0   1   2   3   4   5+

2. Number of glucose tests you do each day:
   0   1   2   3   4   5+

3. Do you write down or download your glucose test results?
   ❑ yes   ❑ no   ❑ occasionally

4. Do you currently adjust your rapid-acting insulin for the carbs in snacks and meals?
   ❑ yes   ❑ no

5. Do you currently give extra insulin to correct high glucoses?
   ❑ yes   ❑ no

6. Do you adjust your long-acting insulin doses?
   ❑ yes   ❑ no

7. Do you use carb counting or other method to match a meal with a meal dose?
   ❑ yes   ❑ no   ❑ sometimes

8. Do you regularly review your glucose data to improve your readings?
   ❑ yes   ❑ no   ❑ rarely

9. Do you adjust insulin doses or foods eaten to improve your glucose results?
   ❑ yes   ❑ no   ❑ occasionally

Other Considerations

1. Do you have vision problems or arthritis where a specific pump may help enter selections, fill the reservoir, or insert an infusion set?

   _____

2. Will your health insurance company, HMO, or Medicare cover the cost of pump therapy? Will out-of-pocket expenses fit your budget?

   _____

Questions for Parents to Consider

1. How willing is your child or teen to wear a pump?
   not willing   1   2   3   4   5   6   7   very willing   ❑ too young to decide

2. How willing are you to be involved in your child/teen's pump program?
   not willing   1   2   3   4   5   6   7   very willing

3. Will your child try to hide their pump/diabetes from their peers?
   ❑ yes   ❑ no   ❑ unsure

4. Does your child/teen learn new skills easily?
   ❑ yes   ❑ no   ❑ sometimes

5. Does your child/teen give their own injections, count carbs, determine their own doses, and monitor glucose levels with minimal help?
   ❑ yes   ❑ no   ❑ not yet

6. How do you feel about your child/teen gradually assuming age-appropriate responsibility for their own diabetes care?

   _____

7. Will you have a trained diabetes professional available when you need help?
   ❑ yes   ❑ no   ❑ unsure

If you or your child are not a good pump candidate at this time, say "no" to pump therapy until it fits well with you or your child's desires or lifestyle. Be open about your reservations and discuss them with your doctor, family, and friends before making a final choice.

People Who Became Pumpers

Motivated by circumstances, the four people below now benefit from an insulin pump. Their stories may help you understand your situation and potential benefits.

Amy

Amy is a software engineer and racquetball fanatic in her late 20s. For most of her 12 years with diabetes, she has been plagued by repeated highs and lows. Her glucose variability has been largely triggered by her low daily insulin requirements and by rapid changes in her level of activity.

Amy's average total daily insulin dose (TDD) is only 18 units a day, and her glucose falls about 140 mg/dl (7.8 mmol/L) per unit of insulin (her correction factor). Amy finally switched to an insulin pump after she was found unconscious behind the wheel of her car in a shopping mall parking lot.

She now loves the ability to deliver insulin in hundredths of a unit, rather than using an insulin pen with only half unit increments. By using a temporary basal reduction over several hours before and after she plays racquetball, she can now avoid most of the night lows that had plagued her in the past. She is now able to fine-tune her doses and marvels at the stability of her glucose readings. She is much less fearful of lows now that she wears a CGM. Her husband and coworkers are thrilled with her mellowed personality. She sums it up, saying, "I now feel like a regular person."

2.1 Are Your Expectations Realisistic?	
Realistic	**Not So Realistic**
It'll improve my glucose control.	I'll have perfect control.
By counting carbs, I can eat when I want.	I can eat and not think about it.
I'll check my glucose more often and get better control.	I'll check my glucose less often.
It may help prevent complications.	Complications won't happen.
It will take some effort.	It will be easy.
Knowing my glucoses, basal and bolus doses, I can adjust settings to improve my control.	My pump will take care of my diabetes.

George

George is 66 and retired after selling his plumbing business. He has had Type 2 diabetes for 15 years. George began to use injections after 10 years when three oral drugs would no longer control his morning readings. Over time, his injected doses increased to 96 units a day, but his fasting readings remained above 150 mg/dl (8.3 mmol/L), well above the level he desired to maintain good health.

He considered a pump for more than a year before he finally agreed with his wife to try it. Three months later, with his A1c at 6.2% on only 60 units a day, George says, "Now I don't have to work so hard to have a good day. I wake up in the morning with normal readings. I use half as much insulin, and my triglyceride levels are normal for the first time in years. I can give insulin whenever I need it. I really love my pump."

Josh

Josh is a tile layer who has had Type 1 diabetes for 37 years. He blamed work and family obligations for not visiting his physician. When he developed nerve damage with tingling in his feet and numbness up both calves, he finally admitted to his doctor that he had been making up most of his readings on the rare monitoring logs he had turned in over the years. His A1c test came back from the lab at 10.7% (normal range: 4-6%). He began to take monitoring and self-management seriously when he could no longer get to sleep because of shooting pains in his legs that medication could not completely stop.

Once Josh started managing his diabetes, his doctor recommended that he try an insulin pump. He was told that the improvement in glucose control might help his neuropathy. With a pump, he could also quickly adjust his doses when his work changed from carrying, cutting, and cementing tile to easier periods of grouting and polishing.

After ten months on his pump and many adjustments, his basals and boluses are matched to his true insulin need. Now Josh is able to sleep through the night without a neuropathy medication. "The feeling in my feet and legs is definitely better. This has made all the effort worth it," he says.

Lisa

Lisa, who is five years old, developed diabetes when she was three. With multiple daily injections, her parents were constantly on alert for night lows due to a variable peaking activity of her long-acting insulin and changes in her activity levels. To help with her management, Lisa's parents put her on a CGM. As a picky eater, her parents couldn't give her meal injections until they knew how many grams of carb she had consumed, causing frequent highs after meals. She complained about having to take so many injections, and her parents were frustrated with trying to give her doses in fractions of units. When they tried to give larger pre-meal injections to avoid having to give corrective ones later, Lisa often went low.

Three months after starting on her pump, Lisa's parents noted that she slept more soundly at night and they were also much less fearful of night lows. They can now give boluses quickly and easily when needed before or after meals without the need for an injection. It was easy to give some of her meal bolus before she ate and give an additional bolus once her total carb intake was known.

Her father programmed her pump to alert two hours after each bolus to retest and correct with a small correction bolus or carb snack, if needed at that time to stabilize her blood sugar. This has improved her control greatly and Lisa no longer worries about having to take injections. Lisa and her parents now smile a lot more.

> ### 2.2 Pumping Tips
> - Test often.
> - Keep adjusting basal and bolus doses until your readings are mostly normal.
> - Change your site in the morning.
> - Disconnect at your infusion site before you remove your reservoir, prime the line, or attempt to free a clog.
> - Beware of unexplained highs – it may be your infusion set or pump.
> - Check your pump clock occasionally to ensure appropriate basal delivery.

Summary

If you believe you could benefit from a pump and are willing to put in the effort to make it work for you, discuss different pump choices with your doctor and how to begin. Try to start when your life is stable and not too busy, as you'll want a clear head and some extra time to devote to learning how best to use your pump to manage your diabetes.

Action springs not from thought, but from a readiness for responsibility.

Dietrich Bonhoeffer

Carb Counting for Accurate Boluses

CHAPTER

3

Carb boluses usually make up nearly half of the insulin taken in a day. ***Thus, matching carbs well with insulin accounts for about half the day's glucose control.*** Carbohydrate is the primary nutrient that raises your glucose. Carb counting lets you match the carbs you eat with precise boluses from your pump. If you do not count carbs, this chapter shows how to use this great tool to maximize your success on a pump. If you already count carbs, a review will sharpen your skills.

Accurate carb counts let you cover meals and snacks with the precise boluses you need. Accurate carb boluses reduce post-meal spiking and make it less likely that you will need to chase high readings. Having fewer post-meal spikes and the highs and lows that go with them is a great way to reduce glucose variability.

This chapter describes

- What carbs and grams are
- How to figure your daily carbohydrate need
- Three methods for carb counting
- The bigger nutrition picture
- The glycemic index and glycemic load

Carb counting even allows you to splurge occasionally on foods like ice cream, cake, pie, or candy. You just need to match the total carbs in these foods with a bolus using the bolus calculator in your pump. Pump software and phone applets contain a list of carb counts for different foods to improve your accuracy.

To get an accurate carb bolus, you want to know ***how many grams of carb one unit of insulin covers. This is called your carb factor (CarbF).*** Once a CarbF is entered into the pump, you simply count how many grams you want to eat and enter this into your pump to get the bolus needed to cover them. It is not always easy to estimate a precise carb count for every meal. Even experienced pumpers and dietitians make mistakes.

Carbs are found in:

- Grains (breads, cereals, crackers, and pasta)
- Fruits and vegetables
- Beans, lentils, and peas
- Root crops (carrots, beets, potatoes, sweet potatoes, and yams)
- Beer, wine, brandy and liquors
- Desserts, candy, cookies, cake, and pie
- Milk, yogurt, and cottage cheese
- Regular soft drinks, fruit juices and drinks
- Sugar, honey, syrup, sucrose, and fructose

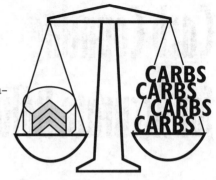

Some foods like meat, eggs, cheese, tofu, or nuts, and fats like oils, margarine, or butter have no carbs.

How Many Carbs Do You Need a Day?

The grams of carb you need a day can be found as a percentage of your daily calorie need. A person who requires 2000 calories a day would ideally get 45% to 55%, or 900 to 1100, of those calories from the carbohydrate in breads, grains, vegetables, fruits, low-fat milk, and so on.

> **3.1 A Three Day Diet Diary**
>
> At your next dietary appointment, bring a three-day diet diary that has brand names, portion sizes, and carb counts. This record will improve your carb counts, and your dietitian can make much better suggestions to improve food choices.

Each gram of carbohydrate contains four calories of energy. This means a person eating 2000 calories a day would usually consume 225 to 275 grams (900 to 1100 calories divided by 4 calories per gram) of carb per day. Other calories come from protein and fat.

To get an idea of how many grams are in your current diet, eat your usual meals for a few days and keep a record of how many carbs you eat. Use this chapter and carb references (books, labels, and perhaps a computer software program) to help you analyze your diet. Sit down with a dietitian and review your diet diary to confirm that it provides a healthy balance of nutrients.

Workspace 3.2 shows the steps to find your recommended daily carb intake. If you are eating fewer carbs than the USDA recommended amount, try increasing your carb intake by 10%, while reducing fat and protein calories by the same amount. Remember that carbs and proteins have four calories per gram, while fat has nine. The same number of fat grams will have more than twice as many calories.

Most foods are not pure carbohydrate, so a food's weight doesn't directly reveal its carb content. For example, even though 224 grams (one cup) of milk, a 160-gram slice of watermelon, a 14-gram rectangular graham cracker (two squares), and 12 grams (one tablespoon) of sugar have different weights, they all contain exactly 12 grams of carbohydrate. Only the sugar is 100% carbs. The other foods contain water and other ingredients. Despite their different weights, these foods require approximately the same carb bolus to cover their identical carb counts.

3.2 Find How Many Carbs You Need a Day in Four Steps

1. Choose a Calorie Factor That Matches Your Activity Level

My Average Daily Activity Level Is:	My Calorie Factor Is: male	female
Very Sedentary: Slow walking, mostly sitting.	13	11.5
Sedentary: Walking, bowling, fishing or similar activities.	14	12.5
Moderately Active: Dancing, 18 hole golf, pleasure swimming, etc.	15	13.5
Active: 20 min. or more of jogging, swimming, or similar activity 3+ times a week.	16	14.5
Super Active: One hour or more of vigorous activity 4 or more days a week: football, weight training, full court basketball.	17	15.5
My Calorie Factor Is: _____		

2. Find Your Daily Calorie Requirement

Multiply your current or desired body weight by your calorie factor.

_____ lbs X _____ = _____ calories/day
    weight   calorie factor   daily calorie need

3. Select a Carb Percentage Factor

The USDA Dietary Guidelines recommend that healthy diets contain 45 to 65% of calories from mostly complex carbs. To convert a daily calorie requirement into grams of carb for a 30% carb diet use a carb % factor of 13.3 in Step 4, for 35% use 11.4, for 40% 10.0, for 45% 8.93, for 50% 8.0, for 55% 7.25, for 60% 6.67, for 65% 6.17, and for 70% use 5.71.

4. Find How Many Grams of Carb You Need a Day

To find the grams of carb you need a day, divide your daily calorie requirement from Step 2 by your Carb % Factor from Step 3.

_____ calories/day ÷ 10 = _____ grams/day
    daily calorie need   carb grams per day

.

How to Count Carbs

Carbs are counted in grams. A gram is a weight unit like an ounce, but its small size makes it more useful to accurately measure foods. One ounce equals 28 grams. Remember that 1 oz. = 28 grams to easily convert ounces on food labels or in books into grams.

Carbs can be counted:

- By reading food labels,
- By looking up the carb content in a book that lists carbs, or
- By using the carb database in your pump or PDA or on a phone app.

For accurate carb counts, carefully weigh and measure your foods and calculate your serving sizes (See 3.7). Carb counting takes a week or two to understand and apply easily. Weighing food, determining serving sizes, and calculating carb content trains your eye to estimate accurately at home and when eating out. You'll be able to look at a piece of fruit, a bowl of pasta, or a plate of stir-fried veggies and rice, and estimate its carb count. For accurate meal boluses, enter your current glucose along with your carb count. Your glucose lets your pump make appropriate adjustments for any bolus insulin still active from recent boluses.

As you look up or measure carbs in foods, make a list of foods you eat often for reference. Once you learn your basic foods, it becomes easier to count carbs in your entire diet.

3.4 What if You Don't Count Carbs?

Not everyone counts carbs. Some people find it easier to eat consistent meals and base meal boluses on how well that bolus worked in the past. This can be a very effective method when someone's meals and lifestyle are consistent from day to day. Keep in mind that carb counting is relatively easy to learn if a personal dosing system is not working.

1. Food Labels

The nutrition labels on packaged foods provide the size of a standard serving and how many grams of carb, fat, protein, calories, and other nutrients contained in that serving. If you eat a single serving, the carb grams listed for that serving is all you need. If you eat a different amount, calculate the exact number of carbs in your serving.

2. Nutrition Books, Cookbooks, Software, and Smart Phone

Nutrition books, cookbooks, and software in a pump or smart phone improve carb count accuracy. They list carb grams in typical servings for different foods. If your serving size differs, weigh or measure your serving and use a calculator to convert what you are eating into grams of carb. Phone apps, carb and calorie books, cookbooks, and software let you easily look up brand name foods, restaurant meals, and food you make at home.

Let's say you want to eat 2 cups of yogurt as part of your meal.

1. Look at the Nutrition Facts label from a yogurt container shown here. The label shows a serving size as 1 cup.

2. A one-cup serving has 18 grams of carbs. Multiply 18 grams by two servings to find the total grams of carb you eat:

1 cup	=	18 grams
x 2		x 2
2 cups	=	36 grams

Nutrition Facts

Serving Size 1 cup (8 oz)
Servings Per Container 8

Amount Per Serving

Calories 130   Calories from Fat 0

% Daily Value

Total Fat 0 g	0%
Saturated Fat 0 g	0%
Cholesterol 0 mg	0%
Sodium 0 mg	0%
Total Carbohydrates 18 g	6%
Dietary Fiber 0 g	0%
Sugars 3 g	
Protein 4 g	

Pay attention to "Dietary Fiber" on nutrition labels. Dietary fiber is not digested, so if a food has 5 grams or more of fiber per serving, subtract the fiber grams from the carb total listed in the serving before you calculate a carb bolus.

Books and cookbooks can be found in the "Nutrition and Diet" section of your local bookstore, library, at online sources like the American Diabetes Association (www.diabetes.org), or ordered from the Diabetes Mall (www.diabetesnet.com/dmall/) where you can call (800) 988-4772 for a 30% discount and suggestions about which books may fit your needs. Online sources and diabetes product guides from diabetes

3.6 Books for Carb Counting and Healthy Eating

- **CalorieKing Calorie Fat & Carbohydrate Counter**
  (Family Health Publications, $8.99) - yearly update of over 14,000 basic foods and those served at fast-food and chain restaurants, plus diet guides for diabetes and weight control.

- **The Diabetes Carbohydrate & Fat Gram Guide**
  by Lea Ann Holzmeister (American Diabetes Association, $16.95) - includes carb and fat grams, exchanges, and many fast food or restaurant items.

- **ADA Complete Guide To Carb Counting**
  by H. Warshaw and K. Kulkarni (American Diabetes Association, $18.95) a guide to help you master the food part of control by learning to count carbs.

Look for these at bookstores, or at www.diabetesnet.com/dmall/ for 30% off.

magazines, such as *Diabetes Health* and *Diabetes Forecast*, provide helpful lists of phone apps, software and books.

3. Weigh and Measure

For foods with no food label, such as cooked pasta, unsliced bread, soups, and casseroles, you can find their carb count in a reference book once you accurately measure your serving size. A measuring cup, teaspoon, tablespoon, and a gram scale are all the tools you need to measure serving sizes. A glass measuring cup with marked lines that you can sight across is helpful for measuring liquids. On a gram scale, a food's total weight is measured in grams, of which a certain percentage will be carbs, while cups and spoons measure the serving size. Once you know your serving size, you can determine the grams of carb in your serving.

Appendix A in this book gives a list of carb foods with the typical percentage of their weight that comes from carbs. You can simply weigh one of them on a gram scale and multiply its weight by its carb percentage to find out how many grams of carb you

---

3.7 Use a Gram Scale to Count the Carbs in Cooked Spaghetti

With a standard gram scale and carb percentage list (Appendix A):

1. Place plate on scale, press the tare button to zero out the plate's weight, and then place the amount of cooked spaghetti you want to eat on the plate.

2. Let's say your portion weighs 200 grams on the scale. From Appendix A, you find that cooked plain spaghetti has 26 percent of its weight as carbohydrate.

3. Multiply the spaghetti's total weight by its percentage of carbs.

> **Example**
>
> | 200 g | x | 0.26 | = | 52 g |
> |-------|---|------|---|------|
> | weight of spaghetti | | carb % | | total carbs in portion |

4. When you eat 200 grams of cooked spaghetti, you eat 52 grams of carbohydrate.

With a computer gram scale:

1. Computerized gram scales already contain programmed information about the nutrition content of spaghetti and other foods.

2. Tare (zero out) your plate on the scale

3. Enter the food code for spaghetti into the scale.

4. Place the amount of spaghetti you want to eat onto your plate.

5. Press the carb key on the scale to find out how many grams of carbohydrate are in the spaghetti.

Gram scales are available online, and at most kitchen supply and many retail stores.

will eat. Another easy way is to use a computerized gram scale with built-in nutritive breakdowns for a variety of foods. Enter a food code or scroll to find a food in the database, and then a computer scale provides the carbs, calories, fat, and protein in the portion being weighed.

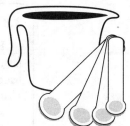

Occasionally, carry your gram scale and list of carb percentages with you to restaurants. Weigh your food to calculate the grams of carbohydrate in the meal. Don't worry. People do strange things in restaurants. Pretend you are a food inspector or food critic. Your self-consciousness will be more than offset by your improved control and the extra service you receive from the waiter.

Most foods have a big difference between volume and weight. For example, 1 1/4 cups of Cheerios® equals 10 ounces in volume (300 ml) but it weighs only 1 ounce (28 grams). For convenience, nutrition labels and food composition tables give serving size in both measures, so you can use either a measuring cup or scale to determine the carb count.

All carb counting is done in grams. Keep the metric conversions in Table 3.3 handy so you can convert ounces to grams.

Cafeteria Style and Combination Foods

Combination foods are somewhat difficult because they can vary greatly in their carb content depending on the recipe. Table 3.11 provides an estimate of the carbs per portion size for a variety of combination foods. You can also conduct your own test. Eat the same amount of a particular food made from the same recipe several times and take a carb bolus based on its estimated carb count. Test your blood sugar at 2 hours and again at 4 hours. Keep a record and use your best estimate from then on.

The Bigger Nutrition Picture – Eating Healthy

Mastering carb counting is not the only health goal you have. If you eat foods high in calories, fat, and sugar, this makes glucose control more difficult. A healthy and balanced diet protects your health, reduces the need for insulin, and improves your A1c. It also lowers your risk for heart disease, stroke, high blood pressure, and some cancers.

It is not necessary to be a food purist. Instead, gradually eliminate poor food choices over time and select healthier foods – vegetables, fruits, and whole grains – that ease your path toward optimum control. Add fiber and lower glycemic index carbs (a GI below 60 in Table 3.13) to reduce spiking of the glucose after meals.

Your overall health depends on:

- Eating a wide variety of nutrient-rich foods
- Keeping fat and protein at reasonable amounts
- Balancing carb intake with carb boluses or exercise

3.8 More on Fats and Proteins

Energy, measured as calories, is derived from three main ingredients: carbohydrates, fats, and proteins. Although the whole story is more complex, carbs and fats are largely used for fuel, while proteins are primarily used to build enzymes for metabolism and structural elements for cells and blood vessels.

Although carbs produce about 90% of the impact on your glucose, fat and protein each have effects, as well. The fat in certain foods may delay the absorption of carbohydrate from the intestine and cause a smaller or slower than expected rise in the glucose.[44,45] For example, milk fat gives ice cream a low glycemic index.

On the other hand, certain high fat meals can make you more resistant to insulin for 8 to 16 hours and make your glucose rise more than expected.[46, 47] The fats found in many chips and pizzas can cause a rise that is higher and longer lasting than expected.

Normal portions of protein have little impact on glucose, but large amounts can make the glucose rise. Half of these protein calories slowly convert to glucose over several hours.[48] A high-protein dinner (eight-ounce steak or a bean burrito) can cause glucose levels to rise 4 to 12 hours later with an unexpected high reading the next morning.

In a healthy diet, most carbs will be eaten as nutrient-dense foods like whole grains, fruits, legumes, vegetables, nonfat or low fat milk, and yogurt. These foods contain a high volume of micronutrients, such as vitamins, minerals, fiber, and protein in proportion to their caloric content. Fiber and nutrients slow digestion and reduce "carb craving" for many people. A huge advantage to eating healthy carb foods is that they tend to be lower on the glycemic index and cause less spiking of the glucose.

Nutrient-poor foods like candy and regular sodas contain carbs from simple sugars but lack the other nutrients your cells require for health. These carbs rank high on the glycemic index, are likely to spike the blood sugar, and are best eaten in small amounts. Nutrient-dense foods like brown rice and broccoli are more filling and are better for your health and your blood sugars. Most vegetables contain so few carbs that they can be ignored unless the carbs add up to more than 15 grams, or you find that your glucose rises after eating them. Some, like corn and peas, usually require a carb bolus.

3.9 Carb and Nutrition Resources Online

A great resource for carb and nutrition information is the USDA National Nutrient Database at www.nal.usda.gov/fnic/foodcomp/Data/. The database can be searched, or you can download an alphabetical list of every food you can think of along with its carb content.

The amount and type of fat in the diet is important. Diets with more fish oil (omega-3 fatty acids), monounsaturated fats (olive oil and avocados), and polyunsaturated fats (vegetable oils) are associated with less heart disease. In contrast, trans or hydrogenated fats, and saturated fats increase risks for heart disease and cancer.

3.10 Grams of Carb Divided through the Day

Meal	Example 1	Example 2	Example 3	My Carbs
Breakfast	75 grams	30 grams	75 grams	____ grams
Morning Snack		15 grams		____ grams
Lunch	75 grams	45 grams	70 grams	____ grams
Afternoon Snack		30 grams		____ grams
Dinner	75 grams	75 grams	40 grams	____ grams
Bedtime Snack		30 grams	40 grams	____ grams
Total Carbs	225	225	225	____ grams

Example 1 divides 225 carbs evenly into 3 meals. Example 2 starts with a light breakfast and lunch, with snacks between meals, and ends with a big dinner. Example 3 starts with a large breakfast and lunch and finishes with a light dinner and bedtime snack.

Find how many carbs you need a day from Workspace 3.2, then divide then your total carbs per day into different meals.

© 2012 Diabetes Services, Inc .

People with diabetes develop heart disease two to six times more often than people without diabetes. The American Heart Association and the Academy of Nutrition and Dietetics recommend a fat intake of less than 20% to 30% of total calories.

To lower your risk of heart disease, lower or eliminate your intake of chips and crackers made with hydrogenated fat or margarine. It also helps to reduce intake of sour cream, cheese, and fried foods. Switch to monounsaturated oils (olive oil, avocado), polyunsaturated seed oils (safflower oil, sunflower oil) corn oil and nuts. Choose protein foods that are lower in fat or that contain better types of fat, such as fish, skinless chicken, nonfat milk, and nonfat cheese products. Instead of margarine on waffles or pancakes, try apple butter (has no fat) and add flavorful nuts.

About one of every three people with Type 1 diabetes develops kidney disease. Eating less animal protein in the diet lessens this risk and slows its progression if it is present. Smaller red meat portions lower the intake of harmful saturated fats and protect kidney function. A vegetarian-heavy diet with small amounts of egg whites, fish and chicken and less red meat may be your best answer. If you have kidney disease, talk with your dietitian about the best diet choices.

No one benefits from an excess of high-calorie, low-nutrient foods, yet small amounts of sweets add flavor and, when chosen wisely, make avoiding fatty foods easier. Today's diabetes diet does not ban sugar from coffee, jelly from toast, nor an occasional small piece of pie from the dinner table. Today's rapid-acting insulins can more easily balance a reasonable amount of carbs in desserts, ice cream, and candy, especially when a bolus is taken early. Be careful though: sugar often travels with saturated fat. Those sweet chocolate candy bars get about 60 percent of their calories from saturated fat!

If you have an addictive sweet craving and a little is never enough, eliminate processed foods made with simple sugars entirely for six to eight weeks and eat more whole grain foods. Then, gradually reintroduce small amounts of refined carbs into your diet. Eating fruit helps satisfy sweet cravings.

Whether you include sweets in your meals or not is not the important issue. The key to glucose control is to determine the amount of carbs in your food and cover them with an appropriate bolus. Counting carbs and eating a nutrient-rich, low-fat, low-protein diet is a vital part of any healthy lifestyle with diabetes.

Eating a similar number of carbs at the same meal each day helps when you first go on a pump or anytime you

3.11 Sample Values in Combination Style Foods			
Homemade and restaurant recipes vary greatly. Don't rely on the carb values below until you eat and test them.			
Food	**Cals**	**Fat**	**Carbs**
Beef Stroganoff, 5 oz	195	13	7
Beef Stroganoff with 4 oz noodles	350	14	36
Chicken Lasagna, 1 piece	300	11	32
Chicken Chop Suey with 4 oz rice	245	4	37
Deep Dish Burrito, 7 oz	265	13	20
Ground Beef Casser., 2 scoop, 6 oz	245	13	17
Ital. Meat Sauce (5 oz) for Spaghetti	150	9	9
with 5 oz Spaghetti	350	10	49
Lasagna, 1 piece	275	11	25
Meatloaf, 3 oz	205	13	4
Ranch Beans, 2 scoops, 6 oz	350	11	45
Red Beans & Rice, 7 oz	280	9	37
Scalloped Pot./Ham, 2 scoop, 6 oz	160	6	20
Stuffed Shells in Sauce (1)	105	3	17
Swedish Meatballs (3)	205	12	9
Sweet & Sour Pork/Rice, 9 oz	240	3	40
Swiss Steak, Mushroom Gravy, 5 oz	280	11	4
Tator Tot Casserole, 2 scoops, 6 oz	260	15	20
Tenderloin Tips Gravy, 5 oz	210	13	3
w 5 oz noodles	395	15	38
Tuna Noodle Casser., 2 scoop, 6 oz	180	6	17
Turkey Tetrazzini, 2 scoop, 6 oz	195	7	17
Vegetable Lasagna, 1 piece	250	13	21

want to bring readings into better control. Some people find glucose control is easier when they eat the same number of carbs for each meal and snack of the day and cover these with fixed carb boluses. It can also help to eat smaller amounts of carbs more often during the day.

Glycemic Index and Glycemic Load

Just like long-acting insulins, there are long-acting or slow (low-GI) carbs. Carbs that digest slowly can be used at bedtime or during lengthy exercise to keep your glucose steady and prevent it from

3.12 Don't Skip Meals

When someone eats only one or two meals a day, the body stores extra fat in the abdomen for quick release due to the longer time between these meals. Unfortunately, during sleep, these larger abdominal fat stores raise circulating free fatty acid and triglyceride levels in the blood that may increase insulin resistance and accelerate damage to blood vessels.

Eat reasonable amounts of complex, low glycemic index carbs through the day to reduce fat release into the blood and assist weight maintenance. A healthy "nibbling" diet lowers triglycerides and LDL cholesterol levels, and may keep your glucose in better control.

rising quickly after you eat and then falling quickly. Slow carbs with a low GI include beans (lima, pinto, etc.), green apples, Power Bars, raw cornstarch, pasta *al dente*, barley, cracked wheat, parboiled long grain and whole grain rice, and whole-grain rye bread.

The glycemic index table lists various carbohydrate foods based on how quickly they digest and affect the blood sugar.[47,48] Glucose, the fastest-acting carbohydrate, is given a value of 100. A food's glycemic index is derived when the same number of carbs is eaten while a researcher measures how that particular food affects the glucose.

Ripeness, cooking time, fiber, fat content, and what other foods are combined with it all impact how a food affects the glucose. Glycemic index ranking may vary somewhat in daily use. If you have access to a CGM, you can create your own glycemic index through repeat testing and record keeping. Personal testing pays off well in better glucose management.

Choose a fast carb with a high GI number to raise a low glucose, cover moderate or strenuous exercise, or quickly rebuild glycogen stores immediately after exercise. When your glucose is low or rapidly dropping due to exercise, high glycemic index carbs are best. If you want to eat a high GI food and your glucose is near your target, you might bolus early, eat the food toward the end of the meal, or simply eat less of it.

Slow carbs that have lower glycemic index numbers minimize unwanted spikes after meals and help keep glucose steadier during long periods of activity. They are better choices for maintaining day-to-day control. If your glucose often spikes after breakfast, change to a cereal or bread that has a lower glycemic index, eat less of it, or combine it with another carb that has a low GI. A low GI food reduces the impact that other carbs in the meal may have on your glucose. A low glycemic index snack at bedtime can help stabilize the glucose during the night.

3.13 Glycemic Index

Foods are compared to glucose, which ranks 100. Higher numbers indicate faster absorption and a faster rise in the blood sugar, while lower numbers indicate a slower rise.

Cereals		Snacks		Fruit	
All Bran™	51	chocolate bar	49	apple	38
Bran Buds +psyll	45	corn chips	72	apricots	57
Bran Flakes™	74	croissant	67	banana	56
Cheerios™	74	doughnut	76	cantaloupe	65
Corn Chex™	83	Graham crackers	74	cherries	22
Cornflakes™	83	jelly beans	80	dates	103
Cream of Wheat	66	Life Savers™	70	grapefruit	25
Frosted Flakes™	55	oatmeal cookie	57	grapes	46
Grapenuts™	67	pizza, cheese & tom.	60	kiwi	52
Life™	66	Pizza Hut™, supreme	33	mango	55
muesli, natural	54	popcorn, light micro	55	orange	43
Nutri-grain™	66	potato chips	56	papaya	58
oatmeal, old fash	48	pound cake	54	peach	42
Puffed Wheat™	67	Power Bars™	58	pear	58
Raisin Bran™	73	pretzels	83	pineapple	66
Rice Chex™	89	rice cakes	82	plums	39
Rice Krispies™	82	saltine crackers	74	prunes	15
Shredded Wheat™	67	shortbread cookies	64	raisins	64
Special K™	54	Snickers™ bar	41	watermelon	72
Total™	76	strawberry jam	51	**Pasta**	
Root Crops		vanilla wafers	77	cheese tortellini	50
french fries	75	**Crackers**		fettucini	32
potato, new, boiled	59	Graham	74	linguini	50
potato, red, baked	93	rice cakes	80	macaroni	46
potato, sweet	52	rye	68	spaghetti, 5m boil	33
potato, wht, boiled	63	soda	72	spaghetti, 15m boil	44
potato, wht, mash	70	water	78	spaghetti, prot enriched	28
yam	54	Wheat Thins™	67	vermicelli	35

3.13 Glycemic Index - continued

Breads		Beans		Soups/Vegetables	
bagel, plain	72	baked	44	beets, canned	64
banana bread	47	black beans, boil	30	black bean soup	64
baguette, French	95	butter, boiled	33	carrots, fresh, boiled	49
croissant	67	cannellini beans	31	corn, sweet	56
dark rye	76	garbanzo, boiled	34	green pea soup	66
hamburger bun	61	kidney, boiled	29	green pea, frozen	47
muffins		kidney, canned	52	lentil soup	44
apple, cinnamon	44	lentils, gr or br	30	parsnips, boiled	97
blueberry	59	lima, boiled or frozen	32	peas, fresh, boiled	48
oat & raisin	54	navy	38	split pea and ham	66
pita	57	pinto, boiled	39	tomato soup	38
pizza, cheese	60	red lentils, boiled	27	**Cereal Grains**	
pumpernickel	49	soy, boiled	16	barley	25
sourdough	54	**Milk Products**		basmati white rice	58
rye	64	chocolate milk	35	bulgar	48
white	70	custard	43	couscous	65
wheat	68	ice cream, vanilla	60	cornmeal	68
Drinks		ice milk, vanilla	50	millet	71
apple juice	40	skim milk	32	**Sugars**	
colas	65	soy milk	31	fructose	22
Gatorade™	78	tofu frozen dessert	115	honey	62
grapefruit juice	48	whole milk	30	maltose	105
orange juice	46	yogurt, fruit	36	sucrose	61
pineapple juice	46	yogurt, plain	14	table sugar	64

See **The New GI Handbook** for information on glycemic index & glycemic load. Available at bookstores, or at www.diabetesnet.com/dmall/ at a 30% discount.

A more precise way to measure a food's effect on your glucose is the glycemic load. *The glycemic load is a food's glycemic index times the number of carb grams in each serving of that food.* The resulting number provides a good guide for how one serving of a food will impact the blood sugar. For instance, the glycemic load of a small

3.14 Alcohol and Diabetes

Excess insulin and alcohol block the liver from releasing or making glucose, respectively. This means your body may not be able to raise your glucose if you go low. For example, four standard drinks lowers glucose production to about half of normal, and is a major cause of nighttime hypoglycemia.[49] Excess alcohol also impairs judgment, reduces accuracy in carb counts and bolus doses, and makes it harder to recognize lows. Never drink to excess or on an empty stomach!

If you do plan to go out drinking with a designated driver, Ulrike Thurm, RN, CDE, of Germany recommends a "Berlin Basal." To reduce the risk of hypoglycemia, she recommends to her young patients that they use a temp basal reduction from the time they leave to go out until noon or so the next day. A temp basal reduction of 20%, or 80% of normal, can be tried.

Hypoglycemia symptoms are strikingly similar to those of intoxication. If you go low after drinking, a police officer may not recognize the real problem due to the smell of alcohol, delaying treatment. You may be placed in a drunk tank rather than receive the carbs you need. If you choose to have a drink, mix alcohol and insulin with care.

Make the best decisions about drinking:

- Know the laws in your state.
- Remember, you can say "No!"
- If you plan to drink, eat carbs first. Do not skip meals or snacks.
- Limit the amount of alcohol by drinking one or two drinks slowly or alternating alcoholic with nonalcoholic beverages.
- Wine, beer and straight alcohol like gin or tequila may not need a bolus. Mixed drinks, liqueurs, and margueritas with sugar usually do.
- Never drink before you drive and never drive after drinking.
- Wear diabetes medical ID tags.
- Let friends know you have diabetes, how hypoglycemia might make you look or act, and that you can pass out from a low. Let them know a low cannot be slept off and you need carbs if you do not respond appropriately for any reason.
- Test your glucose before going to sleep and eat an extra bedtime snack.

serving of a high glycemic index food like hard candy may raise your glucose as much as a medium-sized serving of a low glycemic index food like popcorn.

Summary

Learn and use carb counting. You want to be able to match the meals you eat with appropriate boluses. Carb counting lets you do this, and accurate carb counting pays high dividends through improved control. Review and sharpen your carb counting skills periodically. Carb counting is critical to good control and most people tend to undercount their carbs.

All About CGMs

A *continuous glucose monitor or CGM* reads out a constant stream of glucose data every 1 to 5 minutes and gives 1440 readings a day compared to the 4 to 8 fingerstick readings you rely on with a meter. Not just a snapshot of the moment, a CGM shows whether your glucose is rising, falling, or steady before any changes become full-blown problems.

Clinical research shows that using a CGM reduces the severity, frequency, and length of hypoglycemia. It helps you spend less time hyperglycemic and more time in your target zone.[50-52] While a CGM can assist tight control on injections or MDI, adding it to a pump enhances the best features of both devices.

This chapter describes
- CGM components
- Essential steps for wear
- Site selection
- Warm up and calibration
- Setting the alarms, alerts and arrows
- Treatment guidelines
- Accuracy and other issues
- Using CGM data for pattern detection and pump adjustments

A CGM provides a wealth of real-time information that lets you see trends in your glucose over the previous 1 to 24 hours, shows the direction and speed of your glucose, and gives you alerts when high or low thresholds are reached. Together, these help you detect and avoid impending highs and lows. In adults, CGMs have been shown to lower A1c levels with no increase in hypoglycemia.[52]

A CGM acts like a diabetes coach who shows you how boluses, exercise, carb intake, and treatment of lows and highs affect glucose readings. CGM wearers can easily see if a bolus given just before eating causes the glucose to spike 1-2 hours later. Once undesirable patterns are identified, you can work toward preventing them with insulin and lifestyle adjustments. Low readings that were previously unnoticed during the night can be avoided.

A CGM provides a higher level of security with alarms, trend lines, arrows and a constant flow of readings. Users and their friends, family, colleagues, and healthcare professionals feel a greater level of confidence and peace of mind that glucoses are under control.

Combining a CGM with a pump's precise delivery provides the best method to manage blood glucose levels. The pump delivers insulin very accurately while the CGM helps the wearer fine-tune pump settings so that insulin delivery regulates the glucose well.

CGMs give valuable feedback and insight into situations that affect pump dose decisions. Information on the screen helps detect dislodged infusion sets and missed meal boluses. They also help test basal rates and boluses, monitor the effect of exercise and stress, and help wearers make better decisions on when to override bolus recommendations. While all these *real-time* uses provide the most benefit to wearers, data downloaded *retrospectively* from the CGM is also valuable. Downloaded data provides the details to analyze patterns over the last few days or weeks to quickly improve basal and bolus doses.

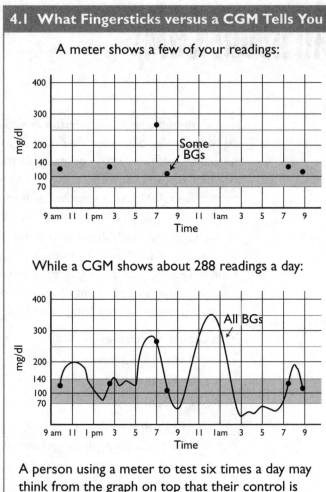

4.1 What Fingersticks versus a CGM Tells You

A meter shows a few of your readings:

While a CGM shows about 288 readings a day:

A person using a meter to test six times a day may think from the graph on top that their control is good. In contrast, the trend line on a CGM used the same day on the bottom shows how often the glucose was above and below their target range.

While CGMs have a wealth of uses, don't think you need to use every application if this is overwhelming. Some people may resist thinking about and responding to all the information a CGM provides. The most important ways that people use a CGM are the simple real-time ones – looking at the *trendline* or direction of their glucose to guide eating carbs or taking more insulin, and letting the *alerts* warn of hypo- and hyperglycemia. Avoiding hypoglycemia and reducing the fear of going low is essential to those who have hypoglycemia unawareness, frequent lows, or who keep glucoses high to lessen the risk of having a low. Alerts help those who live alone, during pregnancy when glucose levels have to be closely maintained, and with higher-risk jobs like long distance driving and fire fighting.

Pump wearers have been early adopters of CGM technology, but now more and more people using MDI are trying a CGM first and then adding a pump when they want the additional benefits for control. Some wearers of both feel that if they had to choose between a pump and a CGM, their CGM is more critical to their care.

CGM Components

CGMs have three basic components: a sensor, a transmitter and a receiver.

Sensor

A *sensor* is a thin, flexible wire inserted beneath the skin with a needle and an insertion device. The sensor rests in the fatty layer below the skin and is usually not felt by the person wearing it. Once the sensor is in place, the inserter and needle are removed. Some sensors can also be inserted by hand. Sensor wires vary from 1/4 to 3/5 inch (6 to 15 mm) in length. Current introducer needles vary from less than 26 gauge to 22 gauge. Sensors contain enzymes that react with glucose in the interstitial fluid around cells. A chemical reaction produces an electric signal that the transmitter sends to the CGM receiver where it is interpreted as a glucose level.

Transmitter

Once the sensor is inserted, a reusable waterproof *transmitter* is seated into a plastic pod on top of the sensor or clicked into the side of the sensor. Transmitters vary in size and shape from 1/4 to ½ inch (6 to 12 mm) thick and from a thumbnail to a half dollar in circumference.

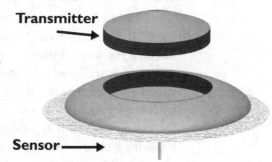

Transmitter

Sensor ⟶

A long-lasting battery that lasts over 12 months powers the Dexcom transmitter. The Medtronic transmitter is recharged about every 3 days and also stores more than 30 minutes of data when the receiver is out of range. It sends the data to the receiver when it is again within range.

Transmitters vary in how far they can send readings, currently about 5 to 10 feet (2 to 3 meters). Cell phones and other electronic devices can occasionally interfere with transmission of data.

4.3 Immediate CGM Information	
Your CGM Data	**What You Gain**
Glucose Values	Glucose values are updated every 5 minutes. Glucose history over the past few hours can be quickly reviewed.
Trend Lines	Direction of change in glucose values
Trend Arrows	Rate of change in glucose values
Alarms	**Threshold alerts** indicate when a high or low glucose value has been reached. **Prediction alerts** indicate that a high or low glucose value is likely to be reached in the future. **Direction and rate of immediate glucose change** indicates when glucose levels are changing rapidly, i.e. more than 1, 2 or 3 mg/dl (0.06-0.2 mmol/L) per minute.

Receiver

A battery-powered *receiver* or a display on the pump or pump controller displays glucose information received from the transmitter. Separate receivers are about the size of a small cell phone and can be carried in a pocket, backpack, or purse, or worn on a belt. With pump receivers, the user does not carry a separate receiver.

Current U.S. insulin pumps don't use CGM readings to adjust insulin delivery, but clinical trials are underway that will gradually add more closed loop features to pumps. Some trials are trying to close the loop with the wearer giving an approximate bolus for a meal to reduce post-meal glucose spiking. This allows slower bolus insulin to get started before the meal, with the CGM and pump handling the smaller dose adjustments that would then be required.

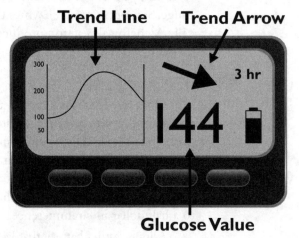

The receiver displays glucose values every five minutes, shows trend graphs of past glucose values over the last several hours (1 to 24 hours), and has arrows and trend lines that show whether the glucose is rising or falling. The receiver can be customized with alarms, covered in Box 4.3 and on pages 41-43.

4.4 Meaning of Trend Arrows for Dexcom and Medtronic CGMs				
Medtronic	**What It Means**	**Dexcom**	**What It Means**	
		↑↑	Rapidly Rising: over 3 mg/dl per min (180 mg/dl per hr)[4]	
↑↑	Rapid Rise: 2-3 mg/dl per min (120-180 mg/dl per hr)[3]	↑	Rising: 2-3 mg/dl per min (120-180 mg/dl per hr)[3]	
↑	Moderate Rise: 1-2 mg/dl per min (60-120 mg/dl per hr)[2]	↗	Slowly Rising: 1-2 mg/dl per min (60-120 mg/dl per hr)[2]	
blank	Stable: less than 1 mg/dl per min (60 mg/dl per hr)[1]	→	Constant: less than 1 mg/dl per min (60 mg/dl per hr)[1]	
↓	Moderate Fall: 1-2 mg/dl per min (60-120 mg/dl per hr)[2]	↘	Slowly Falling: 1-2 mg/dl per min (60-120 mg/dl per hr)[2]	
↓↓	Rapid Fall: 2-3 mg/dl per min (120-180 mg/dl per hr)[3]	↓	Falling: 2-3 mg/dl per min (120-180 mg/dl per hr)[3]	
		↓↓	Rapidly Falling: over 3 mg/dl per min (180 mg/dl per hr)[4]	

1 Change in glucose is less than 0.06 mmol/L per min (3.3 mmol/L per hour)
2 Rise or fall of 0.06 to 0.11 mmol/L per min, (3.3-6.7 mmol/L per hour)
3 Rise or fall of 0.11 to 0.17 mmol/L per min (6.7-10 mmol/L per hour)
4 Rise or fall of 0.17 mmol/L per min (10 mmol/L per hour)

The receiver and transmitter are durable devices that are reused each time the sensor is changed. Sensors are disposable and approved for 3 to 7 days of use depending on the manufacturer. In practice, sensor life varies from person to person and sensors can sometimes be used beyond their stated life.

Steps to Start and Stop a Sensor

The details below show how to put the sensor on, calibrate it, set alarms and remove it when the sensor life is over.

Sites and Sensor Insertion

Any site at least two or three inches away from both the last sensor site and the infusion set can be used. Choose any fleshy site without scars or bruises. Swab the site with alcohol and insert the sensor. Some sensors can be inserted by hand and all sensors come with automatic inserters. Unlike pump infusion sites, infections are rare with sensor sites because nothing is infused into the body. Bleeding can occur, so check the site for bleeding and wipe it clean if needed. If significant bleeding occurs, use another sensor in a different site. Check periodically for redness, tenderness, or swelling.

4.5 CGM Site Tips

- Approved for the abdominal area, many people wear their CGM on the back of the arms, outer thighs, upper buttocks, or love handles.
- Avoid scar tissue, shave areas where hair may prevent good adhesion.
- Pinch up the skin a bit during insertion to prevent the insertion needle from going too deep, BUT make sure it goes deep enough to get into fat tissue.
- If you use an adhesive barrier under the sensor, such as IV 3000, make sure to cut a hole where the sensor goes through.
- If you use Skin Tac or IV Prep pads to improve adhesion, make sure to avoid gumming up the skin near the point where the sensor will go into the skin.

Connect the transmitter to the sensor. A shower protector or adhesive placed over the sensor may improve adhesion and length of use. For more site information for infusion sets and CGMs, see page 85 for special site needs, and page 238 regarding adhesive allergies.

Warm-Up

Readings are not available during the warm-up period for the first two hours or so after sensor insertion. The warm-up period allows the sensor to settle into the interstitial fluid that surrounds cells and allows minor tissue trauma to resolve.

Calibration

After the warm-up period, the CGM requests one or two fingerstick glucose meter readings to calibrate the sensor. CGM accuracy improves after the first 12 to 24 hours as skin trauma subsides and additional calibrations are done. When possible, giving the sensor a low reading and a high reading, such as after eating, in the first 24 hours helps tune it up quicker. The glucose trend line and arrows are reliable during this time but don't rely on CGM glucose values until they are usually within 20 to 30 mg/dl (1.1 to 1.7 mmol/L) of your meter.

A CGM uses formulas to translate glucose values in the interstitial fluid around cells into blood glucose values but variations between the two will exist. Interstitial glucose values lag behind those in the blood.[53,54] Lag times have been reported to be 16 to 21 minutes for one brand of CGM, and 5 to 8 minutes for another.[55-58] The newest CGMs are expected to have lag times of 5 to 12 minutes.[59,60] *During a rapid rise or fall in glucose, lag times increase and larger differences can occur between meter and CGM readings.* On average, a CGM glucose value reads within 15% above or below the blood glucose value at a lab.

CGM error increases when a CGM is calibrated with a glucose meter that has its own accuracy issues. Glucose meter accuracy keeps improving, with some new meters approaching accuracies of ±15 mg/dl below 100 mg/dl (5.6 mmol/L) and ±10% above 100 mg/dl. Always calibrate with the most accurate meter available to minimize the error in your CGM readings.[61, 62] Always wash your hands before testing, and use strips that are not expired and have not been exposed to excessive temperatures.[61]

Sensor accuracy drifts, so calibrations are repeated every 12 to 24 hours, depending on CGM brand. Calibrating more often than requested may improve accuracy, especially when CGM readings differ by more than 30 mg/dl (1.7 mmol/L) from your meter readings. Bedtime calibration helps avoid the annoyance of an alert to calibrate during the night. Do not use alternate test sites like the forearm for calibration.

Accuracy will degrade if you do not calibrate routinely. Some CGMs stop giving readings if you wait too long to calibrate. Pay attention to the frequency your manufacturer recommends for calibration. Glucose accuracy, needle size, and ease of insertion improve with each new generation of sensors.

Set the Alarms and Alerts

CGMs can be set to alert you by an alarm or vibration or both when the glucose goes too high or low, when it is likely to go too high or low, or when there is a rapid rise or fall in glucose. These three alarms are called ***threshold***, ***prediction*** and ***rate of change***. Choose your setting on each of these to control the frequency and accuracy of the alarms and to avoid alarm burnout. Pressing a button on the receiver turns off an alarm.

Threshold alarms warn the user when a preset high or low glucose level called a threshold is reached. Because CGM readings may be somewhat inaccurate and tend to lag behind blood glucose values, choose the lowest upper threshold that warns you early of rising glucoses but does not cause too many alerts to tolerate, such as 140, 160, or 180 mg/dl (7.8, 8.9, or 10.0 mmol/L). For the lower threshold, select a level, like 80 mg/dl (4.4 mmol/L), that is high enough to catch most lows.

With a lower high and higher low, all potential highs and lows will be caught but alarms will sound more often. A trade-off exists between being annoyed by alarms, some of which may not be accurate, versus not being warned and missing an alarm for a real event. Alarm overload can cause some wearers to reset their thresholds further apart. Unfortunately this means that more highs and lows will be missed. To avoid alarm burnout, set your CGM alarms for highs to repeat at least a couple of hours apart.

	Set CGM Target Glucose Alarms To:	
A narrow range like 80 to 140 mg/dl (4.4 to 7.8 mmol/L)	**Pros:** You'll be warned of most high and low glucoses as they happen	**Cons:** More false alarms and disrupted sleep Greater risk of alarm burnout and ignoring alarms
A wider range like 70 to 200 mg/dl (3.9 to 11.1 mmol/L)	**Pros:** Fewer alarms Less risk of alarm burnout	**Cons:** Delayed warning of high and low glucose levels Less ability to correct early

With patience, glucose fluctuations lessen and control improves as CGM readings are used to adjust insulin and carbs. As management improves, thresholds can be adjusted toward more ideal levels, while still reducing the frequency of alarms.

With 80 mg/dl (4.4 mmol/L) as the low threshold and a general accuracy of ±20 mg/dl (±1.1 mmol/L), your glucose is likely to be between 60 and 100 mg/dl (3.3 and 5.5 mmol/L) when a low alert occurs. Lower or higher values can be programmed for pregnancy, hypoglycemia unawareness, and other special needs.

Prediction alarms warn the user that a low or high glucose is likely to occur in 10, 20 or 30 minutes, depending upon the setting the user chooses. Predictions are based on threshold levels and the rate of change. The CGM uses recent glucose measurements to predict a rise above or fall below the threshold. Better accuracy occurs with 10 and 20 minute predictions so try these initially and switch to 30 minutes as glucose control improves. Currently, only the insulin pump tracks bolus on board (BOB) activity. In the future, both pump and CGM information will be used to predict and control the glucose.

Rate of change alarms warn the user that the glucose is changing rapidly. The user can set them at 2 or 3 mg/dl (0.1 to 0.2 mmol/L) per minute, equivalent to at least a 120 to 180 mg/dl (6.7 to 10 mmol/L) change in glucose per hour. This alarm sounds regardless of how close to the thresholds of high or low the glucose reads. It is helpful for quickly detecting a missed meal bolus, high GI foods, or an inadequate bolus that leads to a rapidly rising glucose. It is also helpful for detecting a rapid fall from too large a correction bolus, especially if unrecognized excess BOB exists.

Snooze settings let you set how often a low or high glucose alarm will go off when the low or high reading has not been corrected. The low glucose snooze setting is especially important during sleep. When someone is awakened at night by a low glucose that they verify with a fingerstick reading, if a snooze is set to 15 minutes, the alarm may reawaken them because the CGM takes time to turn direction and catch up with the rising glucose after treatment. However, if they shut off the alarm and simply fall back asleep, a longer snooze may not be wise. Work with your CGM to find settings that work for you.

Removal

Current sensors are approved for up to 7 days of use. Sensor accuracy tends to improve on the second or third day of wear. The CGM will alert you when it is time to change. Sensors typically last longer if the user knows how to "trick" the receiver. (Check online blogs for these tricks.) Extended use is off-label from the Food and Drug Administration (FDA), so check with your provider. Sensor capacity and wound healing time usually allows longer use than the manufacturer's recommended times.

The main concern with longer use is infection, but the risk of this appears to be low compared to infusion sets. At some point during extended use, readings will become less accurate. When inaccurate readings occur, you can try calibrating the sensor a couple of times over an hour or so, but don't continue to use it if readings remain inaccurate. Be sure to discuss this with your physician. Irritation at the site from the sensor or tape is unusual, but check for this on removal.

Treatment Guidelines

CGM data cannot replace fingerstick values. If a high or low reading is seen on the CGM, current FDA guidelines require verification by a fingerstick reading before the glucose is treated. Using the CGM reading alone to determine treatment with a bolus dose may eventually become an approved practice once CGM accuracy provides readings within 20 or 30 mg/dl (1.1 or 1.7 mmol/L) of fingerstick values. The number of fingerstick tests you do each day may or may not decrease on a CGM. Keep in mind that your

---

4.8 A CGM Reading Needs to be Verified with a Fingerstick Test

- During the first 12 to 24 hours of use.

- When CGM and meter tests have been differing by over 30 mg/dl (1.7 mmol/L).

- If the CGM reading is erratic or does not seem right.

- When the CGM reading is high. Do a fingerstick before correcting with a bolus.

- When the CGM reading is low. Do a fingerstick before correcting with carbs if there is time to do so.

- Before driving, verify the CGM reading with a fingerstick, especially if it shows a falling arrow or falling trend line.

- When the CGM reading remains low 15 or 20 minutes after a low was treated in order to decide whether additional carbs are needed. The CGM's slow turn-around time can lead to unnecessary over-treatment.

- If Medtronic MAD (mean absolute difference) is above 20%

---

meter tests become more valuable when they are guided by the trend lines on your CGM. During the daytime, check readings on your receiver about once an hour for the best information from which to make decisions.

CGM Accuracy and Other Issues

CGM sensor accuracy varies from brand to brand and from sensor to sensor. Most sensors perform very well. A few may have some readings that are inaccurate or completely wrong, and an occasional sensor may not work at all. During sensor insertion, some mild trauma can

4.9 Clever CGM Trick – Amplify the Alert

If you're a sound sleeper, Dr. Bruce Buckingham, a pediatrician and researcher at Stanford University, suggests putting the CGM receiver on vibrate and placing it into an open metal or glass saucer beside the bed to amplify its sound. This can help parents of a child on a CGM or someone who lives alone. There are also earthquake detection apps for smartphones. Rubberband your receiver to your phone with the volume up and the app activated – guaranteed to wake you!

A receiver can also be worn in the pocket of sleepwear, on a belt around your waist, or placed near your head while sleeping. Parents of a child wearing a CGM can use a bedroom monitor to listen for alarms at night. Medtronic also offers a Sentry device to alert sleeping parents.

occur under the skin that produces readings with more error until the inflammation dies down. CGM readings are less reliable during the first 12 to 24 hours of use, even though trend lines and arrows are usually fine.

The sensor is a small metal or plastic fiber that can bend or kink while being inserted after hitting muscle, or as the needle that guides it during insertion is pulled out. If this happens, a sensor may not read correctly. Reading errors will also occur if a sensor is used beyond its effective life. Discontinue use as soon as readings start to drift.

Skips in data look like gaps or open spaces in the trend line. They can occur when the receiver is not close enough to the sensor and transmitter, such as when the receiver is left in a bag or jacket pocket that is more than 5 to 10 feet (2 to 3 meters) from the transmitter on the body. Skips may also occur when the wearer is sleeping on the sensor. One CGM user once commented "the dang thing can read through the wall into the next room but not through my body." This loss of signal may be caused by compression of skin and tissues under the transmitter when the wearer sleeps on it. Skips in data may also occur when the glucose is rapidly rising or falling.

The Medtronic receiver gives a **MAD** or mean (average) actual difference value calculated from the difference between fingerstick and CGM readings. If the MAD is above 20%, the CGM values should not be trusted. An erratic trend line or trend arrows that switch direction every few minutes also indicate that the CGM readings should not be relied upon.

One blogger recounts how he was at first disappointed and unsure whether to trust the readings from his CGM because they differed from his glucose meter. Finally, he focused his attention on using the trends and alarms. He still prefers accurate readings, but he now highly values knowing the direction his glucose is headed. Remember that even when CGM readings vary by as much as 30 mg/dl (1.7 mmol/L) from meter readings, this has relatively little impact on your bolus dose decisions.

Using CGM Data to Improve Glucose Control

A CGM will ideally help the user adjust insulin doses, insulin timing, food selections, and activity immediately, based on the displayed glucose levels on the receiver and later from downloaded data.

Rapid Adjustments from Information on the Receiver

Most people use the CGM to make rapid adjustments from the readings, trend lines, and arrows and alarms that warn of highs and lows. These let you adjust insulin, carbs and exercise to stay in your desired glucose target range most of the time. Carb boluses can be adjusted for specific meals, the right number of carbs can be consumed to prevent or treat lows, and correction boluses can be taken sooner for fast-rising readings.

Combine the CGM's approximate glucose, its trend, and the BOB still lowering your glucose to determine more accurate carb and correction doses for specific situations. Some overnight basal adjustments can be made based on the 6- or 12-hour trend lines.

The lag time on a CGM is most noticeable when your glucose is changing directions. With current systems, a downward glucose trend can take 20 minutes or more to change direction once carbs are consumed. If you are unsure, do a fingerstick to find out if your glucose has started to rise. When your glucose is high and climbing, a correction bolus will often take an hour or more before it starts to turn your glucose around. *Be patient with your CGM readings when your glucose is changing directions.*

After you eat carbs for a low or take a correction bolus for a high, watch the trend line to ensure that the treatment is working and ensure that a high or low glucose does not follow. When you are high, wait at least 2 hours between boluses to reduce insulin stacking. When you are low, manage your carb intake carefully, and wait at least 30 minutes when possible before eating again to avoid over-treatment. Insulin always seems slow when you try to bring down a high glucose, and although carbs work faster, they always seem slow when you treat a low glucose. Remember that impatience only makes your readings more erratic.

No CGM can be totally relied on to warn you of highs or lows. If your CGM accuracy is off, it may sound a false alarm or sound no alarm at all when one is needed. Regular glucose tests and calibration of the CGM is essential to catch most glucose problems and verify the CGM's accuracy.

Use Your CGM to Prevent and Correct Lows and Highs

An existing or predicted low glucose on a CGM needs immediate attention. Eat carbs right away or confirm with a fingerstick and eat carbs if needed. Use your trend lines and arrows to prevent lows when you can.

When a glucose is still normal but the trend line and arrows are going down or you have BOB present, eating carbs is the best answer. Confirm with a fingerstick and eat the carbs determined from Box 10.4, taking into account how low your glucose is and how fast the glucose is falling on the CGM.

If you are low before a meal, do not enter the carbs you need to treat the low into your bolus calculator (BC). Some insulin pumps ignore BOB and cover all carbs entered, so the pump's recommended bolus may be too large. Use Workspace 8.11 to check how your pump handles carb coverage and BOB.

Be sure to adjust your pump bolus recommendations based not only on your current glucose, but also the CGM trend line, your BOB, and any upcoming exercise or activity. If the trend arrow is stable and there's little or no BOB, the recommended BC dose should work. If the arrow shows a moderate or rapid fall, decrease the dose. If the trendline is rising, consider increasing the recommended dose while considering your glucose and BOB.

For example, when taking a correction dose for a high glucose on your CGM, verify the reading with a fingerstick and enter it into the pump. You would take the recommended bolus if another bolus has not been given in the last two hours (any BOB will be subtracted from the correction bolus) and the trend lines and arrows indicate the glucose is stable or changing gradually. If the trend arrows show a moderate or rapid fall and there is enough BOB to bring the current glucose down to target, the pump will recommend no correction bolus. Watch the trend line to ensure your glucose keeps coming down but does not go low. If the trendline is pointed upward and there is not enough BOB, consider raising the pump's recommended bolus.

If a reading remains high 3 or 4 hours after a correction dose has already been given, check your infusion set for problems, and consider replacing it. Check for ketones. If the trend line or arrows show a moderate or rapid rise in glucose from carbs, increase the recommended bolus. If there is an illness, stress, an upcoming menstrual cycle, or another reason for the high readings, consider adding a temporary basal increase. Track the glucose with the CGM to see when to end the temporary basal increase.

How to Use CGM Data Downloads

Real-time data is best used for indicating immediate temporary changes, while the patterns found over several days or weeks of data are best for making permanent changes in your basal or bolus setting, such as the CarbF for dinner or the overnight basal rate.

A full analysis of recent data is the best way to adjust settings to lower your A1c or prevent lows. Download CGM data to your computer or over the internet and select the last 14 to 30 days to analyze. The data will be shown as trend reports, data tables, or pie charts. Different graphs and reports will help you see important single events and patterns.

Trend graphs, data tables, and pie charts provide information in a different ways that may appeal to people differently.

4.10 Trend Graph

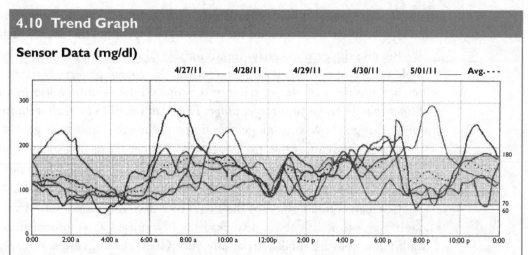

Sensor Data (mg/dl)

4/27/11 _____ 4/28/11 _____ 4/29/11 _____ 4/30/11 _____ 5/01/11 _____ Avg.- - -

This Trend Graph shows overlaid glucose tracks over several days. Here, the glucose tends to rise after eating, with larger excursions after what are likely larger carb meals, Consider bolusing earlier before the meal and lowering the CarbF or insulin-to-carb ratio. The daytime basal, from about 3 am to 3 pm, might also be raised slightly.

Trend Graphs

Trend graphs show the up and down swings of the blood glucose as simple lines. Each 24-hour day is one colored line across the graph. A band of color across the graph is the

4.11 Summary Trend Graph

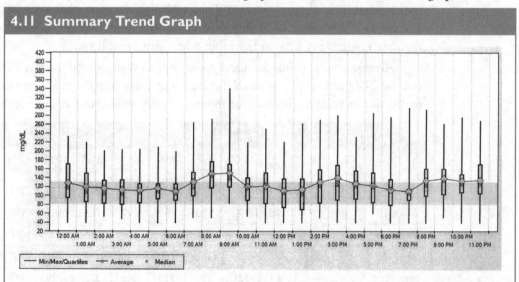

Min/Max/Quartiles · Average · Median

The Summary Trend Graph shows the glucose range at each hour of the day over several days or weeks. The bar represents the middle 50% for readings at that time. The average glucose is the diamond and horizontal line. The line above the bar shows the highest 25% of readings with the top of the line being the highest glucose. The line below the bar shows the lowest 25% with the bottom of the line being the lowest glucose.

target glucose range set by the user. Times are horizontal across the bottom of the graph and glucose levels are vertical on the side. A legend identifies the date of each colored line.

Because the graph overlays trends for several days, it may appear to be a confusing tangle of lines at first. Keep calm and look at the overall pattern, especially when the lines are outside of the target range at the top and the bottom. *Focus first on any groups of lines that go below your target range. These lows need to be dealt with first.* Next look at lines that go above your range, focusing on when the most lines go out of the range.

The trend graph is best for showing a single event or repeated patterns of highs and lows over several days in the context in which they occur. Many people find this graph to be the quickest and easiest way to spot problems that need adjustment.

Compare a trend graph of the first 4 to 7 days you wear a CGM with the same graph over 4 to 7 days about 3 weeks later. If you use CGM information to change insulin doses or carb intake, make sure your CGM readings are reasonably accurate before doing so. You may see much less swing after 3 weeks as graph lines bunch closer together near your target range and fewer lines rise above and below this range.

Data Tables

Data tables give a lot of information about blood glucoses, but it can be difficult to focus on the most relevant data. Important data in the table includes the glucose average at specific times of day, how much variability or swing there is in the glucoses (the standard deviation or SD), and what percent of your values are above, below and within your desired glucose range. Data tables collect data over a range of dates. Usually, the last 14 to 30 days of data provides a very good picture of your control. Be sure the date range is marked on the table when you print it out.

Average glucose values are ideally kept within your desired glucose range throughout the 24-hour period, although this may take a few months to accomplish. To find the problems you want to fix, look for the time of day when your average glucose is highest,

4.12 Data Table

Stats	Total	12:00 am	2:00 am	4:00 am	6:00 am	8:00 am	10:00 am	12:00 pm	2:00 pm	4:00 pm
# of Readings	6716	279	285	286	270	273	273	271	256	281
Average	178	192	180	152	147	166	191	176	206	174
Minimum	39	49	59	56	39	57	71	39	86	70
Median	173	186	162	160	153	154	186	159	196	174
Maximum	401	321	391	325	265	335	329	347	364	303
Standard Deviation	66	61	77	59	50	66	56	65	67	56
Interquartile Range	86	78	98	91	81	86	88	82	96	83
SE Mean	1	4	5	4	3	4	3	4	4	3
% Coefficient of Variation	37	32	43	39	34	40	29	37	32	32

when your standard deviation (variability) is largest, and when low readings are happening. Keep in mind that an average glucose can look deceptively good and still hide extreme highs and lows that average each other into a desired target range. You want not only great average glucose values but also glucose stability with few swings in your readings.

Highest and lowest glucose values show the amount of swing in the glucoses and how extreme the values calculated into the glucose average are.

Percent (%) of glucose values above, below, and within target shows how well the glucose is managed relative to your desired glucose range. Typical target ranges are 70 to 140 mg/dl (3.9 to 7.8 mmol/L) or 80 to 160 mg/dl (4.4 to 8.9 mmol/L). As a goal, work to get at least 50% of your glucose values in your target range and less than 5% of values below. Lows should be worked on first, especially if they are frequent or extreme. Circle them, try to explain them and work on avoiding them.

Standard deviation (SD) shows how much variability exists in your glucose readings. The higher the SD number is, the more variability there is in your readings. A high SD says the average glucose contains numerous ups and downs. Some healthcare professionals suggest that long-term glucose variability, as shown by a high SD number, contributes to diabetes complications. In addition, quality of life suffers when wide swings in the glucose cause irritability. For ideal control, aim for a lower SD such as less than 40% of your average glucose (i.e., for an average glucose of 150, aim for an SD of 60 or less [150 x 0.40 = 60]), with most readings in your target range. A SD of 60 with an average glucose of 150 means that about 95% of readings will be between about 90 mg/dl (150 - 60) and 210 mg/dl (150 + 60). Keep in mind that 30 or more glucose readings are needed before you can get an accurate SD or variability measurement.

Pie Charts

Pie charts give a color-coded picture of glucose values that some people prefer over data tables or line graphs. They are great for showing percentages – the percentage of your glucose readings inside your target range, the percent of highs and lows outside this range, and the time of day this occurs. With pie charts you can quickly spot the time of day when a larger percentage of your glucose values are out of range. Try to get at least 50% inside your range, no more than 5% low and less than 40% high. Pie charts can be viewed only on downloaded data, not on the receiver.

Pie charts give a good overview but are not good for specifics. For example, lows are identified as a percentage that shows how many values are in the low range. This helps adjust doses but does not help spot specific lows. In contrast, trend graphs and data tables give specific glucose values and tell how high and low the values are.

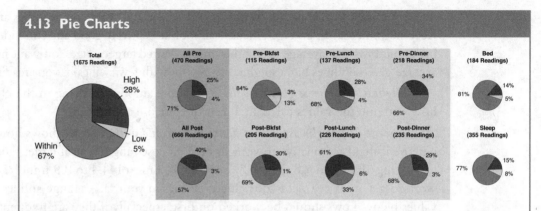

4.13 Pie Charts

These pie charts show the split between low (white), in target (grey), and high (dark) glucose levels averaged over several entire days (large circle), pre- and post-meal readings, and readings before and after breakfast, lunch, and dinner, and at bedtime. These glucoses tend to be highest before dinner, while the before breakfast readings tend to have more lows. Here, one might consider a larger carb bolus at lunch, and retesting the overnight basal rate.

Events

Recording events helps to identify the causes of high and low readings. Events can be entered into all CGMs. It is especially important to enter meal times, carb intake, and bolus doses on integrated CGM/pump systems to get a full picture of what is happening. Add exercise, stress, illness, etc. as they occur. If needed, write more information about these events on the printout of the downloaded data.

Basal and Bolus Testing with Trend Graphs

Basal testing with a CGM is as simple as determining whether the blood glucose trend line stays level when nothing is eaten and no BOB is active. If the glucose drifts up or down, the timing of the drift alerts the user to the time a basal adjustment is needed. Bolus testing is as easy because you can watch the trend line until the action of the bolus insulin has ended. A drift up or down after a carb bolus can show the time of day that food choices, bolus timing, type of bolus, or the carb factor (CarbF) needs to change.

The trend line following a combo or dual wave bolus indicates whether the immediate portion or timing of these boluses needs to change for certain foods. Likewise, after giving correction boluses over time, a look back at the trend lines shows whether a correction factor (CorrF) needs to be changed to give larger or smaller correction boluses to treat high readings. Steps to test your basal and bolus settings are included in Chapters 11-13.

How Often to Wear a CGM

How often you wear a CGM determines how much benefit you gain. CGM research shows that less hypoglycemia and a lower A1c result when a CGM is worn all the time, so daily wear is recommended. If this is too much, wear it when increased stress, a change in schedule or travel, or a change in insulin doses or medications call for the use of a CGM to track the effect these factors have on your glucose. If lows are a problem, wear it to get the low alarms you need, rather than for total control.

Tips for Success on a CGM

CGMs have many benefits, especially as you retrain yourself to make decisions based on more information. Here are tips to help you develop new instincts and attitudes:

- Don't throw your CGM out if your meter and CGM numbers differ. Differences occur, especially in the first 12 to 24 hours as the sensor settles in. Use your trend line for guidance and don't overreact to specific glucose values.
- To bring CGM readings closer to fingerstick readings, re-calibrate your CGM if it is off track.
- Use your CGM like a watch and look at it at least once an hour for the best results.
- Before you take or change a bolus, verify your CGM reading with a fingerstick reading, especially if your CGM accuracy has been suspect or shows a fast glucose drop or rise.
- Always take into account the BOB on your pump before you give more insulin or carbs based on your CGM reading or trend line or arrows.
- Never rely totally on a CGM to catch lows or highs.
- Use on-screen CGM information to quickly change the timing or amount of insulin, the timing, type and amount of carbs, or to adjust exercise or activity.
- Use your trend line to test and adjust basal rates and carb and correction boluses.
- Use retrospective downloads to spot and improve unwanted glucose patterns, such as times and reasons you typically go high or low, your average glucose, and SD.

Always double-check your pump BC's recommended bolus and take a dose only if it makes sense to you.

Summary

Like any other diabetes therapy, current CGM technology isn't perfect. False alarms, alarm overload, inaccurate readings, sensor failure, and calibration requirements are all concerns. Despite these shortcomings, most users are enthusiastic because they know their approximate blood glucose at any time, where it has been, and where it's going. In addition, they get valuable and relevant information regarding when to take action to avoid highs and lows.

The best mind altering drug is the truth.
Lily Tomlin

Future CGM Advances

Many companies are involved in the research efforts to improve CGM technology and eventually combine a CGM with an insulin pump to create an artificial pancreas, often called the closed loop. Current Medtronic and Dexcom CGM sensors use glucose oxidase sensors. Accuracy is gradually improving, but reliability remains an issue. One way that researchers are trying to improve these two areas is to place two glucose oxidase sensors under the skin so the sensors can check on each other and ensure that at least one sensor will be working.

New sensing technology is also under development. One promising approach uses molecules that fluoresce when they come in contact with glucose. Fluorescent sensors have the potential for very good accuracy, rapid detection of glucose changes, very small size, and very low power requirements. Another area of research involves miniaturization and implantation of long-lasting glucose oxidase or fluorescent sensors under the skin. Although the gold standard would be a non-invasive sensor, these devices are larger and less accurate than current CGMs.

The gradual evolution of an artificial pancreas may involve:

- Faster insulin action from new insulins, delivery of insulin into the abdominal (peritoneal) cavity for faster uptake, or use of microneedles for faster delivery
- Dual CGM sensors to minimize sensor error
- An implanted CGM sensor with better accuracy and reliability
- Dual delivery of insulin in tandem with glucagon to prevent hypoglycemia
- Automatic shifting between basal and bolus insulin delivery, such as with the delivery of a variation of a Super Bolus (see page 153).
- Control algorithms that rapidly adjust for exercise, menses, dieting, illness, etc.

Health professionals and people with diabetes look forward to combining insulin pumps and CGMs on the way to a closed loop that takes on more and more of the glucose regulation in the body.

No matter how cynical I get, I just can't keep up.

Lily Tomlin

Data – The Key to Better Control

CHAPTER

5

Good information is key to improving your well being and health. Frequent glucose monitoring is critical for achieving relatively normal and stable glucose levels.

Most of the daily decisions that impact your glucose are forgotten when these important details are not recorded. Nothing beats written records or those entered into a device or phone applet. They can then be analyzed alongside the glucose and insulin data from your insulin pump, meter, and CGM. You and your doctor no longer need to guess what happened.

Much useful information can also be downloaded over the internet using software like CareLink™, DiaSend®, or Sweet Spot. Wearing a CGM also speeds useful connections, especially when accompanied by a written record of events as they happen.

This chapter reviews

- Benefits of graphing your glucose
- What to record to maintain control
- Sample charts and analyses

Frequent glucose checks by themselves do not guarantee a great A1c. In the APP Study, the 132 pump wearers in the group with a lower average glucose of 144 mg/dl (8.0 mmol/L) tested 4.7 times a day, while the group with a higher average glucose of 227 mg/dl (12.6 mmol/L) tested 4.0 times a day with the testing showing a "significant" but rather weak relationship to glucose outcomes.[63] *Frequent monitoring has to be followed with clinical interventions that involve both insulin and lifestyle adjustments to lower the A1c to optimal levels of 7.0% or 6.5% and below.*

Regular data downloads or written records are key to having a minimum of highs and lows. Records provide the critical information you and your medical providers need in order to solve glucose control issues. *Always bring all your glucose data and any lab results that may have been done elsewhere to every doctor's visit.*

Compared to the longer view of an A1c test or the glucose average on your meter, daily records let you lessen glucose variability by revealing what really affects your glucose from day to day. Interactions between your basal rates, boluses, food choices, carb counts, exercise, and glucose readings can be seen. Any time you have a high or low reading, you have the details in a format that makes cause and effect easier to see when

5.1 When to Test and Why

Check your glucose at these times (or wear a CGM) to identify connections and patterns:

Before breakfast - A good breakfast reading lets you control the rest of the day.

Before lunch and dinner - Lets you know how well your carb bolus covered the carbs eaten at breakfast and lunch, respectively.

1-2 hours after meals - Tells whether you covered the carbs well and lets you correct sooner if a reading is going high or low.

3 hours after lunch - Helps avoid afternoon lows.

At Bedtime - Lets you know how well you covered carbs at dinner. Most importantly, helps prevent night lows and lets you wake up with your glucose in your target range.

Occasional 2 am - Prevents night lows, helps test your night basal, and lets you make adjustments for better breakfast readings.

Before driving and hourly during longer trips - Keeps you and others safe.

Before, during, and after exercise or activity that lasts longer than 1 hour - Maximizes performance and safety. Be sure to check at 2 am that night!

Any time you think you are low or high - Speeds up stopping excess lows.

Before and after drinking alcohol - More safety and less embarrassment. Be sure to check during the night when lows are most likely.

After a change in basal or bolus doses - Shows whether the change helped.

Bring your written records and meter and pump downloads to all clinic visits. If your current glucose is not great, checking helps you turn your next reading into a better one. A CGM helps correct your glucose and gives alerts so you can prevent problems.

you use a record like the *Smart Chart* in Fig. 5.6. Charting lets you gradually make the dose adjustments so you can eat, work and exercise the way you want.

When you start on a pump, keep good records for several weeks before and after your start. Then later, whenever you have control problems, be sure to gather all relevant data so you and your doctor can quickly change the timing or amounts of basal rates, boluses, or pump settings.

Software downloads from your pump, meter, and CGM display your data in clear, graphic formats and let you quickly analyze insulin doses, average glucoses at different times of day, and how variable your readings are. This data can be sent over the internet or by phone to a central location or directly to a parent or health care professional.

During basal and bolus testing, it is especially important to record the items in Box 5.2. Wearing a CGM displays your current glucose and its trend for the past few hours. Seeing these immediate glucose trends helps you take action to prevent many highs and lows. A CGM also allows you to record events like carb intake, bolus sizes, and activity, for quicker discovery of glucose patterns and their causes. Your data lets you see whether you are getting where you want to go and whether the changes you make really help.

Evaluate Your Overall Management

Having more stable readings and more of them in your target range is your goal. An A1c test or the average glucose on a meter provides an overview of your success. However, even a "good" A1c may be achieved through numerous up and down readings that makes daily life miserable and places you at a greater risk for a severe low. Glucose variability, the opposite of glucose stability, can be estimated from the *standard deviation (SD)* of your glucose readings. So look at your A1c together with your SD.

An A1c test shows your average glucose exposure over the most recent 60 to 90 days with the last 4 to 6 weeks having a greater impact on this average. Normal A1c values range from 4% to 6% at most labs.

A1c Goals

For a goal, the American Diabetes Association (ADA) recommends that adults with diabetes keep their A1c below 7.0% without significant hypoglycemia,[17] while the American Association of Clinical Endocrinologists (AACE) recommends keeping the A1c below 6.5%.[18] The International Diabetes Federation recommends levels below 6.5% in Type 2 diabetes to prevent complications and heart problems.[64] The International Society for Pediatric and Adolescent Diabetes recommends that the A1c be kept below 7.5% for everyone, again while avoiding severe, as well as frequent hypoglycemia.[65]

Ask your doctor for an A1c test every 3 to 4 months unless excellent control allows you to wait 6 months. You can also do your own A1c test with a variety of at home A1c test kits. Between A1c tests, record the 14 or 30-day average glucose from your meter or CGM to guide you in lowering elevated glucose readings. Table 5.3 translates the 30-day glucose average on your meter into an approximate A1c.

There has been controversy among diabetes specialists about whether glucose variability, besides making daily life miserable, also adds to the risk of having complications.[66,67] One physician who had previously argued strongly against this connection, found in an analysis of the DCCT trial data that *people who have more variability in their A1c level over time have a much higher risk for both eye damage (2.2 times higher) and kidney disease (1.8 times higher).*[68]

However, variability in daily glucose values is very similar to variability in A1c values over time. Both higher A1c values and higher average glucose values involve a higher degree of glucose variability. Imagine that you manage a china shop and someone brings in two dogs, a large one and a small one. Both dogs are excited to be there and wag their tails. Unfortunately for you, the big dog's tail with its bigger wag will cause a lot more damage. Daily glucose variability would be having the dog owner coming to your shop every day, while variability in your A1c is having them come in every other month. One would expect more damage from daily visits, so do what you can to keep the big dog out of your shop.

5.3 Estimated A1c from the Average Glucose on Your Meter	
Average Meter Glucose*	**Est. A1c**
126 mg/dl (7.0 mmol/L)	6%
140 mg/dl (7.8 mmol/L)	6.5%
154 mg/dl (8.6 mmol/L)	7%
183 mg/dl (10.1 mmol/L)	8%
212 mg/dl (11.8 mmol/L)	9%
240 mg/dl (13.4 mmol/L)	10%
269 mg/dl (14.9 mmol/L)	11%
298 mg/dl (16.4 mmol/L)	12%

*Your average glucose may appear lower than it really is if you test only before meals or you test more often when your glucose is low.

A1C-Derived Average Glucose (ADAG) Study, Diabetes Care August 2008 vol. 31 no. 8 1473-1478

A major benefit of both an insulin pump and multiple daily injections is that when insulin is given more frequently throughout the day, it tends to make glucose levels more stable. Both pumps and MDI are associated with major reductions in retinopathy in adolescents compared to 1 or 2 injections a day, and pumps may have some advantage, as discussed in Box 1.7.[19]

Your SD can be found on some meter, CGM, and pump screens, and in almost all data downloads from these devices. Aim to keep your meter SD as low as possible, such as less than 40% of the average glucose on your meter. For example, if your average meter reading is 200 mg/dl (11.1 mmol/L), a desirable SD would be 80 mg/dl (4.4 mmol/L) or less, while for an average glucose of 150 mg/dl (8.3 mmol/L), your SD would be 60 mg/dl (3.3 mmol/L) or less. A CGM with its frequent readings will ideally help the wearer have an even lower SD.

Set Reasonable Glucose Management Goals

Setting personal glucose goals is a vital part of your diabetes management plan. Select reasonable goals that you can reach and a reasonable time to reach them. Start by reviewing your current glucose readings and control, and then select a goal or two that will gradually improve your health. Write all your goals down and date them.

5.4 Glucose and A1c Goals for Adults (20+)

Goal	Normal Values	ADA* Goals	AACE** Goals
Avg Meter BG:	< 126 mg/dl < 7 mmol/L	< 154 mg/dl < 8.6 mmol/L	< 140 mg/dl < 7.8 mmol/L
A1c:	< 6.0%	< 7.0% without significant hypoglycemia	< 6.5%
Fasting BG	< 100 mg/dl	70–130 mg/dl	< 110 mg/dl
Before Meal BG	<110 mg/dl	70–130 mg/dl	< 110 mg/dl
After Meal BG	70–140 mg/dl	180 mg/dl peak	< 140 (2 hrs after meal)
Bedtime BG	< 110 mg/dl	90-150 mg/dl	–

* Diabetes Care. 2009 Jan; 32 Suppl 1: S 13–61

** American Association of Clinical Endocrinologists (AACE, 2007) Medical Guidelines for Clinical Practice for the Management of Diabetes Mellitus.

Reasonable goals might be to:

- Raise the average number of glucose tests per day on your meter by one more test a day by the first of next month.
- Lower the average glucose on your meter by 10 mg/dl (0.6 mmol/L) in 2 weeks,
- Increase the number of readings inside your target range by 10% in one month,
- Lower your A1c below 8.5% on your next test in 3 months
- Check your glucose two hours after breakfast at least 3 days this week
- Cut in half the number of low glucose readings below 60 mg/dl (3.3 mmol/L) that you have each week within one month.

Tailor your glucose goals to your age, lifestyle, and circumstances. For example, a child, someone in a higher-risk profession like a charge nurse or firefighter, a person who lives alone, and anyone who has hypoglycemia unawareness requires higher glucose goals. Suggested adult glucose goals are shown in Table 5.4. A child's desired glucose levels, shown in Table 23.1, may need to be higher than an adult's because they are smaller, are often more sensitive to insulin, and have greater variability in their eating and activity.

Analyze Your Data

Once you select a goal, create a plan to track and record how it is working. For example, you might record each week the average glucose from your meter and how many lows you had below a certain value on your calendar, *Smart Charts*, or logbook.

Record things that might change your glucose, like those in Table 5.2. Your pump automatically tracks basal and bolus doses. This information will be very important in the chapters that follow. Your doses can be found on a history screen on your pump or on a download. You can mark a variety of events in many meters, CGMs, and applets. Knowing this information will help you when you start on a pump and whenever your control is not optimal. Successful pumpers often record many of these details on an ongoing basis to stay in control.

Bring all charts, downloads, and other information to each clinic visit. Ask that your data be reviewed. Be sure to point out and discuss things that you believe are an issue or that you have questions about. A kitchen table conference with family and friends often clarifies the changes you want to try.

If you are unsure about how to correct an unwanted pattern and need advice, contact your physician or health care team. A health care professional who works with diabetes can often see things you may miss. Use their knowledge and experience to simplify your path toward normal readings and to build on your current understanding and ability to control your own glucose.

What to Record

The more information you gather about what impacts your glucose, the easier it becomes to control it. We'll use a written record to show some things to keep in mind.

- Write things down as they happen or wear a CGM to connect glucoses to events in real time. A written record like *Smart Charts*, phone applets, and even event markers in a pump, meter, or CGM can help you remember what led to particular highs and lows. Keep one of these handy to make data entry easy.

- Mark high and low readings with symbols or colored markers to highlight unwanted patterns. In software, set your glucose range so it sorts out acceptable readings from those you don't want.

- When a high or low reading occurs, treat it and record what you think caused it. Tie each one to a food, insulin dose, activity, or event.

Key items to record are shown in Sam's Sample Chart, Fig. 5.5:

Activity – A

With an ink pen or felt pen, block in the time and intensity of activity, exercise, or work that is greater than normal in the activity area at the top of the graph. Add a word or two to specify what it was that you did.

Fill in the grid at the top of the *Smart Chart* to rank your activity on a personal 1 to 5 scale. A "1" would be a mild increase in activity, while a "5" would be an activ-

5.5 Sam's Sample Smart Chart

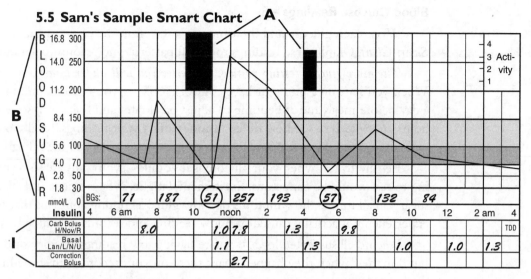

		Breakfast			Lunch			Dinner	
Time	Food	Carb Grams	Time	Food	Carb Grams	Time	Food	Carb Grams
7:00	Cheerios	40	1:00	1 c nonfat milk	13	6:00	pasta and clams	64
	1 c nonfat milk	13		tuna sandwich	34		green salad	11
	strawberries	10		apple—154 gms	23		Chardonnay	6
	2 rye toast	30			70		vanilla ice cream	17
	applebutter	8						98
	poached egg	0						
	Morning Snacks	101		Afternoon Snacks			Evening Snacks	
11:00	2 blueberry muffins	70		crackers	12			
	banana	25		cheese	4			
	diet soda	0		glucose tabs	10			
		95			26			

Day: **Saturday**   Wt: _____   Comments: *Ate too much after morning bike ride! 4 pm - helped*
Date: **03/ 10 /12**   *Fred load dirt into his trailer.*

© 1994, 2012 Diabetes Services, Inc.

A - Activity and exercise B - Blood glucose readings   I - Insulin doses

F - Foods and carbs   C - Comments

ity that is strenuous and close to your maximum effort. For instance, if you usually sit behind a desk but you spend the day moving your files and records to a new office, you would block in an area probably between 2 and 5 during these hours, based on the extra activity this required.

If you start a running program and become quite winded as you run, you would mark a 5 on your chart. After you run the same route for a few days, the same activity may no longer be as strenuous and would be listed progressively as a 4 and then a 3 as your training progresses. Area A in Figure 5.5 shows Sam's exercise and gives an example of how to chart physical activity.

Blood Glucose Readings – B

Write each glucose and the time it was taken in the blood sugar section of the *Smart Chart*. Graph these readings to reveal patterns and readjust basal rates and boluses.

The more glucose testing you do, the better you will understand your insulin needs. When you start on a pump or have control problems, you need a minimum of four tests a day before meals and at bedtime to adjust basal rates and boluses. Test before and two hours after meals to see how different foods affect your readings. Ideally, 6 or 7 tests a day with an occasional test at 2 a.m. to prevent night lows gives you the information you need.

Be sure to test when your glucose is low, unless symptoms are so severe that waiting to test would be dangerous. Excitement, fatigue, stress, anxiety, and even a high blood sugar can all mimic the symptoms of a low glucose. Testing confirms that what you are experiencing is actually caused by a low reading and records its timing in your meter.

Record all suspected lows. If you're having low readings at work or during the night but don't test when they happen, mark these on your record with something like SL for suspected low so you and your physician can appropriately adjust your doses. Highlight all verified and suspected lows on your charts with a circle, an arrow, or a specific color. Show the severity of each low blood sugar by the size of the mark. For instance, if symptoms are mild, use a small circle or arrow, while, if severe, use a large one.

Show all your highs and lows. If your physician has only an elevated A1c test from which to judge your control, he or she may not realize that many of your highs are caused by an excess of insulin that comes from overtreating lows that are not recorded, or that you are simply forgetting to bolus before meals. Problem solving is hard enough when all the facts are known. Without the facts, it can be impossible.

Area B shows a graphic of Sam's glucose results with his readings listed below on the BG line. The dots between his glucose tests are connected to show glucose trends.

Insulin Doses – I

The three rows below the graph area near the middle of the *Smart Chart* are used to record basal and bolus doses. On the top row, record how many carb bolus units you take for each meal and snack. Basal insulin doses can be recorded every few days on the middle row. The third row is for recording correction boluses used to lower high readings. Log your correction boluses separately from carb boluses so you know how much extra insulin you are using each day to correct highs. Note the exact time each bolus is given by placing a dash or crosshatch on the time line when that bolus is given.

Area I shows Sam's insulin doses and when they are taken.

Foods and Carb Counts – F

Carb counting lets you measure how much a meal or snack raises your glucose. How to count carbs is covered in Chapter 3. It is easier than you think and is a very important step to good control, especially when using a smart pump. Start by recording the foods you eat and the number of carbs in them, being as specific as you can.

A general word like "cereal" won't do. All cereals are not equal. Cheerios®, Grape Nuts®, Cornflakes®, and oatmeal affect your glucose differently. A sandwich has very different effects when it is a whole wheat/tuna/tomato sandwich with 32 carb grams, a white bun/hamburger/tomato sandwich with 45 carb grams, or an ice cream sandwich with 68 grams.

5.6 Smart Chart

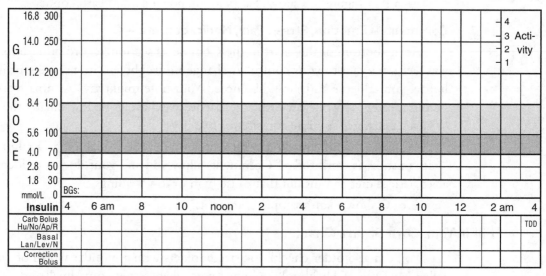

	Breakfast			Lunch			Dinner	
Time	Food	Carb Grams	Time	Food	Carb Grams	Time	Food	Carb Grams
	Morning Snacks			Afternoon Snacks			Evening Snacks	

Day: _____   Wt: ___   Comments: _____

Date: _____

Record all carbs. If you don't record the four full-sized graham crackers (44 grams) and 16 ounces of milk (24 grams) that you took for a nighttime low, you won't know later why your blood sugar rose to 306 mg/dl (17 mmol/L) before breakfast. As you record food effects for a while, you may find some that affect your glucose for reasons other than their carb content, such as fat and protein content, glycemic index of foods, etc.

Area F in Figure 5.5 shows Sam's foods, portions, and carb counts.

Comments – Emotion, Stress, Pain, Medication, etc. – C

At the bottom of the chart in the Comments section, record other information you feel is relevant to your control. A change in weight, emotions, stress, or illness can impact your glucose and should be noted. Your note might say "Asthma worse – used steroid inhaler," "I woke up with a headache, may have gone low during the night," or "I haven't changed my infusion site for five days."

An unusually high reading before dinner might be explained by a comment like "a lot of stress at work today." Comments allow you and your doctor to identify variables besides diet and insulin that cause high or low readings.

Area C shows Sam's sample comments.

Fill in Your Own Smart Chart:

You can also order checkbook size booklets with a month's worth of *Smart Charts*, called My Other Checkbook, online at www.diabetesnet.com/dmall/.

Enhanced Logbook

A simple *Enhanced Logbook* is shown in Fig. 5.7. It lets you quickly spot and add up numbers that fall outside your target range. There is space to record glucose test results before each meal, one to two hours after each meal, and at bedtime, along with the times they occur. Even though space is limited, record food choices and timing, grams of carb, length and type of exercise, and comments about things like stress or illness. Note the time and duration of exercise in the margin. Even short notes help.

Look for the patterns in your readings so you can make the decisions that will improve your control. The logbook has a section at the bottom that helps you spot glucose patterns. At the very bottom of the logbook, fill in your target glucose ranges for different times of day. After you test and record for seven days, circle all the highs above the target range in one color and all the lows below the target range in another color. Total up all the highs and lows for each time of day and write them down in the pattern section at the bottom of the *Enhanced Logbook*.

When a reading falls outside your target range, write an explanation for it in the margin of your logbook or on the back of the page, using numbers to key each note to the log. Write down anything that might have influenced your glucose that day, such as extra stress, unusual exercise or activity, high carb meals, or delayed eating. Place notes close to the time it happens or draw a line to the margin where you have more room to write.

5.7 Enhanced Logbook		Breakfast		Lunch		Dinner		Night	
		Before	After	Before	After	Before	After	Bedtime	2 a.m.
Sunday ___/___/___ walk/run/bike at _____ am/pm	BG								
	Time								
	Carbs								
	Bolus								
Monday ___/___/___ walk/run/bike at _____ am/pm	BG								
	Time								
	Carbs								
	Bolus								
Tuesday ___/___/___ walk/run/bike at _____ am/pm	BG								
	Time								
	Carbs								
	Bolus								
Wednesday ___/___/___ walk/run/bike at _____ am/pm	BG								
	Time								
	Carbs								
	Bolus								
Thursday ___/___/___ walk/run/bike at _____ am/pm	BG								
	Time								
	Carbs								
	Bolus								
Friday ___/___/___ walk/run/bike at _____ am/pm	BG								
	Time								
	Carbs								
	Bolus								
Saturday ___/___/___ walk/run/bike at _____ am/pm	BG								
	Time								
	Carbs								
	Bolus								
# below target					PATTERNS				
# above target									

Targets:

before meals: _____ to _____   bedtime: _____ to _____

after meals: _____ to _____   2 am: _____ to _____

Basals:

_____ u/hr at 12 am   _____ u/hr at _____ am/pm

_____ u/hr at _____ am/pm   _____ u/hr at _____ am/pm

_____ u/hr at _____ am/pm   _____ u/hr at _____ am/pm

When you have high readings at the same time of day on three or more days or low readings on two or more days a week, you have a *glucose pattern* for which you want to seek reasons. Unwanted patterns can often be corrected by adjusting basal rates and carb boluses, but use every tool you have to improve your control. Are you eating too many or too few carbs, engaging in more or less activity than usual, feeling more or less stress than usual, or in the midst of an illness? Is your insulin out of date or is there a problem with your infusion set or pump? Chapter 15 discusses a variety of reasons for control problems like clogs and leaks that are unrelated to your insulin doses.

> ### 5.8 Test When High or Low
>
> Don't skip a glucose check if you suspect you are high or low. These are the most valuable times to test. A high reading can be converted into a better reading the next time you check. With lows, always record your glucose and the timing with a meter check so you and your doctor know when they happen. Only your actual glucose readings will improve your basal and bolus doses.

Summary

As you download your data, or fill out records, *Smart Charts*, or logbooks, you may at first have some difficulty recording all the information you need. Recording gets easier with practice and charting becomes a small distraction that has a big payoff by preventing lows and lessening the time spent with high blood sugars. Review Chapter 4 for how to understand downloaded CGM data and how to make it work for you. This is another helpful way to spot patterns and remedy them.

Common patterns will stand out as you flip *Smart Chart* pages back and forth or you review the readings that are above and below your target range in the *Enhanced Logbook* at the end of each week. Patterns that repeat but do not occur every day, such as low-to-high, will show up in weekly reviews rather than daily ones. By identifying unwanted patterns, you can correct them, and as your confidence increases, you will better manage your diabetes.

Look over your records regularly for patterns and share them with your physician and health care team. Once you stabilize your readings with more appropriate basal rates and better-matched boluses, using a simple logbook or a regular download of your meter or pump to your PC or to a site on the internet may do. Take a cold, hard look at your glucose readings periodically. Any time that your control begins to slip, go back to recording the full data you need via device downloads, *Smart Charts* or a logbook. You want to get back the control you need quickly, and systematic records let you do that.

5.9 Sam's Sample Enhanced Logbook		Breakfast Before	Breakfast After	Lunch Before	Lunch After	Dinner Before	Dinner After	Night Bedtime	Night 2 a.m.
Sunday 5/18/03 walk(circled)/run/bike at 7 am/pm(pm circled)	BG	167 △				181 △		93	
	Time	9:30				7:00		10:30	
	Carbs	88				66			
	Bolus	8+2				6			
Monday 5/19/03 walk/run/bike at ___ am/pm	BG	137 △	172 △	113		103		118	
	Time	8 am	10:30	1:00		6:00		10:00	
	Carbs	75		44		83		26	
	Bolus	7+1		4		7.5		2	
Tuesday 5/20/03 walk/run/bike at ___ am/pm	BG	201 △		173 △		49 (circled)		148 △	
	Time	8:00		12:00		5:30		10:00	
	Carbs	62		48		90		26	
	Bolus	5.5		4+2				2+1	
Wednesday 5/21/03 walk/run/bike at ___ am/pm	BG	172 △	187 △	67 (circled)	279 △	54 (circled)		136	153
	Time	8:00	11:00	12:00		6:00		10:00	2:00 am
	Carbs	76		47	24	89		0	0
	Bolus	7+2		4	2	8+2		*night basal test*	
Thursday 5/22/03 walk/run/bike at ___ am/pm	BG	203 △	168	71	132	106		136 △	153
	Time	7:00	10:00	12:00	4:00	6:00		10:00	1:00 am
	Carbs	65		45	16	96		20	
	Bolus	6+3		4	1	9H+7UL		1+2H	
Friday 5/23/03 walk(circled)/run/bike at 4 am/pm(pm circled)	BG	203 △	196 △	128		87	135	102	
	Time	7:30	10:00	12:30		6:15	8:30	10:30	
	Carbs	55		60		83		20	
	Bolus	5+1	1H	5.5		7+7UL		1H+3L	
Saturday 5/24/03 walk/run/bike(circled) at 7 am(circled)/pm	BG	148 △		77		111		86	
	Time	8:00		12:30		6:00		10:30	
	Carbs	89		52		80		30	
	Bolus	8+1H		4H	7H+7UL	2H+3L			
# below target				1		2			
# above target		7 (circled)	3 (circled)	1	1	1		2	

Targets:
before meals: 70 to 130   bedtime: 90 to 140
after meals: 120 to 180   2 am: 90 to 140

Basals:
___ u/hr at 12 am   ___ u/hr at ___ am/pm
___ u/hr at ___ am/pm   ___ u/hr at ___ am/pm
___ u/hr at ___ am/pm   ___ u/hr at ___ am/pm

PATTERNS

5.10 Going Off Your Pump

Situations like water skiing, river rafting, or pump failure may necessitate going off a pump for awhile. These suggestions help maintain control when you go off a pump for certain lengths of time. Less insulin than the suggested amounts below may be needed if you will be more active. Carefully discuss how to do this with your physician.

Time off:	Try this:
Less than 1 hour	Nothing if BG is OK. Before you detach, give a bolus if your BG is high or you plan to eat carbs soon.
1 to 5 hours	Cover 80% of the basal during your time off the pump with a bolus before you disconnect. Cover any carbs you eat during your time off the pump by reconnecting and bolusing or by taking an injection.
More than 5 hours or overnight	Use a bolus before disconnecting or take an injection of rapid insulin to cover meal carbs plus the next 4 hours of basal insulin. Every 4 to 5 hours, replace the basal insulin with an injection of rapid insulin and cover any meal carbs as needed. For overnight basal coverage, an alternative to injecting rapid insulin every 4 to 5 hours is to take NPH®/Lantus®/Levemir® equal to the next 12 hours of basal insulin at bedtime.
More than a day	Determine the average units of basal insulin given per day from your pump history. Give the same number of units as one injection or half this amount as two evenly split injections of Lantus®/Levemir® per day. Use injections of rapid insulin as needed to cover carb and correction doses.

I feel that luck is
preparation meeting opportunity.

Oprah Winfrey

Select a Pump, Infusion Set, and Insulin

Whether choosing your first insulin pump or a replacement, take the time you need to select the pump that best fits your needs. Pumps typically last four to five years, so discuss different pumps with your doctor and health care team to select the features that will be most helpful for you now and for the next few years.

What this chapter covers

- Questions to ask when choosing a pump
- Infusion set choices
- Insulin for your pump

When choosing a pump, contact different pump companies and get a local pump representative to demonstrate their pump. Review the marketing information you receive, information that is listed at each company's web site and listed at web sites like www.diabetesnet.com/diabetes_technology/insulin_pump_models.php.

Ask lots of questions and find out what advantages each pump may have and the support that each company provides. Talk with a representative of each company in which you are interested. In any sales encounter, don't make quick decisions and don't feel pressured to decide. There are a number of pump support groups and diabetes conferences where pumpers are present and pump vendors are showing their products. The internet, diabetes forums, and blogs have lots of opinions and facts, so read carefully.

Make a final decision once you've collected your information and talked this over with your health care professional. This takes time but lets you make an informed decision.

Pump Features

Many features, like lists of carb counts per serving for different foods, are available in most pumps to get more accurate carb boluses and track the foods you eat. You can also preprogram quick boluses for favorite foods.

Different reminders and alerts can be customized for safety and improved control. For instance, a post-meal reminder can be set to alert you to recheck your glucose an hour and a half or two hours after a bolus has been given. See Table 6.5 for a list of pump reminders and alerts.

Most pumps have an associated meter that will send glucose readings directly to the pump for bolus calculations. CGMs are rapidly being integrated as well. Today's pump-meter and pump-CGM combos provide much of the data you need to evaluate and improve your glucose readings. Your pump history quickly reveals helpful things like your TDD relative to your glucose results, your basal-bolus balance, and your correction bolus percentage. For example, if your A1c is high and you have few lows, or your correction boluses make up a large part of your TDD, you or your doctor can make appropriate adjustments to your basal rates and carb boluses.

Bolus accuracy improves greatly when all glucose readings are automatically entered into the pump from a meter. This reduces manual entry errors, speeds bolus calculations, and ensures that every blood glucose reading is used by the pump to recommend an appropriate bolus. This lets your pump adjust carb and correction boluses for any BOB to minimize insulin stacking.

CGM results are not currently used by the pump for bolus calculations. The CGM lets you see your current glucose trend, provides an alert for impending lows and highs, and gives a wealth of glucose data to evaluate your insulin doses. The combination of pumps with CGMs will gradually provide more features on the path toward an artificial pancreas. Ease of use, better glucose accuracy, and improved control software are first being integrated into an automated control system that requires user assistance for meal coverage. Later systems might be fully automated if faster acting insulins become available.

Compare Line and Patch Pumps

Insulin pumps can deliver insulin either through an infusion line to a small infusion site attached to the skin. Larger patch pumps are directly applied to the skin and deliver insulin through a short cannula on the bottom of the pump.

Line pumps can be disconnected for water sports, showers, and other activities, but not all patch pumps can do this. When an infusion set gets detached with a standard pump, only the infusion set needs to be replaced. With some patch pumps, a new pod must be used at a higher expense to the user or their insurer. Stronger adhesives are used with a patch pump to reduce pod loss during swimming or other longer water exposures. Some upcoming patch pumps have a modular design where only a plastic base with an infusion catheter needs to be replaced. The pump body itself can be reused to reduce expense.

Some patch pumps can't give a bolus unless a separate controller to give these boluses is present. If the wearer goes to school or work and forgets their controller, bolus doses cannot be given until they retrieve it. Newer patch pumps will have a button or two on the pump body to deliver boluses independently of the controller.

6.1 Things to Consider when Choosing a Pump

1. What appeals to you about the pump? Look, feel, and color, features, accessories?

2. How easy is the pump to program and use? Is the screen bright enough to see?

3. How easy are the buttons to push? A bolus should be easy to give, but not accidentally while gesturing, reaching into a pocket, or displaying the pump to inquisitive friends.

4. What reminders and alarms does the pump have?

5. If you need a low basal rate, how finely can it be programmed and how many times each hour will this low rate be delivered?

6. How easy is it to stop a bolus if you change your mind?

7. If the pump is for a child, can a caregiver easily learn to operate the pump?

8. Can you hear or feel the pump alarms when insulin delivery is interrupted or a low glucose is detected by a CGM?

9. How easy are the history screens to access and how much information is given? Can you check if you got distracted and never gave a bolus? Can you check on your current bolus on board? Can a parent verify that their child is giving boluses at school and for afternoon snacks?

10. How does the pump BC handle BOB and glucose target ranges? These are important features for preventing hypoglycemia.

11. Can the pump survive rough use? Is it waterproof? Is it easy to disconnect for showering or swimming?

12. How many different infusion sets can you choose from?

13. For patch pumps, will the adhesive keep it from getting knocked off? Can you deliver a bolus if you forget your controller?

14. How good is 24-hour customer support? Assistance with insurance coverage? Warranty? Trial period? How soon will a replacement arrive if needed? Can you get a loaner pump to borrow while on vacation in case something happens to your pump?

Questions to Ask

Your Doctor and Diabetes Educator

1. How many pumps have they prescribed in the last year?

2. Which of the current pumps and infusion sets do they prefer and why?

3. How familiar are they with the pump you may prefer?

4. What successes or issues have users had with different pumps?

5. Is a loaner pump available to try?

Your Insurance Company or Medicare

Most insurance companies provide coverage for insulin pumps and many are covering CGMs as well. Find out:

1. What are the requirements to start on a pump or CGM?

2. Which insulin pump or pumps will they cover? Many HMOs have a contract with only one or two pump companies.

3. If you prefer a pump that is not currently approved under your insurance plan, how can you obtain coverage for this pump?

4. How much of the expenses for a pump or CGM and supplies are covered by your DME (durable medical equipment) coverage?

Other Pumpers

Other pumpers often have experience that they are willing to share.

1. Is there a local pump club or someone in your church, school, or community that you can talk with about their pump experiences? You may want to join forums or chat rooms on the internet where users share information and opinions.

2. Some pumpers have worn several pumps. Which pump would they recommend?

3. What features do experienced pumpers feel are most important?

4. What advice would they give you from their experience?

5. Have they had particular pump issues that created control problems?

6. Have they needed to contact the pump company's 24-hour support line? What necessitated the call? Was it difficult to get the support they needed?

Once you choose a pump and infusion set and have your doctor's approval, a letter of medical necessity is submitted to your insurer or Medicare. The letter helps you get insurance approval and sometimes makes it easier to choose a pump that may not be on your insurance provider's preferred list. The pump company will prepare the paperwork to submit to your insurance carrier or Medicare to cover their share of the pump and supplies. They can also help you deal with any insurance problems that may arise.

When approved, your pump and pump supplies will be delivered to your door or to your doctor's office. A certified pump trainer from the pump company or from your doctor's office will train you on using the pump. Your doctor will review and assess your skills and guide you in setting initial basal rates and bolus factors, as well as the programmable pump features with which you choose to start.

Your pump trainer and doctor's office will be available by phone or appointment to help with any unexpected problems that may arise. They realize that starting on a pump may be confusing at first and will help you succeed. Ask for an emergency phone number and use it when you need help.

If your request for a pump is turned down, ask your physician and pump representative for advice on how to reapply. If your current insurance company's pump coverage is poor, are you able to switch to another insurance company in the near future that would provide better coverage? Sometimes it pays to wait until you have better coverage before starting on a new pump.

Infusion Set Choices

The most important step you can take toward a successful pump experience is to choose an infusion set that works well for you. Infusion sites and sets have been called the Achilles heel of pumps. Site and set problems are the most common pump-related cause for unexplained high readings and ketoacidosis, followed, on occasion, by incorrect pump programming or bad insulin. Insulin delivery problems can be detected before they reach a critical stage with frequent monitoring or the use of a CGM.

6.2 Types of Teflon Sets

Slanted infusion set

Straight-in infusion set

Reliability is the most important feature for any infusion set. If a set gets loose and leaks when the line is tugged, detaches when you swim or sweat, or kinks the Teflon catheter when you use an autoinserter or insert by hand, this can rapidly raise your glucose over a 4 to 5 hour period. If you have problems with a particular set, talk with your physician or diabetes educator about how to correct this. Ask about other sets that may be more reliable for you. Never wear a set that fails more than once a year.

Table 6.3 shows a partial list of infusion sets. See also www.diabetesnet.com/diabetes_technology/infusion_sets.php for more information. Infusion sets delivery insulin through a small metal needle or a slightly larger Teflon catheter under the skin. Many pumps use a standard Luer™ connection to connect the insulin reservoir with the infusion set that allows more than 20 different infusion set options. Other pumps have a proprietary connection between the reservoir and the infusion set that limits your choice to the infusion sets offered by that company. The Fifty50 company makes a reservoir for Medtronic pumps that allows the pump to accept Luer lock sets.

If you or your physician does not request a specific set, your insulin pump will arrive with a Teflon infusion set manufactured by your pump company or for it. This may or may not turn out to be your best choice. You may want to try different infusion sets to determine which is most comfortable, easy to use, and stays in place. Some pump companies will send samples of their products to try if you call.

When Selecting an Infusion Set, Consider:

- How much body fat do you have and which body sites are best to use?
- Do your activities limit the sites you can use?
- Which type and size of infusion set works best for the body locations you prefer?
- Can you detach the pump easily for showering? Is disconnecting difficult?
- Is a connector at the infusion site or one located a few inches away better?
- Do you need an insertion device for this infusion set?

Automatic spring-loaded insertion devices usually have a higher failure rate than sets that are inserted by hand. Some autoinserters have an adhesive between the inserter and the set that can cause the set to be partially pulled out when the inserter is lifted from the set. When the set is then tamped down to adhere it, the Teflon catheter can get kinked and lead to leakage or blockage of insulin. Better autoinserters do not have adhesive between the inserter and the infusion set and they have a strong spring to insert the set. Autoinserters are not recommended for insertion of slanted Teflon sets due to their high failure rate. If you use an autoinserter, be sure to use it exactly as directed.

Both metal needles and Teflon catheters are available in infusion sets. Today's fine gauge 6 mm long 90-degree metal needle sets are as comfortable as Teflon infusion sets, are usually easier to insert, and tend to cause the fewest infusion site issues. Metal set may cause less trauma under the skin and are preferred for children and lean adults. Some new 1.5 mm micro metal needle sets are under development to speed up insulin action and provide better post meal control.

How to troubleshoot infusion set problems is covered in Chapter 15. Keep in mind that critical pump supplies like infusion sets and reservoirs are not available at local pharmacies. Order supplies ahead of time!

Insulin for Your Pump

In contrast to multiple injections with rapid-acting and long-acting insulins, a pump uses only rapid-acting insulin. A slow release of this insulin through the day provides the background or basal insulin that replaces your injected long-acting insulin. Boluses of rapid-acting insulin are used to cover carbs and lower any high readings.

Today's rapid-acting insulins are very similar in action:

- Novolog® (aspart) by Novo Nordisk was released with pump approval in 2001
- Humalog® (lispro) by Eli Lilly and Company was released for injections in 1996 and approved for pump use in 2004.
- Apidra® (glulisine) by Aventis was released and approved for pump use in 2004

Some faster insulins are being developed, as well as other ways to speed up insulin action, so stay tuned.

6.3 Wide Variety of Infusion Sets to Choose From

	Name	Needle Type & Size	Connection	Tubing
	Ultraflex®	Teflon, Straight 8, 10 mm 25 gauge cannula	Pinch & pull at site Luer lock	24, 31, 43 inches
	Quick-Set®	Teflon, Straight 6, 9 mm 25 gauge cannula	Pinch, twist & lift at site* Luer lock & Paradigm	23, 43 inches
	Inset®, Mio®	Teflon, Straight 6, 9 mm 25 gauge cannula	Pinch & pull at site* Luer lock for Inset Paradigm for Mio	23, 43 inches
	Inset® 30	Teflon, 30-45 degree 13 mm 25 gauge cannula	Pinch & pull at site Luer lock	24, 42 inches
	Silhouette®, Tender®, Comfort®	Teflon, 30-45 degree 13, 17 mm 25 gauge cannula	Pinch & pull at site* Luer lock for all Paradigm for Silhouette	23, 31, 43 inches
	Rapid D®	Metal, Straight 6, 8, 10 mm 28 gauge needle	Twist & pull on line Luer lock	24, 31, 43 inches
	Contact Detach®, Sure-T®	Metal, Straight 6, 8, 10 mm 27/28 gauge needle	Pinch & pull at site Luer lock,	24, 31, 43 inches

See also www.diabetesnet.com/diabetes-technology/infusion-sets

* Inserter Available

6.4 Tips for Using Rapid Insulin in a Pump

- Keep fast carbs, such as glucose tablets, available to treat lows.

- **_Do not stop your pump to treat a low glucose._** Stopping a pump doesn't have any effect on the glucose until 60 to 90 minutes later, plus this may cause your glucose to spike afterward. Quick carbs are much faster and more reliable.

- Be safe, not sorry. Use an injection if you have two consecutive readings above 250 mg/dl (13.9 mmol/L). Inject the insulin you need, hydrate, and then search for any pump or infusion set problem you may have.

- Call your pump manufacturer if you suspect faulty insulin delivery. Their trouble-shooters can calm your anxiety and help you resolve delivery issues.

Insulin Storage Tips

If you have unexplained highs, don't just assume it's something you ate. It could be bad insulin, an infusion set problem, or something else that is raising your glucose.

1. Keep insulin out of direct sunlight.

2. The insulin bottle you use to refill your pump may be stored for 30 days at room temperature. Refrigerate extra unopened insulin bottles above 36° F (2.2° C).

3. A Frio® pack is a convenient way to keep insulin cool.

4. If your insulin is shipped to you, make sure it is insulated and cooled against temperature extremes during shipment.

5. Never leave insulin in a car during freezing or hot weather.

6.5 Reminders and Alerts (vary from pump to pump)

Reminder or Alert	Function	Approx. Range
Low Battery	Warns when battery needs changing.	24 hrs
Low Cartridge	Alerts when a selected # of units are left in reservoir.	5 – 50u
Special Features	Alerts when alternate bolus, temporary basal, or auto-off are active.	24 hrs
Delivery Limit**	Warns when more than selected number of units of insulin are given.	1 – 150u
Glucose Reminder*	Reminder to test glucose at time selected after a bolus.	1 – 4 hr in 15 min increments
Low Glucose**	Reminder to test glucose at selected time after a low glucose reading.	Time: 5 min – 1 hr BG: 50 – 100 mg/dl
High Glucose**	Reminder to test glucose at selected time following a high glucose reading.	Time: 30 min–2 hrs BG: 150–300 mg/dl
Automatic Off*	Safety feature turns pump off if no pump button is pushed during this time.	1 – 24 hrs
Site Reminder**	Reminder to change infusion set.	Alerts at certain time of day in 2–4 days.
Missed Meal Bolus**	Alerts when a meal bolus was not given at a certain time of day.	Time range, such as 11:30 am to noon

*These alerts and reminders often have a default of "OFF" and must be set to "ON".
** Not available in all pumps.

6.6 Responsibilities for Success on a Pump

You:

- Learn and use good techniques with your pump and infusion sets.
- Count carbs to improve control or use an equivalent diet method.
- Check glucose at least 6 times a day or wear a CGM, note all hypoglycemic events and their relation to insulin dosages, exercise, and carb counts.
- Keep all records requested and download devices as needed to improve your control.
- Test basal rates and boluses as instructed.
- Match basal rates and boluses to your insulin need by studying your records or contacting your health professional to identify patterns and troubleshoot problems.

Your health care professional:

- Teaches the technical skills you need to use your pump.
- Sets the duration of insulin action, target values, alarms, and reminders in pump.
- Sets your starting basals, carb factor, and correction factor and shows how to test and adjust them.
- Teaches problem-solving techniques so you can make needed adjustments for patterns of highs or lows.
- Provides 24-hour contact for problems that a new pumper may encounter.
- Gradually trains you about complete glucose management.

A hospital bed is a parked taxi with the meter running.

Groucho Marx

Get Ready for Your Pump Start

When you start on a pump or switch to a new pump, always work with an experienced health care team. Your pump company will also have training and support personnel to help you understand how your pump operates and guide you through any challenges on your path to good control.

Talk with other pump wearers and your medical team about any issues that arise. Your successes and failures will eventually improve your knowledge and success. Don't give up before you reach the best control you have ever had.

What this chapter covers

- What to practice with your pump before you start
- How to switch from injections
- What to bring for your start day
- What you'll learn on start day
- Choosing an infusion site and inserting the set
- Monitoring the infusion site
- Follow-up

Starting on a pump involves pre-pump visits and training with your health care team. You will learn how a pump differs from taking injections and how to operate your pump. This is followed by your pump start and clinic visits after your start. Ideally, this involves several visits with a multi-skilled health care team, including a physician, a nurse or diabetes educator, dietitian, and pharmacist with expertise in diabetes. Ask questions about any terms or procedures you do not understand.

How to Prepare

Knowing how to press the buttons or screens on your pump is easy. Knowing how to use your pump to optimize your control takes time. Read this and the next chapter carefully before you start on your pump. In addition, become familiar with your pump manual, any other material that your health care team or pump trainer gives you, along with any internet training that is provided by your pump company. *Your best preparation for a pump start is to take good care of your diabetes before you start.*

To quickly evaluate your readiness, ask yourself if you:

1. Know how to count carbs or have an alternate diet plan?

2. Know your CarbF (insulin-to-carb ratio) and how to use it for meals?

3. Know your CorrF and can use it to bring down high readings successfully?

4. Know what to do if your glucose keeps climbing on a pump?

5. Have the supplies and know how to tell if you have ketoacidosis?

Learn to count carbs and cover them with insulin in doses that work for you. Record the information that you and your doctor need in order to adjust your basal rates, carb and correction boluses. Use basal/bolus therapy and learn to adjust your doses on MDI therapy before you start on a pump. Understand how your long-acting (or basal) insulin serves a different purpose than the rapid insulin used to cover carbs and correct high readings.

Make an appointment with a dietitian to learn or improve carb counting. Bring with you a three day diet diary with all the foods you eat, their quantities, and your best estimate of their carb content. Be frank about your food choices and amounts to get the help you need. Listen carefully to the dietitian's recommendations and write down any changes you need to make.

Take a local or online class or workshop on diabetes management skills, carb counting, and pump techniques taught by a diabetes educator and a dietitian. Make it a habit to chart your blood glucose tests, carbs, insulin doses, exercise, and stress, so you and your doctor can see what affects your glucose. Use a CGM for even more information to guide your insulin dosing. The ***Smart Chart*** shown in Figures 5.5 and 5.6 lets you see the information you need on one page in a graphic format.

As Soon as Your Pump Arrives

Don't come to your pump training or, even worse, your pump start with an unopened box but never start on a pump on your own! As soon as it arrives, take everything out of the box and get familiar with your new pump. Read the manual and insert or charge the battery. You can't harm the pump, but you can harm yourself if you aren't familiar with it when you start. The more you do before and during your training, the more quickly you will use your pump with confidence.

With the pump in front of you, watch the training CD or DVD in your pump package or available online at your pump company's website. Get comfortable with the buttons and how to change settings. Try your infusion sets out. Following the instructions in the set box, insert an infusion set or two into an orange or apple. Practice as much as you can, even before you get hands-on training from an experienced diabetes professional.

Table 7.1 lists steps to practice and become familiar with before you start. Practice each step a few times. Set the time and date, program some practice basal rates and boluses, clear alarms, and review your glucose and dosing history. Use an old bottle of insulin, saline, or tap water in your reservoir to practice with an infusion set. DO NOT infuse any of these under your skin.

Complete as many of the practice steps below as you can. Check when done. Any programming you do can be changed later at your pump start.

Preparation

☐ Insert or charge the battery.

☐ Set the date and the time.

☐ Fill a reservoir with saline or water and load the reservoir.

☐ Attach an infusion set to the reservoir and prime the infusion line.

☐ Wash your hands, then cleanse your skin with IV prep or other antiseptic.

☐ Insert an infusion set under your skin (or into a nearby fruit) by following the instructions that came with your infusion set.

☐ Place a two inch length of 1" tape across the infusion line.

☐ Suspend and reactivate the pump a couple of times.

☐ Change your default duration of insulin action (DIA) time to a new time between 4.5 to 6 hours.

Program Your Pump

☐ Program a target glucose of 120 mg/dL (6.7 mmol/L) or a narrow target range of 100 mg/dL to 120 mg/dL (5.6 to 6.7 mmol/L).

☐ Program start times and basal rates for pretend basals: 0.6 u/hr at 12 am, 0.8 u/hr at 3:30 am, and 0.7 u/hr at 10 am. Check that your total basal equals 17.1 u.

☐ Program a CarbF (insulin-to-carb ratio) of 1 unit for each 12 grams of carb.

☐ Program a CorrF (or ISF) of 1 unit for 80 mg/dL (4.4 mmol/L) point drop.

Practice Using Your Pump

☐ Give a carb bolus for 48 grams of carb (should equal 4 units). Deliver, then check how much BOB you have (should be 4 units).

☐ Give a correction bolus for 280 mg/dL (15.6 mmol/L). The pump subtracts your target of 120 from 280 to give 160 mg/dL (8.9 mmol/L) as your desired drop. 160 divided by 80 = 2 units, but the recommended bolus should be 0 units if you have 4 units of BOB. (Just practice, not the normal way you would bolus.)

☐ Set a temporary basal rate at 80% of your usual rate for 4 hours, then cancel it.

☐ Review the pump's history – basal rates, boluses, alarms, and daily insulin totals. These have little data, but you want to know where this information is located.

☐ Get familiar with the list of alarms in your pump manual and any messages your pump may give and how to respond to them.

2012 © Diabetes Services, Inc.

Other things you want to know:

- What your basal rates and boluses do
- How to test your starting basal rates
- How to test your CarbF (carb boluses) and CorrF (correction boluses)
- How long bolus insulin lowers your glucose
- How to use Bolus On Board (BOB) and where to find BOB on your pump
- When to use temporary and alternate basal rates
- How to identify glucose patterns and eliminate those you don't want

Know When to Stop Your Long-Acting Insulin

The glucose-lowering activity of Lantus® and Levemir® usually disappears about 20 to 26 hours after the last injection, while NPH disappears 14 to 18 hours after the last injection. If Lantus® or Levemir® is injected once a day in the morning, this dose can be taken the morning before your start but usually not on the day you start. Rapid-acting insulin can then be taken as needed on the morning of the pump start to cover basal need, carbs, and to correct any high reading until your pump start.

If Lantus®, Levemir®, or NPH® is injected at bedtime, this dose can be cut in half on the night before your start. Small doses of rapid-acting insulin may be needed to replace the lost insulin during the night and at breakfast the next morning until the pump start. Wake up in the middle of the night to take rapid-acting insulin as needed to cover any glucose elevation and perhaps replace some of the long-acting insulin that was not taken.

7.2 When to Stop Long-Acting Insulin for a Pump Start											
Typical Long-Acting Doses				**On Day Before Start**				**Start Day**			
B	**L**	**D**	**Bed**	**B**	**L**	**D**	**Bed**	**B**	**L**	**D**	**Bed**
✓				✓				X			
		✓					half² dose				
✓		✓		✓		✓¹		X		X	
✓			✓	✓			half² dose				X

✓ = take
X = skip

1. If your usual dose of long-acting insulin is taken on the day before your pump start, some of this insulin will still be working. A temporary basal rate can be used until all the long-acting insulin is gone.
2. If half your usual dose of long-acting insulin is taken on the day before your pump start, small doses of rapid-acting insulin may be needed to supplement the lower dose, as well as a temp basal rate on start day.

Discuss appropriate doses for each insulin with your physician.

7.3 What to Bring for Your Pump Start

Wear comfortable 2-piece clothing for your pump training and start. Bring:

- The pump
- Fast-acting carbs to treat lows
- Glucose test supplies – meter, strips, lancets, lancing device, plus CGM if available
- A written glucose record or a download from your meter or CGM
- 3 or more pump reservoirs and infusion sets
- A new bottle of rapid insulin
- Alcohol pads
- A roll of 1" tape (3M Micropore™, Durapore™, Transpore™, Blenderm™, or Smith and Nephew Hypafix™)
- Skin disinfectant pads (IV Prep®, Hibiclens®, etc.) to kill bacteria on the skin if you are a staph carrier or have had skin infections in the past
- An additional adhesive dressing, if requested, like IV 3000®, Tegaderm HP™, Polyskin™ II, DuoDerm®, or Opsite®
- A list of all your questions and concerns

Alternatively, you may be instructed to take your usual dose of long-acting insulin the previous night. In this case, a temporary basal reduction can be programmed into your pump for a few hours until all of the long-acting insulin is gone. Your health care professional will guide you on this.

Start Day

An insulin pump is usually started at your doctor's office as a regular office visit or group medical visit where other people also start on a pump. After this training, return to your normal daily activities while your new basal rates and boluses are adjusted to match your lifestyle. Occasionally, a physician may prefer to hospitalize a new pump user for a couple of days to evaluate their pump settings and teach carb counting in an environment where professional help is readily available.

Training will be provided for each step in the operation of your pump by a diabetes educator in your physician's office or by a clinical representative from your pump company. Your physician will provide the initial pump settings for your pump.

Settings you and your doctor will program into your pump for your start.

- Time and date
- Other bolus calculator settings
- Basal rates
- Carb factor

- Correction factor
- Glucose correction target range
- Duration of insulin action
- Alarms and warnings

Review the steps you will be taking in the next few chapters in the Pump Tune-Up Checklist on page 14 before you start.

> ### 7.4 Avoid Champagne
>
> When cold insulin is used to fill a reservoir, small fizzy champagne bubbles often appear as the insulin gradually reaches room temperature. Avoid harmless champagne bubbles by filling your reservoir from an insulin bottle kept at room temperature.

Pump Start Techniques

Train and practice the following pump start techniques.

Fill the Reservoir (or Cartridge) with Insulin and Load

Some pumps have a reservoir or cartridge into which insulin is drawn directly from an insulin bottle. Others have a bladder into which insulin is injected through a port, a chamber that is loaded with insulin and then placed into the pump, or space for a standard 3 ml insulin pen cartridge to be placed into the pump. Refer to your pump manual for instructions on how to put insulin into your pump reservoir or bladder, and how to prime the infusion line.

1. For pumps with syringe-type reservoirs, lubricate the O-rings as shown in Box 7.5.

2. Insert an amount of air from the reservoir equal to the amount of insulin you will withdraw into the air inside an upright insulin bottle.

7.5 Prepare the O-Rings

Some pumps have a plastic reservoir or cartridge that is coated with a lubricant to give a tight seal between the O-rings and the barrel of the reservoir. When a reservoir is stored for a while, the lubricant may pool at the bottom of the reservoir. This increases the chance of insulin leaking into the area between the O-rings.

The picture to the right shows an O-ring leak. Even a small leak can cause a rapid loss of control. Replace the reservoir with another one if liquid, mist or bubbles are ever seen between the O-rings.

The area betwen the O-rings should be empty. An insulin leak like this can cause unexpected highs or DKA.

To avoid O-ring leaks, recoat the reservoir wall with lubricant prior to use. Free the plunger and push it completely into the barrel. Rotate the plunger a couple of times to recoat the O-rings; then carefully pull it back and forth 2 or 3 times in the reservoir to recoat the barrel. This redistributes the lubricant onto the O-rings and reservoir wall to help prevent this type of leak.

---

3. Then turn the insulin bottle upside down and draw into the reservoir enough insulin to last until your next infusion set change, plus enough to prime the infusion line and another 20 units or so extra, just in case.

4. Keep your thumb on the back of the plunger and release slowly to avoid champagne bubbles. Remove air bubbles by tapping them loose and working them out of the reservoir into the insulin bottle.

5. Insert the reservoir into the pump, following the procedure in your pump manual or audiovisual guide. Prime the infusion line after firmly tightening the connection between the infusion line and the reservoir.

Select a Site for an Infusion Set or Patch Pump

1. Any place you can "pinch an inch" can be used to insert an infusion set. The abdomen usually gives the fastest and most consistent absorption. Pinchable areas in the abdomen extend from just below the rib cage to just above the pubic area on both sides of the navel. The upper buttocks, thighs, and back of the upper arms also can be used, as shown in the graphic below. The buttock area often works best for young children because it is a large skin area that is out of sight. An area you can easily see is best when first starting on a pump or if you are having site issues.

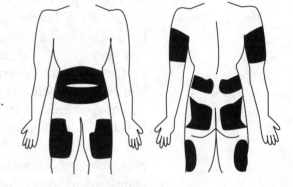

A patch pump can be placed in many of the same locations but stay away from skin folds where the pump may get detached if you bend over or twist sideways.

2. Stay at least two finger widths away from the navel for good absorption, and above or below the belt line.

3. Different Teflon and metal needle lengths are available. To absorb insulin, a short 6 mm length for 90-degree sets or 13 mm for slanted sets is usually all that is needed. Longer versions of these are sometimes preferred for extra security during pregnancy, etc. To minimize set failure, always anchor the infusion line with tape. See Table 6.3 for more information on infusion set choices.

4. Change the infusion set and site every 2 to 4 days, at least 4 hours before bed, and at least 24 hours before your glucose typically rises if you have set problems. You want to prevent infection, damage to the skin, scarring below the skin, and fat buildup from excessive use of one area, called *lipohypertrophy*.

5. Close to 10% of Teflon sets can become kinked when some autoinserter are used. If you use one, check your glucose 2 to 3 hours after inserting a new set to detect kinks.

6. Rotate areas, such as right upper quadrant of the abdomen to right lower to left lower to left upper. Sites may also be rotated in small steps, such as moving each new site about 2 inches from the last one. To remember to change your infusion site, put just enough insulin in the reservoir to last until the next site change. Most pumps have reminders that you can set to alert when it is time to change.

Prepare the Skin Site for an Infusion Set or Patch Pump

To prevent infections and the need for antibiotics or surgical drainage or hospitalization, always use *sterile technique* when setting up a skin site:

1. Wash your hands thoroughly with soap and water. Do not touch the reservoir needle, open end of the reservoir, end of the infusion set, or top of the insulin bottle.

2. For close viewing, hold your reservoir or infusion set at eye level above your nose. Many germs reside in the nose and breath, so do not breathe or blow directly on the pump, the reservoir, the infusion set or the infusion site.

3. An alcohol pad is adequate to cleanse the skin for many, but it is not strong enough if you carry staph. For staph carriers or if you are not sure, scrub the skin at the new infusion site with an antiseptic product. IV Prep or Betadine™ pads are convenient, or you can use bottled products such as Betadine™ Solution (iodine) or Hibiclens™ (chlorhexidine). Start at the center of the area and rotate the pad or swab in a circular fashion away from the center and do not go back. A cleansed area about three inches in diameter is needed.

> ### 7.6 Always Use Sterile Technique
> 1. Wash your hands well.
> 2. Do not breathe or blow on your infusion set or site.
> 3. Do not touch your face or nose.
> 4. Eliminate bacteria from the skin with IV Prep®, Hibiclens®, or Betadine® prior to inserting the infusion set.
> 5. Place a bio-occlusive material on the sterilized skin and insert the infusion set through it, or place over a low profile metal set.

For staph carriers, discussed on page 86, as well as for extra safety or for those who are allergic to set adhesives, place a bio-occlusive adhesive dressing like IV 3000™ or J&J Bioclusive Transparent Dressing™ over the site as soon as it dries. Unlike a standard adhesive, a bio-occlusive adhesive can seal sterilized skin to prevent bacteria from gaining access to the infusion site. The set or pump is then inserted through the bio-occlusive dressing.

Insert the Infusion Set or Patch Pump

1. Insert the infusion set or patch pump into the skin or through IV3000™ bio-occlusive adhesive already on the skin by hand or with an inserter. Have a qualified instructor show you how to properly insert your set.

2. After inserting a Teflon set, the metal introducer needle is pulled out. The empty space left in the Teflon cannula needs to be filled with a small bolus of insulin. Your pump instructor will tell you or read the product insert that comes with the set to find out how much insulin is needed to fill the space left after the needle is removed, usually 0.3 to 0.8 unit. This space in Teflon cannulas needs to be filled only once after you first insert it. Metal sets do not need a cannula fill.

3. ***Always anchor the infusion line*** with a 2" long piece of 1" Micropore™, Durapore™, or Transpore™ tape placed a couple of inches away from the site. Anchoring the infusion line with tape eliminates MANY erratic control issues that arise when tugs on the line causes a set to become loose or allows insulin to leak along a Teflon cannula back to the skin. Remember to replace the tape anchor after showers, etc.

Special Site Needs

1. If you experience a tape allergy, try coating the skin with Skin Prep™ before applying the infusion set or patch pump. You can also place an adhesive patch, like IV3000™, Tegaderm™, etc., onto your skin before inserting the infusion set through it.

2. Several products help keep an infusion set or patch pump from detaching when you sweat or swim. These include Mastisol™/Detachol™, Skin Tac H™, Applicare's Compound Benzoin Swabstick™, Drysol™, or an odorless antiperspirant (not a deodorant) spray. For excessive perspiration, try using a fragrance-free antiperspirant spray on top of the IV Prep. For excessive sweating or swimming, try Mastisol™ to keep the infu-

---

7.7 Reduce Insertion Pain

Some people feel pain or discomfort when inserting needles or catheters. Numby Stuff® and LMX™ 4 cream can be used to reduce sensation, or EMLA, a prescription numbing cream, can be applied to the skin about an hour before inserting the infusion set. A handy solution for children and adults with a needle phobia is to place an ice cube or cold spoon on the site before insertion to trick the nerve endings into feeling cold instead of pain.

Metal needles are preferred by parents of small toddlers and young children for their ease of insertion and very minimal pain. Auto insertion devices can minimize pain as the device touches the skin around where the needle enters so the nervous system gets distracted. The small gauge of metal needles makes them painless for most users.

If one infusion set causes pain, try another.

sion set or patch pump adhered to the skin. Mastisol can be removed from the skin with a cleaner called Detachol.™ Another product called Benzoin may also help.

Load Insulin and Prime the Line

For line pumps, there are a few basic steps that will get your pump operating:

1. Load a battery or charge your pump ahead of the clinic visit.

2. Insert and load the insulin reservoir

3. Attach and prime the infusion line with insulin

4. With a Teflon set, an extra step is needed to fill the Teflon cannula with insulin after the insertion needle is removed. This is not needed with metal needle sets.

See your pump manual for specific steps to load your pump.

Monitor Your Infusion Site

1. *Infusion site or set failures are a common source for unexplained highs.* Check your site regularly for irritation, redness, swelling or bleeding. Change the infusion set immediately if you have unexplained high readings or moderate or large ketones.

2. If your glucose is high twice in a row for no obvious reason, give a correction dose by injection and change your infusion set and rotate to a new site right away.

3. Retest your glucose within two hours of changing your set and monitor regularly over the next few hours to ensure that your glucose is coming down.

4. There is no perfect infusion set for everyone. If you experience unexplained highs that seem to disappear after the set is changed, ask to try a different infusion set or be sure to anchor your infusion line.

Prevent Site Infections

Compared to injections where infections are rare, infusion sites and patch pumps are more prone to infection because they stay in place for 3 days or so. Bacteria can be found on the hands, breath, skin, counter tops, clothing, and anything touched. A dangerous bacteria called staph aureus is the most common culprit in site infections. Even a small skin infection in the past or history of inflammation and redness around skin cuts or wounds suggests that a person carries staph. Over 20% of people carry staph on their body at all times and another 25% intermittently carry it. People with diabetes are more likely to be carriers.

Staph carriers have a much higher risk for site infection. Staph bacteria are usually present in the nasal cavity and on the skin, especially in the armpits and between the legs or buttocks. Carriers can often decontaminate themselves by treating the inside of the nose with a triple antibiotic cream on a Q-tip and by cleansing the skin with an antiseptic cleanser like Dial soap about three times in one week. This may have to be repeated once or twice over a few weeks to totally eliminate staph and be at less risk of infection. Any sign of infection from a cut in the skin or at an infusion site suggests that staph has returned. If this happens, repeat the decontamination process.

Follow-Up after Your Start

Close follow-up is essential for success. Your health car team will schedule phone calls and appointments to follow your glucose readings and adjust your pump settings.

1. Changes in pump settings may be needed within a few days of your pump start, so have a 24-hour phone contact number available.

2. A follow-up visit in the first week and one or two more in the first month are needed to adjust basals and bolus does. Your doctor may find that a pump adjustment is needed, so do not cancel an appointment even if you think things are going well. Communicate clearly about problems and why they may be happening.

3. Keep good records of boluses, carbs eaten, glucose readings, activity and stress.

   a) Check your pump for your TDD, basal percentage, basal rates, CarbF, CorrF, and duration of insulin action (DIA). Download information from your meter, pump, and CGM before all clinic visits to show your trends and patterns.

   b) Bring your meter, CGM, written records, *Smart Charts,* data downloads, etc., to every clinic visit.

   Your physician will use this information during clinic visits or phone calls to make basal rate and bolus factor adjustments.

4. Document all hypoglycemia and hyperglycemia and their treatment.

5. At the doctor's office, show your infusion site and review your pattern of site rotation. Point out any skin or site issues.

6. At clinic visits, write down any recommendations you are given, new basal profiles, carb and correction factors, dates of follow-up appointments, what you need at the next visit, and who to contact. Know what particular high or low glucose results should be reported to your doctor or nurse. See Workspace 7.8.

Your initial settings are tested and adjusted over the first few days and weeks of use. Basal rates are always tested first because boluses cannot be accurately set if your background delivery does not keep your glucose relatively flat through the day. Carb and correction boluses are then tested. To speed up dose adjustments after your pump start, keep your life as routine as you can. Eat familiar and consistently sized carbs at each meal, and exercise and sleep at regular times.

Will My Starting Basal and Bolus Doses Change?

The starting basal rates and carb and correction factors are estimates that often have to be changed during the first week or two of pump use. Both high and low readings on injections can cause glucose toxicity, release stress hormones, and makes you more resistant to insulin. As your control stabilizes on a pump, you may find you need less insulin. Don't be surprised if you have low glucose readings within the first two or three days after your start.

Keep glucose tablets handy and know how many carbs you need to treat each low (See Tables 10.4 and 19.9.). If you happen to also be improving your diet when you start on a pump, don't panic or stop your pump because you start having lows. Instead, get your doctor's help to lower your basal rates and raise your carb factor number to stop them.

When you eat your first meal on your pump, enter the number of carbs and your current glucose to see the carb bolus the pump BC recommends. Give the bolus if you agree with this recommendation. You can always raise or lower a recommended bolus before delivery. If you modify your BC's recommended doses, alert your health care professional so they can help you adjust your settings. Discuss these and any other issues with your health care professional so needed adjustments to your pump settings can be made quickly.

How to Tell if Your Starting Settings Work

After your pump start, check your glucose at least 7 times a day and any time you may be going low or high. Use a CGM if possible. Record any hypo or hyper excursions so your pump settings can be quickly tailored to your needs. Your starting or modified pump settings only work when they give you stable and relatively normal glucose readings.

7.8 Follow-Up Contract for Your Pump Star

Aour pump start, know your glucose targets and who to contact if pump or control issues occur.

My target ranges:

_____ to _____ mg/dl (mmol/L) before meals

_____ to _____ mg/dl (mmol/L) after meals

_____ to _____ mg/dl (mmol/L) at bedtime

I will call _____ at (____)_____ or (____)_____ if I have:

❑ more than _____ results below _____ mg/dl (mmol/L) in any _____ day period.

❑ any glucose value below _____ mg/dl (mmol/L).

❑ more than _____ results above _____ mg/dl in any ____ day period.

_____   _____
      Your signature   Your doctor's signature

Whom Do You Call?

Unexpected questions and problems often arise during the first week of pump use. Each pump manufacturer lists their 24-hour help line on the back of the pump or controller if you encounter questions, problems, or alerts. You and your family or friends will want 24-hour telephone access to your

> ### 7.9 Critical Pump Gear
> - Quick carbs
> - Glucagon injection kit
> - A blood ketone meter (MUCH preferred), like the Abbott Precision Xtra™ or Nova Max™ Plus, or with urine tests like Bayer Ketostix® or foil-wrapped Ketodiastix®

physician or health care team and to your insulin pump manufacturer to deal with any unexpected issues.

Know who and when to call for help if problems occur with your pump or control. Know which red flag situations, such as extremely high or low blood sugars, site problems (itching, infection), and emergencies require a call.

Contact your health provider for glucose control problems or insulin dosing issues. Don't hesitate to call when glucose problems occur. The earlier that control problems are resolved, the better.

Contact your pump company or pump trainer regarding questions or issues related to your pump. Mechanical or technical problems, such as alarms or unclear messages, should be communicated with your ***pump company***. Have your pump or pump controller handy when you call.

Be ready for emergencies. For lows, have plenty of quick carbs on hand. For severe lows, be sure to have a glucagon kit on hand that someone else can give you if you are unconscious. Ask your diabetes educator or physician to show you and a significant other how to inject glucagon.

For severe or unexplained highs above 250 mg/dl (13.9 mmol/L), have ketone testing materials available to monitor your ketone levels. A ketone meter is highly recommended for everyone on a pump. It detects dangerous ketone levels much earlier and shows them dropping much faster that urine ketone testing with Keto-Diastix® strips. The Precision Xtra® meter by Abbott Diabetes Care or Nova Max Plus® meter by Nova Biomedical will test both glucose and ketones in the blood.

On blood ketone tests, a level above 0.5 mg/dl suggests a problem. Levels between 0.6 and 1.5 mmol/L indicate ketosis and that a problem requiring medical assistance is underway. A blood ketone level above 1.5 mmol/L indicates that you are in or at high risk of developing DKA and you should call your doctor. Although urine tests are not as reliable, any urine ketone test that reads moderate or large indicates you have a serious medical problem. Elevated ketones on a blood or urine test suggest that your pump may have a delivery problem. Ketones begin to appear within 4 to 5 hours after an infusion set failure.

Ask your physician for a prescription for a ketone meter or foil-wrapped Keto-Diastix®.

7.10 Fit Your Pump into Your Lifestyle

Showers and Bathing

Detachable infusion sets allow the infusion line to be disconnected from the set so that the pump can be put aside temporarily. Be sure to reattach within 30-45 minutes after a bath or shower. Leave the pump in run mode to reduce the chance of having a clog and so that you do not forget to restart it.

Sleeping

Place the pump free on the bed, under a pillow, in a soft bag hanging from a neck ribbon, in a pajama pocket, or clamped to shorts or a soft belt. A wide variety of pump accessories are available that make wearing a pump at night a convenient experience.

Sex

If you and your partner are comfortable with the pump, put it in one of the above locations and let it take care of itself. Women may want to attach the pump to a garter belt by using the pump's belt clip. With detachable infusion sets, it is easy to detach from the pump for up to 45 minutes. Staying detached longer may cause the glucose to rise, so be sure to reattach your pump before you fall asleep.

Hot Tubs and Saunas

A hot tub or sauna quickly mobilizes any pooled insulin under the skin from an infusion site. Check your BOB before coming in contact with hot water. A large amount of BOB makes a low more likely. Excessive heat can make proteins like insulin lose potency, so disconnect your pump at the infusion site before you enter a sauna, hot tub or hot shower. If a pump or infusion line gets exposed to excess heat, it can turn an enjoyable experience into high glucose readings or ketoacidosis. Check your glucose carefully after a hot tub or sauna to avoid a severe low or unexpected high readings.

If you can't change your fate, change your attitude.

Amy Tan

People get creative in where to wear a pump. There are a wide range of clothing, cases and carriers, including backpacks for kids, sleep and sports clothing with specially designed pockets, cases strapped around the waist, thigh, or calf, and pouches that attach to a bra or garter belt. This head-to-foot list comes from Barb Chafe of Insulin Pumpers Canada™ with input from pumpers all over the world!

- Upside down to keep bubbles out of tubing
- Inside your clothing, only the pump clip shows
- Clipped on bathrobes
- In bicycle shorts that are then worn under pants, skirts and dresses
- In a regular or sports bra in the front middle
- In a baby sock pinned inside clothing
- Clipped onto the back of a bra
- Clipped onto a bra under the arm
- In a shelf bra sewn into the top of a camisole
- Clipped onto a garter belt clipped to underwear
- In a garter
- Inside pump cases like the Waist-It, Thigh Thing, Clip-N-Go, or Leg Thing, or Sports Pak
- In a pocket sewn inside a bathing suit, favorite jammies or on clothing
- Clipped to your belt/waistband - front or back
- In a vest with pockets for electronic gadgets
- Slipped under a pillow at night
- Pinned or clipped to bedsheets
- Strapped to the headboard of the bed
- In a money belt
- In pockets sewn on the outside of clothing so that the pump is easily accessible with the tubing threaded through the back of the pocket.
- Carried in a fanny pack
- On a backpack strap
- Strapped on the arm
- In the pocket of tennis shorts worn under other clothing
- Velcroed or safety-pinned in homemade products
- In Calvin Klein body slimmers under other clothing
- Hanging from a collar
- In your boot
- Strapped to a thigh or calf with elastobandage
- In a Frio pump wallet for extreme cold or heat
- Hanging in a pouch attached to a strap around the neck (useful when trying on clothes at a store)
- Slipped into the top of your sock with the tubing running down the leg
- In a cell phone case
- In a change purse
- In a leather gun holster
- Hanging inside or outside of anything with a carabiner (mountain-climbing clip) or in combination with a key ring and case
- In Tubi-Grip, a stretchy wrap from home health stores that can be put around an arm or leg
- Hanging from your ear – don't know why, but someone has done it

7.12 Future Pump Features

Feature	Benefit
Automatic Basal/Bolus Testing	Basal rates and bolus settings can be automatically evaluated for consistent glucose patterns, such as a rise in glucose from breakfast to lunch. Basal or bolus changes can be suggested to discuss with your physician.
Current Carb or Insulin Need (Hypo Manager™)	Any time a glucose test is done, a pump can recommend what to take: 1) a correction bolus if BG need is greater than than BOB; 2) nothing if BG need and BOB are in balance; or 3) how many carbs may be needed if BOB is greater than that needed for BG.
BOB Alert	If a bolus is being given without a BG but a significant amount of BOB is present, the wearer is alerted that they may want to check their glucose and account for this extra insulin.
Super Bolus	Helps cover high glucoses, high carb meals, and high GI foods. Future basal delivery (next 1 to 3.5 hours) is automatically shifted into the current bolus, accompanied by a temporary basal reduction of the same amount. See pages 153-154.
Delayed Eating Alert for High Glucose	When a glucose is high, this lets you combine a carb and correction bolus to get a faster drop in glucose. Based on the glucose, an alert is given later to retest when the glucose should be lower. Let's you safely delay eating until your glucose is lower.
Basal versus Bolus Check	Following a high or low glucose, you can compare how much basal and how much bolus insulin you got in the previous 5 to 6 hours. Helps to identify which insulin may have caused the high or low glucose.
BG Pattern Identification	Pump regularly displays current glucose patterns to speed up basal and bolus adjustments.
Dose Adjustments for Exercise	User enters how long and how intensely (1-7 scale) they plan to be active. Pump suggests appropriate carb intake and basal or bolus reductions to balance it, considering the current glucose, BOB, and length and intensity of exercise.
Daily Activity Monitor	With an integrated heart rate monitor or motion detector, pump suggests bolus and basal adjustments to prevent night or other lows.
Automatic Glucose Alerts	instant communication of glucose readings between pump wearer and others.

All About the Bolus Calculator

The best way to have stable glucose readings as close to your target as possible is to use your insulin pump's *bolus calculator (BC)*. The BC contains the settings that make bolus recommendations match the carbs you eat, bring down high readings, and minimize insulin stacking. The BC lets your pump give precise doses for life's variables.

This chapter covers the BC's role in getting the best control from your pump:

- Total daily dose of insulin (TDD)
- BC settings:
  - Basal rates
  - Carb factor (CarbF)
  - Correction factor (CorrF)
  - Correction target or target range
  - Duration of insulin action (DIA)
- Bolus on Board (BOB)
- How a BC handles BOB
- BOB's blind spot
- Basal/bolus balance
- Correction bolus percentage
- Limitations of the pump BC

Before the first smart pump, the Deltec Cozmo®, became available in December 2002, users estimated their bolus doses for carbs and glucose readings mentally or used hand-held calculators. The Cozmo is no longer available, but current pumps all have a bolus calculator and BCs are starting to appear in glucose meters and phone applets as well.

When your BC settings, carb counts, and glucose readings are accurate, you get accurate bolus doses for most situations. Unfortunately, setting errors are common in pumps. Also, BCs differ in how they calculate bolus doses, especially in whether and when BOB is subtracted from carb boluses. *As a result, different BCs can recommend different bolus doses for the same situation.* Know how your BC works to get the best bolus doses.

This chapter provides important information about each BC setting. It also reviews how BCs vary, why the duration of insulin action (DIA) time is so critical to bolus accuracy, the different methods used to make bolus recommendations, and when to override them.

Total Daily Insulin Dose

Your average total daily dose of insulin (TDD) is critical to your control. **An accurate TDD, discussed in this and the next two chapters, is key to success on your pump.**

8.1 Overview of Actual Pump Practices (APP) Study

The APP Study was conducted to see how people in relatively good control use their pumps and to find what settings gave the best glucose results. We analyzed anonymous data from several hundred well-functioning Deltec Cozmo insulin pumps (Smiths Medical) that were downloaded during a large, routine software upgrade in 2007. The pumps were prescribed and used around the U.S. by a wide variety of clinicians and wearers. Insulin dosing was analyzed from a subset of 396 pumps where glucose readings were directly entered from an attached meter.

The basal/bolus balance and pump settings for one third of the pumps (132 pumps) that had the lowest average glucose readings were determined. Formulas were then derived for optimal basal rates, carb factor (CarbF), and correction factor (CorrF) relative to individual total daily doses (TDD) of insulin.[63, 69]

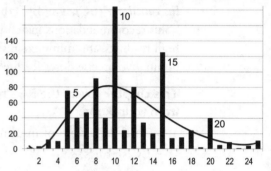

Carb Factor Settings Found In 899 Pumps

Key Findings of the APP Study

- The average glucose was 185 mg/dl (10.3 mmol/L) for all 396 pumps (120,445 glucose readings), equivalent to an estimated A1c of 8.1% or higher.

- Only 27.3% of pump wearers had an average glucose below 154 mg/dl (8.6 mmol/L), roughly equivalent to the ADA's recommended goal of 7%. This indicates that most people currently on pumps do not receive enough insulin.[63]

- Carb factors, shown in the figure above, did not match expected values, shown by the line. Easy to use CarbFs, like 5, 10, and 15, and CorrFs, like 50 and 100 were preferred over precise settings that would likely improve glucose outcomes. In this study, people used their BC to get carb and correction bolus recommendations over 93% of the time.

- 64% of boluses are given within 4.5 hrs of each other, so bolus stacking is common.

- The avg. time for the DIA setting was quite short at 3.1 hours, similar to what is found in most pumps today. This hides insulin stacking and may lead to unexplained hypoglycemia.

- The higher average glucose group used more insulin, not less. Interestingly, the lower and higher glucose groups did not differ in the grams of carb eaten per day nor in the number of carb boluses given a day. A small reduction in the number of glucose tests (4.0 versus 4.7 per day) and the use of higher CarbFs and CorrFs contributed only slightly to higher readings. The major contributor to hyperglycemia was a "relative" insulin deficiency.

- The lower glucose group (avg. BG 144 mg/dl or 8.0 mmol/L) had 2.74 documented glucoses below 50 mg/dl (mmol/L) per month, compared to 1.00 in the highest third (avg. BG 226 mg/dl or 12.7 mmol/L). Low glucoses were more common with better control.

A convenient APP Pump Settings Tool can be found at www.opensourcediabetes.org.

Table 8.2 Sample Glucose Goals			
Time	**DCCT**	**Pregnancy**	**Hypo Unawareness**
Before Meals	70 to 120 mg/dl 3.9 to 6.7 mmol/L	60 to 90 mg/dl 3.3 to 5.0 mmol/L	80 to 150 mg/dl 5.6 to 8.3 mmol/L
2hr after Meals	≤ 180 mg/dl ≤ 10 mmol/L	≤ 120 mg/dl ≤ 6.7 mmol/L	≤ 200 mg/dl ≤ 11.1 mmol/L
2 am	≥ 65 mg/dl ≥ 3.6 mmol/L	60 to 90 mg/dl 3.3 to 5.0 mmol/L	≥ 90 mg/dl ≥ 5.0 mmol/L
HbA1c	≤ 7.0%	5.5% to 6.5% – near or below lab's upper limit for normal	≤ 8.0%

Glucose goals must be modified for your situation. Higher goals are required for children, hypoglycemia unawareness, living alone, operation of heavy machinery, firefighters, etc.

The TDD is the major factor that controls the frequent highs that most pumpers experience and frequent lows that some experience. If your A1c or average glucose is high or you have frequent lows, an ***improved TDD (iTDD)*** is the quickest way to get more stable readings. Using an iTDD covered in Chapter 10, you and your doctor can select very accurate BC settings. Determining an iTDD is not difficult. **Frequent lows mean you need a lower TDD, while a recent A1c over 7.0% or average meter glucose above 154 mg/dl (8.6 mmol/L) usually means your average TDD needs to be raised.**

Most pumps let you average your TDD, total basal, and carb and correction bolus totals over the last 2 to 90 days. This makes finding the causes for lows and highs much easier than it is with injections where doses are often not recorded. The next chapter shows how to find a TDD to start on a pump, while the chapter after that shows how to find an improved TDD (iTDD) from your current TDD on a pump to improve your glucose control.

Bolus Calculator Settings

Basal Rates

Correct basal rates keep your glucose readings flat in a desired range when you sleep, skip meals, or eat a meal late. The correct basal lets you wake up with great readings and maintain better readings with less hypoglycemia. Basal insulin prevents your glucose from "escaping" by preventing your liver from making too much glucose. Basal rates are delivered around the clock in small increments and provide about half of the day's insulin for most people. The basal is about half of your TDD and has a significant impact on overall control. Chapter 11 covers how to select and test basal rates from your TDD (see Table 9.5).

Carb Factor

The *carb factor (CarbF)* or *insulin-to-carb ratio* is how many grams of carbohydrate one unit of insulin covers. An accurate CarbF lets carb boluses cover meals so you can go from a normal glucose before one meal to a normal glucose before the next one. Accurate carb counts are critical to make this happen. *If your glucose routinely goes high or low after meals, either your CarbF needs to be changed or you need to improve your technique for counting carbs or quantifying your food.* If your glucose goes both high and low after meals, paying attention to accurate carb counting will likely help.

The CarbF generates carb boluses making up 40% to 45% of the TDD for most people. A single CarbF may be used for the whole day or different CarbFs for specific meals. Entry of how many grams of carb are in a meal with an accurate CarbF lets the BC calculate and recommend a bolus that generally works. See the Bolus On Board section later in this chapter for situations where you may want to modify your pump's carb bolus recommendation. A starting CarbF can be found in Table 9.5 or from a formula in Chapter 12 obtained from the APP Study. Chapter 12 also reviews CarbF testing and adjustment.

Correction Factor

An accurate *CorrF* or *insulin sensitivity factor (ISF)* lets your pump BC know how much one unit of insulin will lower your glucose. This lets you bring high glucose readings back to your correction target within 5 hours with little risk of going low if no carbs are eaten or boluses given during this time. Once your CorrF and correction target are set in your pump, the BC can recommend the correction bolus you need for a high glucose. Choose your CorrF from Table 9.5 or from a formula in Chapter 13 obtained from the APP Study. Chapter 13 also reviews CorrF testing and adjustments.

Correction Target or Target Range

The *correction target, target glucose*, or *target range* gives the pump BC a glucose target or range to aim for with its correction bolus recommendation. Don't confuse the correction target in your BC with a glucose target range that you desire for ongoing good control. The glucose range for your overall diabetes control is always wider than the more specific glucose target that your pump aims for when it lowers high readings.

A single correction target value like 110 mg/dl (6.1 mmol/L) or a narrow target range like 100 to 120 mg/dl (5.5-6.6 mmol/L) generally works best. *A wide correction target range makes your pump's aim less exact.* For example, if you choose a range of 70 to 180 mg/dl (3.9 to 10 mmol/L), the BC won't recommend a change to your bolus for any value between 70 and 180 mg/dl. Only after your glucose is above 180 mg/dl (10 mmol/L) will a correction dose be recommended, and only when your glucose is below this range, will it recommend that you eat carbs or reduce a bolus.

A wide correction range changes the glucose target differently in different pumps. When your glucose goes above the correction range, most pumps aim for the middle of the range, or 125 mg/dl in this example (70 + 180 = 250/2 = 125). However, the Medtronic pump corrects high readings to the top of the range (to 180 mg/dl in this example) and low values to the bottom of the range. To avoid confusion, always select a single correction target or a narrow correction range.

A higher correction target like 140 mg/dl (7.8 mmol/L) may work better for someone who has hypoglycemia unawareness, while a lower target like 90 mg/dl (5 mmol/L) may be preferred for a woman who is pregnant. A pump can be set up with different correction targets for different times of day. For example, if a higher correction target of 140 mg/dl (7.8 mmol/L) is desired for a 10 p.m. bedtime, start this target at 5 p.m. This allows your BC to reduce boluses given before and after dinner sufficiently so your glucose will reach the desired bedtime target.

Duration of Insulin Action

The *duration of insulin action time* (*DIA*, or *active insulin time*) is how long a bolus will lower your glucose. This is a critical BC setting for your control that is frequently misunderstood. The DIA time in your pump starts as soon as a bolus is given and ends when that bolus is no longer lowering your glucose. Meanwhile, basal insulin keeps your glucose flat and steady through the day during sleep and when a meal is skipped.

An accurate DIA time in your pump allows the BC to accurately calculate how much glucose lowering activity (BOB) remains from recent boluses. After the first bolus of the day, subsequent boluses are likely to involve insulin stacking. The average DIA time, or roughly the pharmacodynamic time, for today's rapid-acting insulins from research studies is 5 to 6 hours.[70-75] DIA time varies to some extent between people, but how much variability in insulin activity actually exists between individuals has not been accurately measured.

Prior experience often makes people believe insulin works faster for them than 5 to 6 hours. For example, after taking a bolus for a meal, their glucose may suddenly have gone low 30 minutes later. It seems logical to blame this low on the bolus that was just taken, but it's more likely that the remaining action of a bolus given some hours earlier will actually be the real cause. An excessive bolus can also be mistaken as fast insulin.

Current insulin pumps allow DIA time to be set between 2 and 8 hours. If a shorter than actual DIA time is chosen, it makes the BOB or active bolus insulin appear to be gone when it is still lowering the glucose. Lutz Heinemann, PhD, the researcher involved in many pharmacodynamic studies of insulin, says about BCs in pumps that "the logic behind current advice systems is obscure" because the time choices for DIA in pumps are so much wider than the actual DIAs for current insulins.[76]

Table 8.5 shows how a short DIA time of 3 hours hides a large amount of glucose-lowering activity from recent boluses. This can lead to unexplained hypoglycemia and incorrect adjustments in other pump settings when a pump wearer or clinician attempts to prevent these lows. The table shows how much BOB your BC will calculate as remaining 3 hours after a 10-unit bolus. When the DIA is set to 3 hours, the BC calculates that no bolus activity remains at 3 hours after a 10-unit bolus, marked as A. If more realistic DIA times of 4.5 to 5.5 hours are used, the BC calculates that 2.5 to 4.0 units of glucose-lowering activity actually remains as shown in box B. These times more closely reflect insulin's true duration of glucose lowering activity in the body.

8.5 The DIA Setting Changes How Much BOB Appears to Be Left

If your DIA is set to:	This much of a 10 unit bolus APPEARS to be left after:				
	1 hr	2 hrs	3 hrs	4 hrs	5 hrs
3.0 hrs	7.0 u	2.6 u	0 u A	0 u	0 u
4.0 hrs	8.3 u	4.7 u	1.8 u	0 u	0 u
4.5 hrs	8.6 u	5.4 u	2.5 u	1.0 u	0 u
5.0 hrs	8.9 u	6.2 u	3.4 u B	1.4 u	0 u
5.5 hrs	9.0 u	6.6 u	4.0 u	2.0 u	0.8 u

8.6 Duration of Insulin Action Is Not the Same as Insulin Action Time

Fig 1 Insulin Action Time (IAT)

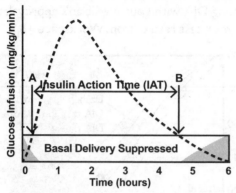

IAT is measured between points A and B while basal insulin delivery is suppressed

Fig 2 Duration of Insulin Action (DIA)

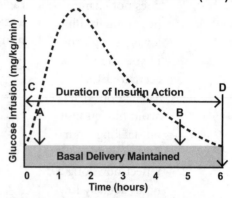

DIA is measured between points A and D while basal insulin delivery is maintained from a pump or with a long-acting insulin.

It's easy to get confused about what DIA time to choose as your pump setting *because DIA has not yet been accurately measured!* Insulin product handouts often quote insulin action time for a rapid insulin is "3 to 5 hours", but *these times are not the same thing as the DIA time for a pump!*

Figure 1 shows how **Insulin Action Time (IAT)** is measured. To measure IAT, researchers give people who usually do not have diabetes an injection of insulin and then measure the duration and amount of glucose that needs to be infused from an IV bag into the person's arm to offset this insulin and keep their glucose flat at 90 mg/dl (5 mmol/L).

IAT is measured from the start (A) to the end (B) of the IV glucose infusion. This type of study is useful for comparing one insulin with another, but *it does not include the time it takes for the injected insulin to suppress nor to recover the normal basal insulin output from a healthy pancreas.* This makes the glucose infusion start later and end earlier and makes IAT appear shorter than it actually is on an insulin pump where basal insulin continues to be delivered after a bolus is given. This type of study also makes smaller injected doses appear to have a shorter action time because a smaller dose is not able to suppresses the healthy person's basal output as long as a larger dose.

In contrast to IAT, **duration of insulin action (DIA)** is measured in Figure 2 from when insulin is injected or bolused (C) up to the time when insulin activity actually ends (D) *while basal insulin is being delivered from a pump or supplied as injections of long-acting insulin.* In 4 different experimental studies, the time between points C and A averaged 38 +/- 4.7 minutes, while the time between B and D is longer, although less insulin activity is involved.

See Fig. 8.7 for suggested DIA times to enter as your pump setting.

Selecting a shorter DIA time setting in a BC does not change how long insulin lowers the glucose in your body. For accurate BOB calculations that avoid hidden insulin stacking, your DIA time has to reflect how long a bolus actually lowers your glucose. Short DIA settings in the pump tend to be more dangerous for those with lower A1cs and anyone having frequent lows.

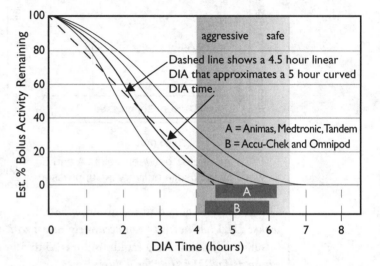

8.7 The Best DIA Times

The grey bars below show the best DIA times for today's rapid insulins in various pumps. Use these guidelines to select a starting DIA with your physician's approval, then modify it using your test results from Workspace 13.9.

Est. % Bolus Activity Remaining

aggressive   safe

Dashed line shows a 4.5 hour linear DIA that approximates a 5 hour curved DIA time.

A = Animas, Medtronic, Tandem
B = Accu-Chek and Omnipod

DIA Time (hours)

Visit www.diabetesnet.com/diabetes_technology/duration_of_insulin_action.php for latest updates on DIAs for new pumps or insulins.   © 2012 Diabetes Services, Inc.

Even if your glucose readings are high, don't shorten your DIA. This makes some boluses larger, but it also makes the real causes for highs harder to find and often leads to incorrect adjustments of the CarbF, CorrF, or basal rates. When you are not getting enough insulin, always fix the real problem by increasing your TDD, raising your basal rates or lowering your CarbF, rather than complicating things by shortening the DIA time. Fig. 8.7 shows our recommendations for DIA time, but *always check with your physician for the best DIA time for you*.

No difference in DIA times has been found between children and adults in research studies. Novo-Nordisk studied 18 children and adolescents between 6 and 18 years of age, concluding that: "The relative differences in....pharmacodynamics in children and adolescents with Type 1 diabetes between NovoLog® and Regular human insulin were similar to those in healthy adult subjects and adults with Type 1 diabetes." [77] Although children use smaller boluses than adults, bolus size relative to weight is not terribly different. For example, a 2 unit bolus for a 50 lb. child and an 8 unit bolus for a 200 lb. adult are equivalent relative to weight, so the DIA of each bolus will be similar.

A study of 9 children between 6 and 12 years old found no difference from adults,[78] and another study at Stanford University of 8 children found DIA to be slightly longer than adults.[79] Sanofi Aventis studied the activity of Apidra insulin in 20 children aged 7 to 16 and found no difference from adults.[80]

Pumps measure the decrease in bolus insulin activity linearly (Accu-Chek and Omnipod) as a steady decline, such as 20% or 25% each hour, or more accurately as a curved line (Animas, Medtronic, and Tandem) as shown in Fig. 8.7. Curved lines better match the delayed tailing action that insulin has. *In linear pumps, DIA times tend to have better accuracy when the DIA is set to 4.25 to 6 hours. Curvilinear pumps work well with DIAs of 4.5 to 6.25 hours.* These ranges are wide, so some trial and error testing is needed to determine the best DIA. Visit www.diabetesnet.com/diabetes_technology/dia. php for suggested DIA times to use in different pumps and to get updates on DIA times for new insulins and new delivery methods that speed insulin up.

Larger boluses increase DIA time,[81] but the way research studies on insulin timing are conducted tends to make smaller boluses seem to last a shorter time than they actually do.[82] (See Box 8.6.) *When boluses are often larger than 12 to 15 units, a DIA time of 6 hours or 6.5 hours may be preferred.* Check with your doctor. Anything that increases blood flow to the skin temporarily like heat and exercise can speed insulin absorption, but it is best not to shorten the DIA time setting for uncommon situations. *How to test your DIA time is shown in Workspace 13.9.*

Bolus On Board (BOB)

BOB, also known as insulin on board or active insulin, is the amount of bolus insulin remaining from recent carb and correction boluses that is still actively lowering your glucose. BOB measures only bolus insulin activity on the assumption that your basal rates have already been accurately set. With the correct DIA setting, BOB measures the insulin activity that remains from any boluses given within the DIA time.

Insulin stacking is a buildup of bolus insulin when two or more boluses overlap. The goal is to track BOB accurately so that insulin stacking does not cause hypoglycemia. In the APP study, 64% of all boluses were given within 4.5 hours of a previous bolus, well within the time in which BOB remains active.[83] BOB rises when a correction bolus is increased to lower a glucose faster and following increased physical activity.

If you give a carb bolus without entering a glucose value in your pump, it will recommend a full carb bolus, regardless of how much BOB remains. Don't give blind boluses – *always enter your current glucose before you bolus.* To ensure accurate bolus doses, use glucose values taken within the last 10 minutes from an accurate meter. Meters that directly enter glucose readings into a pump avoid data entry errors and lapses of memory. Each glucose reading is important to track BOB, minimize insulin stacking, and get accurate boluses.

Future pumps will hopefully alert if a bolus is started while significant BOB is present. This would allow a glucose reading to be entered to minimize insulin stacking.

One of the great advantages of an insulin pump is that it calculates your BOB for you in a reasonably accurate way. BOB is shown on one or more screens. Once the DIA is correctly set, *know where to find your BOB on your pump screens so you can override bolus recommendations when needed.*

How the BC Handles BOB for Bolus Recommendations

Although the DIA time has the greatest impact on whether BOB is measured accurately, how your BC handles BOB can also create some hidden insulin stacking. Because some pump BCs ignore BOB when giving carb boluses, *different pumps can recommend significantly different boluses for the same situation.* An example of this is shown in Box 8.9 where for the same situation one pump will recommend that no bolus be given and another recommends taking 6 units.

Correction Boluses

All pump BCs subtract BOB from any correction bolus given for a high glucose to help avoid insulin stacking. However, BOB can sometimes be greater than the correction bolus needed for the current glucose, or the glucose may already be low when BOB is still present. This excess BOB would ideally be deducted from any carb bolus being given, or trigger an alert showing how many grams of carb are needed to treat the impending low. No current pump does this.

Carb Boluses

A short DIA time is the most common source for insulin stacking. However, how a pump adjusts a carb bolus for excess BOB can also generate hidden insulin stacking. Excess BOB can easily happen with increased physical activity or after taking a larger bolus than the one recommended to bring a high glucose down quickly.

Theoretically, carb bolus recommendations should be reduced when the glucose is low or when there is excess BOB that will make it go low, but this does not always happen. *For example, most pumps do not subtract excess BOB from carb bolus recommendations when the BOB is greater than the units needed to correct the glucose.*

Todays pump BCs use four different methods to adjust or not adjust a carb bolus for excess BOB. Box 8.9 shows an example of this. *Know how your own pump BC works, as well as how to calculate an accurate carb bolus yourself because it is often wise to adjust or override bolus recommendations when needed.* Box 8.10 covers how to find a safer bolus in certain situations.

Four methods are used by pump BCs to handle excess BOB for carb boluses:

1. The Medtronic and Omnipod BCs do not subtract excess BOB from carb bolus recommendations. If a glucose is below the target range, a carb bolus is reduced enough to bring the glucose up to the bottom of the target range. If a glucose is above the bottom of the target range but excess BOB is present, the recommended bolus may be more than you need. See Box 8.9. This approach carries less risk for those who avoid lows by keeping their glucose levels somewhat higher.

2. Animas and Tandem BCs subtract BOB from carb bolus recommendations only when the glucose is below the correction target or target range. If the glucose is lower than the correction target or range, all excess BOB is subtracted from the carb bolus to bring the glucose to the middle of a range (Animas) or to 70 mg/dl (3.9 mmol/L)

8.8 What Do Pumps or Meters Count as BOB and How Is BOB Applied?				
	Is Bolus Included in BOB?		Is BOB Subtracted from Bolus?	
	Carb	Correction	Carb	Correction
Best Practice [1]	Yes	Yes	Yes	Yes
Abbott InsuLinx *	Yes	Yes	Yes	Yes
Accu-Chek Solo **	Yes	Yes	Yes	Yes
Animas	Yes	Yes	No [2]	Yes
Medtronic/ Omnipod	Yes	Yes	No	Yes
Tandem	Yes	Yes	No [3]	Yes

[1] Best practice is the least likely to allow insulin stacking and cause hypoglycemia
[2] Animas subtracts BOB from carb boluses once glucose is below the target range.
[3] Tandem subtracts BOB from carb boluses once glucose is 70 mg/dl (3.9 mmol/L).

* The bolus calculator for the InsuLinx is available only in Europe at this time.
** Expected to be available in the U.S. in 2013 or 2014.

AccuChek Spirit and Combo pumps calculate bolus doses based on glucose values rather than BOB (most situations). Insulin stacking can occur with this method as well.

© 2013 Diabetes Services, Inc.

(Tandem). If the glucose is in or above target, these BCs act like those in #1, and ignore excess BOB.

Bolus recommendations from these pumps can change dramatically depending on whether the glucose is above or below target. For example, someone may have a correction target of 120 mg/dl (5.6 mmol/L) and have 6 units of excess BOB a couple of hours after their last bolus. If they want to eat carbs that normally require a 6 unit carb bolus, no bolus will be recommended when the glucose is 119 mg/dl, but a full 6 unit bolus is recommended if the glucose is 121 mg/dl. These pumps provide some protection against insulin stacking when the glucose is below target or below 70 mg/dl. They work for people in reasonable control who do not experience significant lows.

3. The Accu-Chek Solo and the bolus calculator on the European version of the Abbott InsuLinx Freestyle meter (whole units only) subtract excess BOB from carb boluses regardless of whether the glucose is above or below target. This method was first outlined on page 72 in the first edition (1989) of **Pumping Insulin**.

This carries less risk for causing unexplained lows because hidden insulin stacking is avoided. This pump is best for someone who has frequent or severe lows, hypoglycemia unawareness, or who wants well-controlled readings with less risk of going low.

This method appropriately decreases carb boluses to account for excess BOB even when the current glucose may still be high. If you are having frequent highs after meals, the subtraction of excess BOB from carb and correction boluses is NOT causing these high readings. Check instead whether your carb boluses are too small (CarbF too large), your carb counting is off, or your basal rates are too low.

4. Smiths Medical used the last method, called HypoManager™, in the Deltec Cozmo pump. Although not currently available, it usually provides the safest bolus recommendations. When excess BOB is present, the pump would tell the wearer how many grams of carb they need either now or later to offset the excess BOB and avoid going low later. *Refer to Box 10.4 to see how to do this yourself.*

This method helps avoid over-treatment of lows and guards against an upcoming low glucose by warning the pump wearer that one may occur later because the BOB appears excessive even when the current glucose is normal or elevated.

Insulin stacking is especially worrisome near bedtime. If you bolus for a snack and your glucose is above target, any current BC will ignore any excess in the BOB and recommend a full carb bolus. Before giving a bolus and going to sleep, check whether you need to eat carbs because you have excess BOB or you need to take a correction bolus because not enough BOB remains to cover the current glucose. Consider reducing the bolus recommendation any time that BOB exceeds the correction bolus.

Pump wearers can more easily sort out the true setting adjustments that are needed for highs and lows when a BC has an appropriate DIA time setting, avoids insulin stacking by accounting for BOB, and recommends the carbs needed to offset insulin stacking.

No approach is perfect. For example, after eating a bean burrito, method 4 may recommend that too many free carbs be eaten because the glucose stays flat longer afterward. Some meals contain fats that create insulin resistance. Your glucose may be elevated hours later even though the BOB would normally cover this glucose.

Box 8.11 shows how to check whether your pump subtracts BOB from carb boluses when your glucose is above or below your correction target. In most situations, it is safer to subtract any excess BOB from carb boluses. If your glucose is above 140 or 150 mg/dl (7.8 or 8.3 mmol/L) with excess BOB, you may want to wait to eat carbs needed to cover this BOB until your glucose is lower.

If you are having low glucoses, Box 8.10 shows how to determine a safe bolus yourself. Remember that having frequent highs with few lows suggests that your TDD needs to be raised, along with better food choices if this is needed. Frequent lows suggests that your current TDD is too high.

Never take a recommended bolus that seems too large before checking this recommendation using Box 8.10. You may also want to recheck your glucose to ensure your reading is accurate. Visit www.diabetesnet.com/diabetes_technology/dia.php for more information on the different methods pumps use to calculate BOB.

8.9 Bolus Recommendations Differ from Different Pumps

Even with an accurate DIA time, different pump BCs subtract BOB differently from carb and correction boluses. As an example, Alex is a 46 year old pump wearer whose CarbF = 10 g, CorrF = 30 mg/dl, and correction target = 120 mg/dl. For four nights in a row, he ate the same dinner at the same time and took 12 u for 120 grams of carb.

Two hours after dinner, Alex wants to eat a 50 gram dessert when he still has 5 u of BOB left from a 10 unit carb bolus he gave for dinner. He would usually take 5 u to cover this dessert, but wants to consider his current glucose and BOB to get an accurate bolus dose.

On the first two evenings he played racquetball for 45 minutes just after dinner. On the 3rd he did not. On the 4th, he learned his daughter had become engaged to a twice divorced man who has a $30,000 gambling debt. His glucose before dessert on these four evenings was 119, 121, 210, and 300 mg/dl (6.6, 6.7, 11.7, and 16.7 mmol/L).

Alex's true bolus need is easy to find: the 5 u of BOB still left from his dinner will cover the 5 u he needs for his dessert, so the only bolus needed would be a correction bolus if his glucose is high. The table below shows boluses recommended by each of the methods found in current pumps for these different glucose levels.

If Alex's Glucose Is:	Alex needs	Method 1 says	Method 2 says	Methods 3 & 4 say
Night 1: 119 mg/dl	0 u	6 u	0 u	0 u
Night 2: 121 mg/dl	0 u	6 u	6 u	0 u
Night 3: 210 mg/dl	3 u	6 u	6 u	3 u
Night 5: 300 mg/dl	6 u	6 u	6 u	6 u

Method 1 recommends taking a 5 u bolus on all 4 evenings regardless of the glucose reading. With his glucose at 119 mg/dl (6.6 mmol/L), Method 2 calculates accurately and recommends 0 u, but if his glucose is 121 mg/dl (6.7 mmol/L), it recommends taking 5 u. Methods 3 and 4 give the most conservative (safest) doses.

© 2013 Diabetes Services, Inc.

BOB's Blind Spot

Although carb and correction boluses are usually more accurate when you account for BOB, there are certain times when it is better to simply ignore BOB. *After a meal bolus is given, a "blind spot" exists for about 90 to 120 minutes when the effect of carbs raising the glucose cannot be fully measured against the carb bolus insulin lowering it.* Both you and your BC will have trouble determining an accurate bolus during this time. Any carbs eaten during this blind spot are typically covered with a full carb bolus.

When Do You Override Your BC?

With accurate settings, your BC will give you great bolus recommendations. But always be smarter than your BC and know when to take recommended boluses or when to adjust them for other factors. You know when you will be more active, are more stressed, a cold is coming on, or the last meal had more fat or protein and is digesting slowly. At times like these, you will definitely want to override your pump BC's bolus recommendations.

A CGM adds helpful information on the direction and rate of change of your glucose. When you consider this added information and take into account how much BOB is left, you have much better information on whether to override a BC bolus recommendation.

If you frequently have to override your pump BC recommendations, or you are having frequent highs or lows, then one or more of the settings in your BC or your BC logic may need to be improved. The DIA may be too short, basal/bolus balance skewed, or the CarbF or CorrF too large or too small. You may know adjustments are needed but be unsure what to do. Always choose starting settings from formulas like those from the APP Study, as shown in the next three chapters, then optimize them through testing. Until you and your doctor figure this out, override your BC recommendations as needed.

In a presentation on pumps and CGMs at the American Diabetes Association convention in June, 2011, Dr. Irl Hirsch, an endocrinologist and pump specialist, suggested he was comfortable when his patients overrode their pump BC bolus recommendations about 25% of the time, especially if they wear a CGM. He said that someone who never overrides their bolus recommendations is probably not thinking about what they are doing.

8.11 Check How Your Pump Handles Bolus On Board (BOB)

Excess BOB can occur in many situations. It is more likely when your glucose is well controlled, after being more active, or after a bolus is increased to bring a high glucose down quickly. Unexplained lows can occur if a pump BC that does not subtract excess BOB from carb boluses.

To test whether your pump BC subtracts BOB from carb boluses, pretend the following:

1. Any time you have more than 1 unit of BOB still active from an earlier bolus, enter into your BC the number that equals your carb factor (CarbF) as the number of carbs you intend to eat. For example, if your CarbF is 1 unit for 12 grams, enter 12 grams of carb. This would give 1.0 u as your bolus.

2. Now enter a glucose that is 1 mg/dl (0.1 mmol/L) higher than your correction target (or target range). For example, if your target range is 100 to 120 mg/dl, enter 121 mg/dl as your glucose. (For 5.6 to 6.0 mmol/L, enter 6.1 mmol/L.)

3. If your pump recommends giving a 1.0 unit bolus, your pump BC DOES NOT subtract BOB from carb boluses when your glucose is above your target. **(Don't deliver this bolus!)** If your BC says no bolus is needed, your pump DOES subtract BOB from carb boluses.

4. Next, check whether your BC subtracts excess BOB from carb boluses when your glucose is below your target. Enter the same grams of carb with a glucose value that is 1 mg/dl (0.1 mmol/L) below your correction target or target range. For example, if your correction target range is 100 to 120 mg/dl, enter 99 mg/dl as your glucose. (If 5.6 to 6.0 mmol/L, enter 5.5 mmol/L.) If your BC says no carb bolus is needed, your BC DOES subtract BOB from carb boluses when your glucose is below your target range.

To minimize insulin stacking, keep track of your BOB. If your pump does not subtract BOB from carb boluses, double-check your pump's bolus recommendations, as shown in Box 8.10.

© 2013 Diabetes Services, Inc.

Many pump companies have software that tracks how often you override bolus recommendations. Some software shows the bolus dose that the BC recommended, the dose that was taken and whether the next glucose reading was close to target. This allows the user and clinician to evaluate how well the user is making bolus adjustments.

Basal/Bolus Balance

Basal and bolus doses work best when balanced. For the 132 pump wearers with the lowest average glucose in the APP Study, basal rates made up 48% of the TDD, with 43% given as carb boluses and 9% as correction boluses, as shown in Workspace 8.14.[63] Daily basal totals have averaged 48% to 54% of the TDD in several clinical studies.[9,84] Of interest, basal rates also made up 48% of the TDD in the highest average glucose group in the APP Study, indicating that *the TDD is the primary factor that controls the A1c.*

Although there are exceptions, ***most people do well when basal rates make up 45% to 55% of the TDD***. A child or adult recently diagnosed with Type 1 may retain some insulin production and do well with less than 40% of their TDD as basal. Some thin, older adults with lower stress hormone output may also benefit from a lower basal percentage to avoid night lows. Similarly, someone on a high carb diet uses more TDD for carb boluses, so basal delivery can work well at 40% of the TDD. In contrast, someone on a low carb diet with smaller carb boluses may have basal rates that make up 70% or more of the TDD.

Most pumps have a history screen that shows the basal/bolus balance to help you spot where control problems originate. For example, a woman with Type 2 diabetes thought her carb boluses were too large because she kept having lows after meals, even though she consistently took less than the carb bolus recommended by her pump. However, a check of her basal/bolus balance during a clinic visit revealed that over 80% of her TDD came from her basal rates. She had recently gone on a diet and lost 15 pounds. Her physician recommended lowering her TDD by lowering her single daily basal rate of 2.15 u/hr to 1.8 u/hr. This stopped her lows. She was advised to lower her basal rate again if she lost more weight.

If you have control problems, check your pump history screens to see what percentage of your TDD you currently use for basal rates, carb boluses, and correction boluses. Compare these to the optimal values in Table 8.14. Adjustments of basal rates and bolus factors over time may throw off your basal/bolus balance, so keep an eye on this balance, and discuss this with your physician to keep your ratios in the balance you need.

Correction Bolus Percentage

Most pumps have a history screen that shows how much correction bolus insulin you have averaged over the last 2 to 30 days to lower high readings. Ideally, correction boluses will make up less than 9% of the TDD, or 0.09 times your TDD. ***When over 9% of your TDD is used to bring down high readings, some of this excess insulin needs to be shifted into your basal rates or carb boluses to prevent highs from happening.***

8.13 What if You Don't Use a Bolus Calculator?

Most people find that their BC improves their control, but a pump wearer whose math skills are good or who lives a routine lifestyle may not need to use a BC at all. Some people who started on pumps before BCs first became available do very well relying on the dosing calculations they have used for years.

Other pumpers may never have been trained to use their BC or they mistrust the BC's recommendations because its settings were never optimized. Better training or more accurate BC settings may be all that is needed.

Correction boluses are needed, often daily, to fine-tune your control, but don't routinely use more than 9% of your TDD to correct high readings. Instead, make sure you get enough basal and carb bolus insulin to prevent these highs. Your correction bolus percentage can creep up over time, so check this percentage from time to time.

Tips on Bolus Calculators

- Know how your pump handles BOB in its carb or correction bolus recommendations.
- Know where to find your current BOB (residual bolus insulin, insulin on board, active insulin) on your pump screen.
- Adjust bolus recommendations before and after exercise, during illnesses or infections, during stress, with menses, etc.
- A CGM improves dosing by showing your approximate glucose value and its trend line, backed up by arrows and alarms that indicate impending highs and lows. CGM information helps you know when to override bolus recommendations.
- With a normal glucose, check your BOB before you assume that everything is fine.
- When a reading is low, check your pump to see how much BOB is left so you can get the right amount of carbs to treat it.
- Never give a bolus that doesn't seem right. Double-check your pump settings if this is often the case.

8.14 Innovators in BC Accuracy

Bolus calculator accuracy depends on having accurate BC settings. Dr. Paul Davidson, Mr. Harry Hebblewhite, MS., and others with Atlanta Diabetes Associates did much of the work to derive the formulas required to obtain accurate BC settings. They first introduced a 1500 Rule for the correction factor in 2002[159] and later expanded to rules derived from pump patient data for the basal percentage, CarbF, and CorrF in 2003 and 2007.[160] Much of the benefit you derive from your bolus calculator is based on their pioneering work.

8.15 Check Your Basal/Bolus Balance on a Pump

Compare your current insulin use from your pump to the average and the middle 50% values (the half of all settings nearest the middle) for the basal and bolus doses in the 132 pumpers who were in the best control group in the APP study.[69]

Optimal Doses for the Group with the Best Control

Insulin:	Average % of TDD	Middle 50% or Optimal Range
Basal	47.7%	39.6% to 54.9%
Carb Boluses	43.1%	35.6% to 51.2%
Corr Boluses	9.0%	6.2% to 11.3%

Compare your own values averaged over the last 14 to 30 days to those above:

My average TDD   =   ____ units/day

My average basal   =   ____ units/day   =   ____% of TDD

My average carb bolus = ____ units/day   =   ____% of TDD

My average corr bolus = ____ units/day   =   ____% of TDD

To find percentages if your pump doesn't show this, divide your average total daily basal (or daily carb boluses or daily correction boluses) by your average TDD in a calculator, then multiply by 100 to get your percentage.

For example, if your average basal dose per day is 55.0 units and your average TDD is 100 units, 55/100 = 0.55 or 55%. Here, basal rates average 55% of the TDD.

Reality is the leading cause of stress among those in touch with it.

Lily Tomlin

Copy this worksheet, write in your current values, and bring to each clinic visit:

1. **Average glucose** (14 or 30 days) = _____ mg/dl (mmol/L)

2. **Basal rates:**

   _____ am/pm   _____ u/h   _____ am/pm   _____ u/h

   _____ am/pm   _____ u/h   _____ am/pm   _____ u/h

   _____ am/pm   _____ u/h   _____ am/pm   _____ u/h

   Total basal = _____ units a day

3. **CarbF** = 1 unit for each _____ grams of carb.

4. **CorrF** = 1 unit for each _____ mg/dl (mmol/L) drop in BG

5. **Corr. target** = _____ mg/dl (mmol/L), or _____ to _____ mg/dl (mmol/L)

6. **Basal/Bolus balance** (10-30 day average):

   TDD = _____ u/day

   Basal rates = _____ u/day and _____% of TDD

   Carb boluses = _____ u/day and _____% of TDD

   Correction boluses = _____ u/day and _____% of TDD

7. **Duration of insulin action** = _____ hrs _____ min

8. **Avg. # of carb boluses/day** = _____   **Avg grams of carb/day** = _____

9. **Average # of corr boluses/day** = _____

10. **Avg. % of TDD used for corr. boluses** = _____   © 2012 Diabetes Services, Inc.

Summary

For good glucose outcomes, it is important that your insulin pump bolus calculator (BC) has settings that work for you. Use the core concepts in this chapter as you set, test, and adjust your settings in the chapters that follow. Before you start this phase, make copies of Workspace 8.15, Workspace 11.5 for basal testing, Workspace 12.5 for carb factor testing, Workspace 13.5 for correction factor testing, and Workspace 8.14 for checking your basal/bolus balance. Put these into a folder where you also keep the forms filled out with your basal and bolus test results. Ensure that you know how your BC works, and gradually learn when to override its bolus recommendation.

8.17 The Path to Better Control

- Monitor glucoses frequently (or wear a CGM), match boluses to your carbs and current glucose, bolus for every meal and snack (unless there's a good reason not to do so), and don't overtreat lows with carbs or highs with insulin.

- Stop frequent lows first. Lower your TDD by 5% for frequent, mild lows or by 10% for frequent, severe lows.

- Find an improved TDD (iTDD) from your A1c or average glucose (Table 10.3).

- Get new pump settings from this iTDD (Table 9.5).

- Adjust these starting settings with testing and pattern analysis (Chapters 11-14).

- Keep your average basal rate and carb bolus totals balanced, and compare your insulin use with that of pump wearers in excellent control (Workspace 8.14).

- Keep correction boluses at or below 9% of your TDD (Chapter 13).

- If control issues arise, double check your current pump settings against the optimal values for your TDD (Table 9.5).

- Use a DIA time of 4.5 hours or longer to minimize insulin stacking.

Use doses that give you good control, no matter what best practices may be.

Be careful about reading health books.
You may die of a misprint.

Mark Twain

Get a TDD to Start on a Pump

Your **total daily dose** (**TDD**) of insulin is the total of the basal insulin, carb insulin, and correction insulin doses you use each day. The TDD used with injections often has to be reduced when you start on a pump. This chapter shows how to do this.

If you are already on a pump and want to improve your diabetes management, skip this chapter and go directly to Chapter 10 that covers how to optimize your TDD.

In this chapter, you will find:

- How to find a starting TDD from injections
- How to use your TDD to find the starting settings for your pump

Your average TDD is the major factor that controls your A1c, average glucose, and how often you have lows. Before you find your TDD and optimal insulin doses, make sure you do the other things critical to good control: monitor your glucose at least 6 times a day or wear a CGM, match your injections or boluses to your meal carbs and current glucose, cover all meals and snacks with insulin unless there's a good reason not to, and don't overtreat lows with carbs nor highs with insulin.

Your TDD also lets you closely estimate the BC settings that you need: your basal rates, CarbF (insulin-to-carb ratio), and CorrF. The starting TDD you and your doctor find below will be used to select the settings you enter into your BC for your pump start. You can then work with your health care team to test these settings to ensure they keep your glucose stable and close to your target range. If you encounter ups and downs in your glucose on this starting TDD, more accurate basal and bolus settings can be quickly determined from an **improved TDD** (**iTDD**) found in the next chapter. Pattern management can also be used to fine-tune your control. This involves using smaller setting and dose adjustments using the tools found in Chapter 14.

Find a Starting TDD for Your Pump Start

Your current TDD can be found by adding up an average of your current total daily injection doses. To find your actual TDD on injections, you will want to record how many units you actually inject each day. For accuracy, keep a written record of all the insulin doses you take for at least a week or two prior to your pump start. Once you are on a pump, your pump will record your TDD automatically for you.

A pump uses rapid insulin for both basal and bolus doses, so insulin delivery and uptake are more efficient. This usually means you need less insulin on a pump. Better glucose levels also lessen glucose toxicity and lower the amount of insulin you need. For Type 1 diabetes, a 5 to 12 unit reduction in the TDD is common.[15,16] Reductions can be greater with Type 2 diabetes with the TDD on a pump sometimes cut in half.

Use the 3 steps below to find your starting TDD. Your current TDD on injections is determined in Step 1. A second TDD for a person of your weight who has an average sensitivity to insulin is derived in Step 2. This is used to help bring your injected TDD toward a better value. These two TDD values are averaged and multiplied by 90% in Step 3 to reduce your current TDD even more and create less risk of hypoglycemia as you start on your pump.

1. Determine Your Current TDD on Injections

In Workspace 9.1, enter an average of your usual injected insulin doses. Include an average of the typical correction doses that you take for each meal over the last 2 weeks. Add up these doses to determine your current TDD on injections. If you occasionally forget an injection or two, base your average dose on the insulin you actually take. For example, if you take 10 units for breakfast but miss this dose one day each week, you would lower the average dose of rapid insulin taken for breakfast by 1/7th or 0.14. So rather than enter 10 units for breakfast, you would enter 10u x 0.86 or 8.6 units.

To get your average TDD, don't include "throw-away days", such as days when you were un-

9.1 Determine Current TDD on Injections

1. Enter an average of the insulin doses injected at each time of day over the last 7 or more days. **Rapid** includes your typical meal insulin PLUS an average of the correction doses you take for high readings. **Long** is your background long-acting insulin.

2. Total these doses to find your current average TDD.

Insulin	Rapid	Long	
Breakfast	_____ u	_____ u	
Lunch	_____ u	_____ u	
Dinner	_____ u	_____ u	
Bedtime	_____ u	_____ u	
Total	_____ u + _____ u = _____ u **Current TDD**		

usually high because you had an infection or were taking a steroid medication. If your TDD varies widely from day to day, discuss why it varies so much with your physician before you try to determine an average TDD.

2. Determine an Average TDD for Your Weight

Now find the TDD for someone of your weight in good control with an average sensitivity to insulin. To do this, multiply your current weight in pounds by 0.24 units per pound (or 0.53 units per kilogram). For children prior to puberty, multiply weight by 0.20 units per pound (or 0.44 units per kilogram).

For example, someone who weighs 167 lbs. would typically use 167 lbs. x 0.24 u/lb. or 40 units a day

9.2 Determine Avg. TDD for Your Weight

1. Enter your current weight below.
2. To find the average TDD for your weight, multiply by 0.24 for lbs or 0.53 for kg. *

   My weight = _____ lb (kg)

   x 0.24 (x 0.53 for kg)

3. Avg. TDD for my weight = _____ units/day

* For children prior to puberty, multiply by 0.20 for lbs (0.44 for kgs)

3. Determine Your Starting TDD

Next, add together your current TDD from Workspace 9.1 and the average TDD for your weight from 9.2 into 9.3. After adding them together, multiply by 0.45. This equals 90% of the combination of your current TDD and TDD based on weight and reduces your starting TDD enough so it should not cause hypoglycemia.

As an example, a growing teenager who weighs 167 lbs. and has high growth hormone levels may have a current TDD of 80 units a day on injections. When added to an

9.3 Determine Your Starting TDD

Add your values from Workspace 9.1 and 9.2. Multiply the total by 0.45 to get your starting TDD:

From 9.1:   My current TDD = _____ u/day

From 9.2:   Avg. TDD for my Wt = +_____ u/day

Total of 9.1 + 9.2 = _____ u/day

x 0.45

My Starting TDD = _____ u/day

average TDD of 40 units a day for someone of the same weight who is in good control, the total of 80 plus 40 equals 120 units, which when multiplied by 0.45, gives a TDD for the pump start of 54 units. This insulin reduction creates a starting TDD that is safe and usually effective for maintaining reasonable control.

There are exceptions to using this method to find a starting TDD. If someone on injections has a high A1c like 9.5% (meter average of about 226 mg/dl (12.6 mmol/L)), their current TDD on injections is obviously too low. If this TDD is averaged with an average TDD for their weight that happens to be smaller, the starting TDD calculated above may be too small for their pump start. Here, their physician may suggest starting with a higher TDD than the one in Workspace 9.3.

> **9.4 Helpful Pump, Meter, and CGM Information:**
> 1. Average doses for the TDD, basal rates, carb and correction boluses
> 2. Average blood glucose and standard deviation
> 3. Frequency and timing of high and low glucoses
> 4. Average grams of carb consumed per day
> 5. Timing of carb intake and bolus doses
> 6. Percentage of TDD used for correction boluses

An uncommon exception may occur for someone who is very sensitive to insulin. If the TDD on injections is less than the TDD based on weight, but this TDD is causing frequent lows, the physician may suggest starting on a TDD lower than that found in Workspace 9.3.

If you are having frequent or severe lows on multiple daily injections (MDI), there is no obvious pattern to your readings, or your exact insulin doses on MDI are not clear, your physician may not use 9.1 but instead base your starting TDD on your weight in 9.2.

Whether your starting TDD is too high or too low quickly becomes apparent in the first 2 to 4 days after your pump start as glucose readings go higher or lower than desired. If this happens, you and your health provider can reset your TDD and use it to determine more appropriate basal and bolus settings.

Use Your TDD to Find Your Pump Settings

The TDD you find in Workspace 9.5 is used to find your starting basal rate, CarbF and CorrF. Then go to Chapter 11 to test and adjust your starting basals, followed by testing and adjustment of your CarbF and CorrF in Chapters 12 and 13.

Once these adjusted settings keep your glucose reasonably controlled, you can use pattern management in Chapter 14 to fine-tune them. Testing and tuning of your starting pump settings can usually be done in the first three to six weeks on your pump when this is done in an organized manner.

Your ultimate goal is to keep your glucose reading inside your target range at least 75% of the time. A target range might be between 70 and 120 mg/dl (3.9 and 6.7 mmol/L) before meals and between 140 and 180 mg/dl (7.8 and 10 mmol/L) after meals. Personal glucose targets will differ based on the values you and your health provider agree on. Some target ranges are shown in Table 5.4. Set realistic goals, pace yourself, and celebrate small steps as you move toward a good match between your goals and your new self-management routine.

9.5 Master List for Bolus Calculator Settings: Find Your Basal Rates, CarbF, and CorrF from Your TDD (or iTDD) and Weight

TDD or iTDD u/day	Basal[1] u/day	Basal u/hr	Carb Factor[2] in grams/u									CorrF[3] (mg/dl) / u
			100 lbs 45.4 kg	110 lbs 49.9 kg	120 lbs 54.4 kg	130 lbs 60.0 kg	140 lbs 63.5 kg	150 lbs 68.0 kg	160 lbs 72.6 kg	170 lbs 77.1 kg	180 lbs 81.6 kg	
16	7.7	0.32	16.3	17.9	19.5	21.1	22.8					122
20	9.6	0.40	13.0	14.3	15.6	16.9	18.2	19.5	20.8			98.0
24	11.5	0.48	10.8	11.9	13.0	14.1	15.2	16.3	17.3	19.5	21.7	81.7
28	13.4	0.56	9.3	10.2	11.1	12.1	13.0	13.9	14.9	16.7	18.6	70.0
32	15.4	0.64	8.1	8.9	9.8	10.6	11.4	12.2	13.0	14.6	16.3	61.3
36	17.3	0.72	7.2	7.9	8.7	9.4	10.1	10.8	11.6	13.0	14.4	54.4
40	19.2	0.80	6.5	7.2	7.8	8.5	9.1	9.8	10.4	11.7	13.0	49.0
45	21.6	0.90	5.8	6.4	6.9	7.5	8.1	8.7	9.2	10.4	11.6	43.6
50	24.0	1.00	5.2	5.7	6.2	6.8	7.3	7.8	8.3	9.4	10.4	39.2
55	26.4	1.10	4.7	5.2	5.7	6.1	6.6	7.1	7.6	8.5	9.5	35.6
60	28.8	1.20	4.3	4.8	5.2	5.6	6.1	6.5	6.9	7.8	8.7	32.7
65	31.2	1.30	4.0	4.4	4.8	5.2	5.6	6.0	6.4	7.2	8.0	30.2
70	33.6	1.40	3.7	4.1	4.5	4.8	5.2	5.6	5.9	6.7	7.4	28.0
80	38.4	1.60	3.3	3.6	3.9	4.2	4.6	4.9	5.2	5.9	6.5	24.5
90	43.2	1.80	2.9	3.2	3.5	3.8	4.0	4.3	4.6	5.2	5.8	21.8
100	48.0	2.00	2.6	2.9	3.1	3.4	3.6	3.9	4.2	4.7	5.2	19.6

1 Basal = TDD x 0.48   2 Carb Factor = 10.8 x insulin sensitivity = (2.6 x Wt (lb))/TDD   3 Correction Factor = 1960/TDD

For exact calculations, use the Pump Setting Tool at opensourcediabetes.org

9.6 How Different Factors Impact the TDD

Typical TDDs are shown below for people who weigh 100 to 200 lbs. for level of fitness, puberty, pregnancy, and presence of physical stress or pain. Compare your TDD to that for your weight. For example, a moderately active person who weighs 160 lbs will have a TDD close to 40 units a day. If you weigh 160 lbs and use only 30 units a day, you are sensitive to insulin, still produce some of your own insulin, or are having frequent highs. On the other hand, if you use 60 units a day, your insulin sensitivity may be lower or you are having frequent lows.

Variable	100 lbs (45 kg) TDD units	120 lbs (55 kg) TDD units	140 lbs (64 kg) TDD units	160 lbs (73 kg) TDD units	180 lbs (82 kg) TDD units	200 lbs (91 kg) TDD units
New start Type 2	5-11	6-14	6-16	7-18	8-20	9-23
New start Type 1	13-18	16-22	19-26	22-29	25-33	27-36
Physically fit	20	24	29	33	37	41
Moderately active	25	30	35	40	45	50
Sedentary or adolescent	30	37	44	50	56	62
Moderate physical stress, 2nd trim. pregnancy	36	43	51	58	66	73
Greater physical stress, 3rd trim. pregnancy	40	49	57	65	74	82
Severe phy. stress	45	55	64	73	82	91
Infection, DKA, or steroid medication	50-90	60-108	70-126	80-144	90-162	100-180

Adapted from a presentation by Lois Jovanovic, M.D., at the 2002 annual meeting of the American Association of Clinical Endocrinologists, and from N.S. Pierce: Diabetes and Exercise, Br J Sports Med: 161-173, 1999.

© 2012 Diabetes Services, Inc

Don't own so much clutter that you will be relieved to see your house catch fire.

Wendell Berry

Get an Improved TDD for Better Control

Your TDD (total daily dose of insulin) has a major impact on the frequency of lows, your A1c, and your average glucose. It is the total of all the basal and bolus insulin you take each day. Whenever you have frequent lows or frequent highs, this chapter helps you and your health care provider convert your current TDD to an *improved TDD (iTDD)*.

In this chapter, you will find:

- How to find the current TDD on your pump
- How to adjust your current TDD to an improved TDD

The pump settings you derive from an iTDD should give you more readings in your target range and make your glucose readings more stable. In Chapter 14, you can further refine your settings using the pattern management tools.

An accurate TDD cannot improve control if other important factors are missing. Make sure you are doing the other things that are critical:

- Monitor your glucose at least 6 times a day
- Wear a CGM if possible
- Use carb counting or another meal dose calculation that works
- Determine all recommended carb and correction boluses with your bolus calculator, but double-check and adjust when needed
- Take a bolus for the carbs in every meal and snack
- Don't overtreat lows with food, or highs with insulin

An Improved TDD (iTDD) Stops Highs and Lows

Does your average TDD needs to be adjusted? To find out, simply look at the average glucose level on your meter or a recent A1c, and think about how often you are having lows. Your TDD is optimized when your glucose is often in your target range, you have a great A1c, and you're not having frequent highs or lows.

119

10.1 Not All Average Glucoses Are the Same

To get your average glucose, make sure that the average glucose on your meter represents your true glucose levels. For example, if you check your glucose only when you feel low or you don't check when you feel low but just eat carbs, or you only check your glucose before meals, the average glucose on your meter won't represent your actual glucose levels through the day.

For a more accurate average glucose, check your glucose before and after meals at different times of day. Check when you go low, especially at night. Usually, 4 to 8 tests a day are sufficient if they are spread evenly at different times of day.

Your pump tracks your TDD each day. If your glucose goes up and down a lot, look at your daily total TDD over the last 14 to 30 days. Some variation in your TDD from day to day is normal, but if your TDD varies a great deal for reasons that aren't clear, other issues may be at play, such as an infusion set problem, missing meal boluses, infrequent glucose checks, or pain. These can make your daily insulin requirement vary

Steps to Find Your iTDD:

1. Find your average TDD for the last 14 to 30 days on a history screen in your pump. You can also find your own average TDD over the last 14 days by adding up your last 14 TDDs and dividing this total by 14.

   a. Don't include unusual days in your average, like days when readings were unusually high because of an infection, menses, or an infusion set problem. If your TDDs vary widely, discuss this with your physician before finding an average.

2. Next, find your average glucose for the last 14 or 30 days on your glucose meter. If your diet or activity has changed significantly over the past few days, consider using an average over only those days.

3. *Always stop frequent or severe lows first by lowering your TDD before you try to regain control.*

4. When frequent lows are not present, your basal rates and/or carb boluses can be accurately raised to correct any patterns of frequent highs. Generally, the TDD is raised if the A1c is above 7.5% or the average meter glucose is above 145 to 160 mg/dl (8.0 to 8.9 mmol/L) without frequent lows.

Glucose levels can often be quickly stabilized when you select your basal rate and pump settings from an accurate TDD. It then becomes easier to use pattern management for finer insulin adjustments. If your glucose readings tend to be erratic, you may want to compare your current pump settings to the typical settings expected for your TDD in Table 9.5.

Frequent Lows? Lower Your TDD

With frequent or severe lows, you cannot tell how much excess insulin there is! Start with a 5% or 10% reduction in your current TDD. Repeat as needed. Once lows are not frequent, you can safely address any highs that remain. Remember that your lows also include the ones you treat but don't confirm with your meter. If you have lots of glucose tabs next to your bed, desk, or locker to treat frequent lows but don't have a glucose meter handy to record their timing and severity, keep a written record of these lows and **let your doctor know about ALL the lows you have, not just those on your meter.** A CGM is ideal for picking up the frequency and severity of lows.

If you are having frequent lows, DON'T WAIT until your next clinic visit to lower your doses. Deal with this right away. Frequent lows always mean **you are getting too much insulin.** Call your health care professional promptly for an appointment to make an appropriate dose reduction. If there's an obvious cause for lows, such as taking your carb boluses but not eating meals, deal with this first. Otherwise, lower your TDD.

Frequent lows can occur if you have been "chasing" high readings too aggressively, or you start a diet, or increase your activity. Start by reducing your TDD by 5%, as shown in Table 10.2, and reduce by another 5% every 4 to 7 days until your lows are no longer frequent. If lows are frequent and often go below 50 mg/dl (2.8 mmol/L), start with a 10% reduction in your TDD.

A good goal is to have only a handful of readings below 70 mg/dl (3.9 mmol/L) and none below 55 mg/dl (3.1 mmol/L) each week. If you have hypoglycemia unawareness, set high glucose goals with no more than a handful of readings below 80 mg/dl (4.4 mmol/L) and none below 70 mg/dl (3.9 mmol/L) each week.

Be proactive. Don't keep treating frequent lows before dinner by eat-

10.2 Lower Your TDD for Lows

For frequent lows, discuss reducing your TDD by 5% or 10% with your physician. Find an iTDD from your current avg. TDD in the left column and use Table 9.5 to get new settings.

Current TDD	iTDD 5% Less	iTDD 10% Less
20.0 u	19.0 u	18.0 u
25.0 u	23.8 u	22.5 u
30.0 u	28.5 u	27.0 u
35.0 u	33.3 u	31.5 u
40.0 u	38.1 u	36.0 u
45.0 u	42.9 u	40.5 u
50.0 u	47.6 u	45.0 u
55.0 u	52.4 u	50.5 u
60.0 u	57.1 u	54.0 u
65.0 u	61.9 u	58.5 u
70.0 u	66.7 u	63.5 u
80.0 u	76.2 u	72.0 u
90.0 u	85.7 u	81.0 u
100.0 u	95.0 u	90.0 u

My new iTDD = _____ units/day

ing more carbs and lowering your dinner boluses. This won't stop them and will likely make your bedtime readings higher. Instead, raise your lunch carb factor (CarbF) to get smaller lunch boluses or lower your late morning through mid-afternoon basal rates. Check your basal/bolus balance during the 5 hour period before the lows occur to narrow down their source.

Frequent Lows and Highs? Lower Your TDD (Usually)

When both highs and lows are happening, it can be hard to decide whether your TDD needs to be increased or decreased. If you're not sure whether lows or highs are the primary problem, lower your TDD by 5% *to stop the lows first* before you attempt to improve your overall control. Always get your doctor's advice if you are unsure.

Frequent lows and highs mean you get too much insulin at times and too little at others. If your lows often lead to highs, the rebound highs can artificially raise your average glucose, and your TDD may also be artificially high from the extra correction doses you have to give. If readings often swing between 30 and 300 mg/dl (1.7 and 16.7 mmol/L), lower your TDD to reduce the number of lows, even if your current average glucose seems to be high.

Lower your TDD and use this iTDD to find new basal rates and new carb and correction factors that are less likely to give excess doses. If lows are often followed by highs, get off this rollercoaster by not over-treating your lows! See Box 10.4 to find out how many carbs you actually need to treat your lows. Sorting out your pump settings is easier after your glucose readings are slightly high and less erratic. This makes it easier to find out whether and when you actually need more insulin.

Frequent Highs? Raise Your TDD (Usually)

Was your most recent A1c above 7.0% or is your average glucose (meter or CGM) above 154 mg/dl (8.5 mmol/L)? Do you have frequent highs? If you answer "yes", most people will want to increase their TDD, unless higher glucose goals are required because of age, living alone, or a history of hypoglycemia unawareness.

Of course, if your diet has been chock full of sugared soda and ice cream and you take these off your shopping list, or you are starting on a diet to lose weight, your TDD may not need to be increased at all. For anyone with proliferative retinopathy or cardiovascular disease, your doctor will likely prefer that you lower your glucose gradually over time with small, regularly timed increases in your TDD. Always check with your health care professional regarding the dose adjustments you need.

Table 10.3 gives a close estimate for how much to raise the TDD when most of your readings are on the high side and lows are infrequent. The iTDD is then used to estimate more appropriate basal rates, CarbF, and CorrF from Table 9.4. The increase in TDD suggested in Table 10.3 provides most of the total increase you are likely to need.

10.3 Raise Your TDD when Glucoses Are Mostly High

Use this table ONLY if you are NOT having frequent or severe lows. Find your average TDD on the left and your 14 day average glucose (meter or CGM) or a recent A1c value at the top. Where they intersect gives a good estimate for your iTDD.

To find an improved TDD, raise the current TDD by 1% for each 6 mg/dl that the glucose needs to be lowered, or 1% for each 0.2% lowering of the A1c. Use Table 9.5 to find new basal and bolus doses from this iTDD. Adjust again in 2 weeks, if needed.

Your New Improved TDD (iTDD)

	14 Day BG mg/dl (mmol/L)	155 (8.6)	169 (9.4)	183 (10.2)	197 (10.9)	212 (11.8)	226 (12.6)	240 (13.3)	255 (14.2)	269 (14.9)
	Recent A1c	7.0	7.5	8.0	8.5	9.0	9.5	10.0	10.5	11.0
Your Current TDD	**15 u**	**15.3**	**15.6**	**16.0**	**16.3**	**16.7**	**17.0**	**17.4**	**17.8**	**18.1**
	20 u	**20.3**	**20.8**	**21.3**	**21.7**	**22.2**	**22.7**	**23.2**	**23.7**	**24.1**
	25 u	**25.4**	**26.0**	**26.6**	**27.2**	**27.8**	**28.4**	**29.0**	**29.6**	**30.2**
	30 u	**30.5**	**31.2**	**31.9**	**32.6**	**33.4**	**34.1**	**34.8**	**35.5**	**36.2**
	35 u	**35.6**	**36.4**	**37.2**	**38.0**	**38.9**	**39.7**	**40.5**	**41.4**	**42.2**
	40 u	**40.7**	**41.6**	**42.5**	**43.5**	**44.5**	**45.4**	**46.3**	**47.3**	**48.3**
	45 u	**45.8**	**46.8**	**47.9**	**48.9**	**50.0**	**51.1**	**52.1**	**53.3**	**54.3**
	50 u	**50.8**	**52.0**	**53.2**	**54.3**	**55.6**	**56.8**	**57.9**	**59.2**	**60.3**
	55 u	**55.9**	**57.2**	**58.5**	**59.8**	**61.1**	**62.4**	**63.7**	**65.1**	**66.4**
	60 u	**61.0**	**62.4**	**63.8**	**65.2**	**66.7**	**68.1**	**69.5**	**71.0**	**72.4**
	65 u	**66.1**	**67.6**	**69.1**	**70.6**	**72.3**	**73.8**	**75.3**	**76.9**	**78.4**
	70 u	**71.2**	**72.8**	**74.4**	**76.1**	**77.8**	**79.5**	**81.1**	**82.8**	**84.5**
	75 u	**76.3**	**78.0**	**79.8**	**81.5**	**83.4**	**85.1**	**86.9**	**88.8**	**90.5**
	80 u	**81.3**	**83.2**	**85.1**	**86.9**	**88.9**	**90.8**	**92.7**	**94.7**	**96.5**
	85 u	**86.4**	**88.4**	**90.4**	**92.4**	**94.5**	**96.5**	**98.5**	**100.6**	**102.6**
	90 u	**91.5**	**93.6**	**95.7**	**97.8**	**100.1**	**102.2**	**104.3**	**106.5**	**108.6**
	95 u	**96.6**	**98.8**	**101.0**	**103.2**	**105.6**	**107.8**	**110.0**	**112.4**	**114.6**
	100 u	**101.7**	**104.0**	**106.3**	**108.7**	**111.2**	**113.5**	**115.8**	**118.3**	**120.7**

Derived from the APP Study[69]

© 2013 Diabetes Services, Inc

With frequent highs and few lows, there are some quick ways to find an improved TDD (iTDD) from which to derive more accurate pump settings:

1. **Find an iTDD in Table 10.3** from a recent A1c or from your average glucose over the last 14 to 30 days.

2. **For every 1% you want to lower your A1c, raise your TDD by 5%.** For example, if your A1c is 10.0% and you want it to be 7.0%, a 15% increase in your TDD will help. (10% − 7% = a 3% lowering of the A1c; 3% x 5 = a 15% increase in your TDD) If your current TDD were 40 units a day, your iTDD would be 40u x 1.15 or 46 units a day.

3. **Or raise your TDD by 1% for every 6 mg/dl (0.33 mmol/L) you want to lower your average glucose.** For example, if your average meter glucose is 220 mg/dl (12.2 mmol/L), a 10% increase in your TDD will lower your average glucose about 60 mg/dl (3.3 mmol/L) to 160 mg/dl (8.9 mmol/L). You can always raise your TDD by 5% first to see how it affects your average glucose, and then adjust again as needed. Any large increase in your TDD can always be done in smaller steps.

4. Alternatively, if you check your glucose at least 4 times a day and take correction boluses whenever they are needed, **the average TDD in your pump already includes much of the extra correction doses you will likely need**. In this case, simply take your current TDD (with these correction doses) and use this as your iTDD in Table 9.5 to generate new pump settings. This shifts some of the excess in your correction boluses into higher basal rates and/or larger carb boluses (smaller CarbF) to stop many of the excess highs. (This method won't work if you've been skipping meal boluses and just correcting the high readings that follow.)

A new iTDD found with one of these methods is then used to generate more appropriate basal rates and bolus factors from Table 9.5. Your health care professional can use the Pump Settings Tool at www.opensourcediabetes.org or www.diabetesnet.com as a fast way to find an iTDD and new pump settings that may work better for you. As with any new pump settings, check your glucose frequently or wear a CGM after these changes are made to verify that the new iTDD and pump settings are working.

Monitor Your Progress

To track your progress, write down on a calendar each week the 7-day or 14-day average glucose from your meter, how many glucose tests were done, and whether you had frequent or severe lows during that time. Knowing your progress (or lack of) over time helps you reach your glucose goals. Don't judge any glucose result as undesirable – just keep working to improve them!

Discuss new settings with your doctor or diabetes educator before you use them. Before you change any of your pump settings, make it a practice to calculate how many more or fewer units of insulin your pump will give you each day. As you gradually gain experience, your physician may encourage you to start making basal and bolus changes on your own.

10.4 How Many Grams of Carb Do You Need?

To Treat a Low Glucose

1. *Take 10 grams of carb for weights up to 100 lbs (45 kgs) and add 1 gram for each additional 10 lbs (4.5 kgs).* For example, a 150 lb (68 kg) child or adult would need 15 grams, while a 220 lb (100 kg) adult would need 22 grams. Glucose or glucose tabs work best for treating lows.[98]

2. *Add to this amount the free carbs you need to offset any BOB you have.* Check your BOB and multiply this by your CarbF to determine the extra carbs.

3. *Take this total grams of carb* and recheck your glucose 20 to 30 min. later.*

For example, let's take someone whose glucose is 50 mg/dl (2.7 mmol/L) and their weight is 130 lbs (59 kgs) with 2 units of BOB and a CarbF of 1u/11 grams:

    a) 130 lbs = 13 grams

    b) BOB x CarbF = 2 units x 11 grams/unit = 22 grams

    c) So, they will need 35 grams (13 g + 22 g = 35 g) to treat this low glucose.

    d) Any additional carbs above these amounts would be covered with a bolus right away to avoid having a high glucose later.

    * Extra carbs might also be needed for increased activity – see ExCarbs in Chap. 22.

To Prevent a Low Glucose

As another example, consider someone whose glucose is 100 mg/dl (5.6 mmol/L) at bedtime but has 3 units of BOB still lowering their glucose. If this person's CarbF is 10 grams/unit, how many carbs will they need to prevent a low glucose so they can sleep soundly through the night?

Here, carbs are needed only to cover the remaining BOB:

$$\text{BOB (3 units) x CarbF (10 g/u) = 30 grams of carb}$$

© 2013 Diabetes Services, Inc.

If your weight, activity, or stress level changes, or you have an illness, your TDD, basals, and boluses also need to change. If you start training for a marathon or digging up a spring garden, you'll need to lower your basal and bolus doses. If you start a diet, go on vacation, or change to a more or less active job, adjust your doses. As days shorten and weight rises in the fall, your TDD usually rises. In the spring, the TDD often needs to fall. Always match life changes with simultaneous adjustments in your basal and bolus settings.

10.5 Steps to Successful Doses	
How	**Why**
1) Stop frequent lows first	Safer and it stops many highs
2) Find your improved TDD	For more normal and stable BGs
3) Test and adjust basals	Lets you skip meals and sleep soundly
4) Test and adjust CarbF	Better readings before each meal
5) Stop postmeal spiking	More stable readings
6) Test and adjust CorrF	Brings highs down safely
7) Use pattern management	Corrects consistent lows or highs
Enjoy great readings or return to #1	
Erratic readings or frequent highs? **Typically caused by the wrong pump settings!**	

Summary

Great readings are not guaranteed by wearing a pump. Don't be satisfied with your pump settings until they deliver optimum control. Things change. Keep on top of these changes with adjustments in your pump TDD and settings.

Although finding the right TDD is the most critical step for accurate pump settings, patience and persistence make great allies as you select and adjust the TDD and pump settings to improve your control. The average glucose on your meter and how often you have lows are great guides for when your TDD needs to change.

Pattern management works well for consistent pattern of lows or highs. Otherwise, start by adjusting your TDD and selecting new pump settings from this iTDD. Finer adjustments can then be made from the patterns in your readings and from direct testing of your basal rates and carb and correction boluses. The next three chapters show how to test and adjust your basal rates, CarbF, and CorrF, while Chapter 14 reviews pattern management.

Frequent monitoring (or wearing a CGM) is the best way to detect a problem before it gets serious.

Computers are like Old Testament gods –
lots of rules and no mercy.

Joseph Campbell

Test and Adjust Your Basal Rates

Optimal basal or background insulin rates will keep your readings flat in a desirable range when you fast. This lets you wake up with regulated glucose readings from day to day, skip meals, and eat late without experiencing hypoglycemia. Using the starting TDD from Chapter 9 or an iTDD from Chapter 10, an average hourly basal rate will be selected, tested, and adjusted in this chapter until it keeps your glucose from rising or falling when you are not eating.

This chapter shows how to:

- Use single or multiple basal rates
- Select your average hourly basal rate
- Test and adjust basal rates for optimal control
- Use a CGM for basal testing
- Set temporary and alternate basal rates

Your liver makes and releases glucose around the clock to provide fuel to other cells. To balance this, the normal pancreas releases insulin all day to keep the liver from releasing too much glucose and to move the glucose produced by the liver into muscle, fat, and other cells. On a pump, this background insulin is delivered as small amounts of rapid insulin every few minutes over 24 hours. When a basal rate is too low, the liver makes excess glucose and the glucose rises. A high basal does the opposite.

Although multiple research studies have shown that basal rates provide about half of the insulin required each day, hourly basal doses are far smaller than most bolus doses.[15,16,63] When a basal rate is changed on a pump, it takes more than 4 hours to see its effect on the glucose.[85] Basal and bolus insulin delivered under the skin is far slower to act than insulin delivered from the pancreas into the portal vein directly to the liver.

Accurate basal rates are required before you test and set accurate boluses. If your basal rate is too high, your glucose will fall when you skip a meal. If the basal is too low, larger carb boluses are required to cover carbs and to cover the missing basal, and when a meal is skipped the glucose climbs. You can test and verify your basal rates in this chapter before attempting to find your CarbF or CorrF in the next two chapters.

When basal rates are set too high, pumpers often raise their CarbF and CorrF to make their meal and correction boluses smaller. But when more carbs than usual are consumed, the meal bolus – which has been set to deliver smaller boluses – now can't cover these carbs and the glucose goes high. Likewise, the smaller correction boluses can't cover unusually high glucose readings and correction boluses to not bring the glucose back to target.

When basal rates are set too low, the wearer may select a lower CarbF and CorrF to get larger meal and correction boluses that compensate for the lack of basal insulin. This makes hypoglycemia more likely when a large carb meal is consumed or a high glucose reading needs to be lowered. Accurate basal rates and a proper basal/carb bolus balance are needed in order for the CarbF and CorrF to work over a wide range of carb intakes and glucose elevations.

If you change only your CarbF or only basal rates to solve every control issue, your basal/carb bolus balance is likely to be eventually thrown off and make it harder to manage your glucose. Check the basal/carb bolus balance in your pump history from time to time with Table 8.14. Over a 7- to 14-day period, an optimal range for basal rates in the best control group in the APP Study was 40% to 55% of the TDD, averaging close to 50%. Most of the rest (43%) was given primarily as carb boluses. Most people who are not on a low or high carb diet will want to keep their average basal total close to 50% of the TDD.

Single or Multiple Basal Rates

You may need different basal rates at different times of the day to match your body's needs. For a simple approach to finding your true basal requirements, your physician may recommend that you start with a single basal rate for the entire day as shown in Figure 11.1.

Starting with a single basal is easy and can sometimes be advantageous for a person who flies across time zones frequently or does shift work. A single basal avoids a problem if AM and PM settings are accidentally switched in a pump's 12 hour clock. A single basal keeps the pump from delivering day

11.1 Single and Multiple Basal Rates

A single basal rate for the whole day works for many, especially shift workers, those who frequently fly across times zones, and when first starting on a pump.

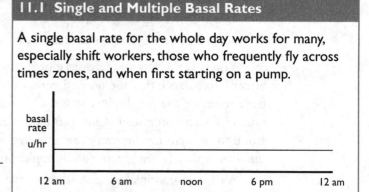

Multiple basal rates are best for people who have a Dawn Phenomenon or are physically active during the day.

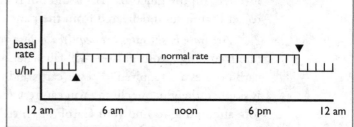

rates at night and vice versa. Your health care professional will help you select a single or multiple rates from your average hourly basal rate in Tables 9.5 or 11.2.

About 90% of experienced pumpers use more than one basal rate a day,[86] so it is not uncommon to be started on more than one basal. However, basal insulin delivery is slow and the insulin continues to lower the glucose for 5 to 6 hours after a rate is changed. *Because of these limitations, having more than 5 basal rates during the day usually provides no benefit.* Focus on using fewer basal rates and make basal changes early.

Because basal rates are adjusted in increments as small as hundredths of a unit rather than full units, they take longer to impact your glucose than boluses do. For example, a basal rate increase of 0.1 unit per hour has to be delivered for 50 hours before it equals a 5.0 unit bolus.

WHEN you change basal rates is often as important as HOW MUCH you change them. In order for the small dose changes involved to make a difference, basal rates need to be changed at least 2 to 3 hours before your glucose starts to rise or fall, and 4 to 8 hours before the high or low reading you are trying to avoid typically occurs. Unlike boluses that may vary a great deal as carb counts change from meal to meal, basal rates do not vary much through the day for most pumpers.

11.2 Starting Basal Rates

Find your starting TDD in the first column and look across that row to find your starting average hourly basal rate. © 2012 Diabetes Services, Inc

Starting TDD	Total Basal per Day	Avg. Basal per Hour
18 units	8.64 u/day	0.36 u/hr
22 units	10.6 u/day	0.44 u/hr
26 units	12.5 u/day	0.52 u/hr
30 units	14.4 u/day	0.60 u/hr
35 units	16.8 u/day	0.70 u/hr
40 units	19.2 u/day	0.80 u/hr
45 units	21.6 u/day	0.90 u/hr
50 units	24.0 u/day	1.00 u/hr
60 units	28.8 u/day	1.20 u/hr
70 units	33.6 u/day	1.40 u/hr
80 units	38.4 u/day	1.60 u/hr
90 units	43.2 u/day	1.80 u/hr
100 units	48.0 u/day	2.00 u/hr

Select Your Basal Rates

Find your starting average basal rate by looking up your starting TDD in the first column of Table 11.2 or Table 9.5, then move across that row to the average basal column to find your average hourly basal rate. Table 9.5 gives the typical basal rate, CarbF, and CorrF for your TDD. The average basal gives you and your health care professional an excellent starting point from which to test and adjust your rate or rates as needed.

Test Your Basal Rates

Any new basal rates need to be tested in the first few days of use to make sure they work. They need to be retested anytime you start to have frequent lows or highs. When starting on a pump, basal testing can begin 30 hours after your last Lantus® (glargine) or Levemir® (detemir) dose, 24 hours after your last NPH dose. If you are already on a pump and changing basal rates, you can begin testing the new ones five hours after they were changed.

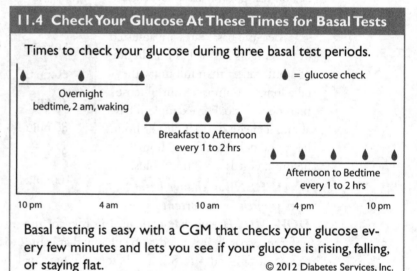

11.4 Check Your Glucose At These Times for Basal Tests

Times to check your glucose during three basal test periods.

● = glucose check

Overnight
bedtime, 2 am, waking

Breakfast to Afternoon
every 1 to 2 hrs

Afternoon to Bedtime
every 1 to 2 hrs

10 pm   4 am   10 am   4 pm   10 pm

Basal testing is easy with a CGM that checks your glucose every few minutes and lets you see if your glucose is rising, falling, or staying flat.   © 2012 Diabetes Services, Inc.

Workspace 11.5 shows the steps for *basal testing*. It includes an area to write down and analyze your test results. Make a few copies of this page for the basal tests that may be needed. For convenience, break your basal testing into three test periods: overnight, breakfast to midafternoon, and midafternoon to bedtime, as shown in Figure 11.4. Test multiple basal rates the same way you test a single rate.

Goal: Basal rates that keep your glucose within 30 mg/dl (1.7 mmol/L) of its starting point without going low.

1. Start your basal test when your glucose is between 100 and 150 mg/dl (5.6 - 8.3 mmol/L) and you have not eaten in the last 3 hours nor taken a bolus in the last 5 hours.

2. Eat no carbs during the test. Small amounts of protein (few nuts, cheese, boiled egg, etc.) are OK.

3. Check your glucose at least every 2 hours or wear a CGM. If your glucose goes below 70 mg/dl (3.9 mmol/L), stop the test and eat carbs.

4. Record and plot the results of the basal test below.

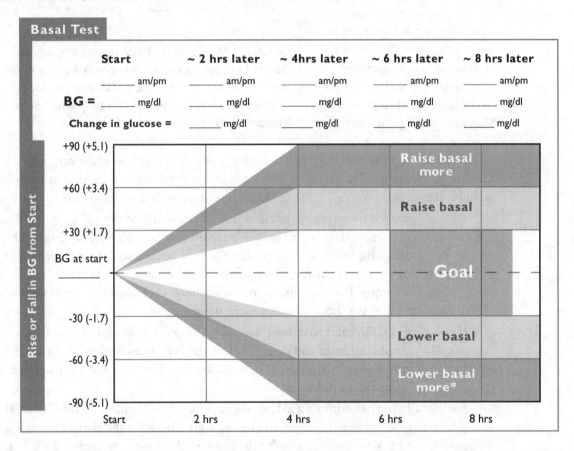

Basal Test

	Start	~ 2 hrs later	~ 4hrs later	~ 6 hrs later	~ 8 hrs later
	_____ am/pm	_____ am/pm	_____ am/pm	_____ am/pm	_____ am/pm
BG =	_____ mg/dl	_____ mg/dl	_____ mg/dl	_____ mg/dl	_____ mg/dl
Change in glucose =		_____ mg/dl	_____ mg/dl	_____ mg/dl	_____ mg/dl

See Basal Adjustments if your glucose rises or falls more than 30 mg/dl (1.7 mmol/L) in this test.

Overnight Basal Test

Overnight basal rates are the easiest to test. Your basal rate is the only thing affecting your glucose as you sleep if your last bolus was taken 5 or more hours before bedtime. The night basal rates are adjusted until you can go to bed and wake up with readings in your target range without going low.

Testing your overnight basal rates first is important to keep your night glucose flat. Waking up with a relatively normal reading makes it easier to control daytime readings.[87,88] Plus you, your spouse, parents, children, friends, roommates,

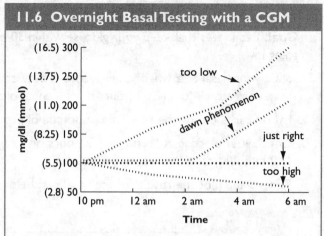

11.6 Overnight Basal Testing with a CGM

A CGM allows precise basal testing and adjustments because its trend line reveals exactly when your glucose starts to rise or fall. Any rise or fall in the trend line lets you see exactly when your glucose starts to drift.

and healthcare team will all sleep better knowing you won't go low while you sleep. An accurate overnight basal rate lets you control over one third of the day's glucose levels. Your night basal rates also provide a great guide for setting your daytime basal rates.

A simple way for many people to check the night basal is to test the glucose 6 hours before waking and at breakfast on a night when no bolus was taken after dinner. This way, no late dinner carb bolus or correction bolus will be interfering with the basal during the early morning hours. If it will not deprive you of sleep, set a timer or an alarm clock to wake you up at least a couple of times to check your glucose, even if you wear a CGM. Wake up every two hours to get a more precise trend line.

If you wear a CGM and have been on your pump for a while, download to a computer or over the internet and take a look at the last 10 to 30 days of data. Check whether your glucose stays flat, rises, or falls during this time. You and your physician can make basal adjustments from this.

For night basal tests with a CGM, set the high and low alarms on your CGM 30 to 40 mg/dl (1.7 to 2.2 mmol/L) above and below your glucose at the start of the test. This will quickly alert you when your glucose drifts too high or too low during sleep. For example, if the starting glucose on your CGM is 126 mg/dl (6.6 mmol/L), set your high alert at 160 mg/dl (+34 mg/dl) and your low alert at 90 mg/dl (−36 mg/dl). Your CGM will then alert if your glucose rises or falls more than 30 mg/dl. Verify with a fingerstick test. Reset your CGM to your standard alert settings once the night test is complete.

Daytime Basal Tests

Daytime testing can be split into two 6- to 8-hour segments done on different days. If a single basal rate is used through the night, use the same rate to start your daytime tests. If more than one basal rate is required during the night, try an average of the lowest and highest overnight rates as your starting daytime rate. For instance, if you use 0.9 to 1.1 u/hr through the night, try 1.0 as your daytime basal.

Daytime tests require that you skip one meal and eat another meal earlier or later on the day of the test. Small amounts of protein foods like cheese or nuts can be eaten during your test, but no carbs unless your glucose goes low. Testing is repeated until your basal rates keep your readings relatively flat on two consecutive tests.

A test from *waking to mid afternoon* covers 6 to 8 hours, and can be started anytime you wake up with a relatively normal reading. Skip breakfast, have a late lunch, and eat your evening meal at the usual time. A *mid-afternoon to bedtime* basal test can be started at least 5 hours after your breakfast bolus and 3 or more hours since eating any carbs. Skip lunch and enjoy a snack or late dinner near bedtime once the test is finished.

For children, it is easier to break daytime testing into three segments: morning (skip breakfast), afternoon (skip lunch) and evening (skip dinner) but always start the test at least 5 hours after the last bolus. For a child, the overnight basals are the easiest to test and an average of the child's hourly basal rates through the night are a good guide for their daytime basal rates. A slightly higher daytime rate sometimes helps cover the frequent snacking that is common among kids. A slightly higher CarbF number may be needed if this is done.

Adjust Your Basal Rates

Keep adjusting your basal rates until they keep your glucose within 30 mg/dl (1.7 mmol/L) of your starting glucose during the 6- to 8-hour test. If your glucose rises or falls during the test, discuss how much to raise or lower your basal rates with your physician. Table 11.7 provides a quick guide on how a basal rate adjustment over an 8-hour period will lower or raise your glucose 9 to 10 hours after it is started. The same basal adjustment, done over 24 hours will raise or lower the average glucose on your meter by about this same amount for the entire day.

Basal adjustments can be fine-tuned in amounts as small as 0.01 to 0.025 u/hr, or a total of 0.024 to 0.6 u/day. If your glucose shows a slow drop on your basal test, a small basal decrease on the order of 0.05 u/hr may work. If your glucose drops rapidly, try a larger and earlier decrease in rates. If your glucose rises rapidly, you will need a larger and earlier basal increase. Remember to adjust the basal at least 2 hours before the rise or fall in your glucose begins.

	11.7 Adjust Your Basal Rates from Your Basal Test			
	If your glucose FALLS (or RISES) a total of:			
	100 mg/dl (5.5 mmol/L)	80 mg/dl (6.1 mmol/L)	60 mg/dl (3.3 mmol/L)	40 mg/dl (2.2 mmol/L)
For this TDD:	**LOWER (or RAISE) your basal for 8 hours by:**			
20 u	0.1 u/hr (0.8 u)	0.075 u/hr (0.66 u)	0.05 u/hr (0.5 u)	0.025 u/hr (0.32 u)
30 u	0.15 u/hr (1.2 u)	0.125 u/hr (1.0 u)	0.075 u/hr (0.75 u)	0.05 u/hr (0.5 u)
40 u	0.2 u/hr (1.6 u)	0.15 u/hr (1.3 u)	0.125 u/hr (1.0 u)	0.075 u/hr (0.6 u)
50 u	0.25 u/hr (2.0 u)	0.225 u/hr (1.6 u)	0.15 u/hr (1.25 u)	0.1 u/hr (0.8 u)
60 u	0.3 u/hr (2.4 u)	0.25 u/hr (2.0 u)	0.175 u/hr (1.5 u)	0.125 u/hr (1.0 u)
80 u	0.4 u/hr (3.2 u)	0.325 u/hr (2.6 u)	0.25 u/hr (2.0 u)	0.15 u/hr (1.3 u)
100 u	0.5 u/hr (4.0 u)	0.4 u/hr (3.3 u)	0.3 u/hr (2.5 u)	0.2 u/hr (1.6 u)

These adjustments may be slightly more or less than you actually need.
Example: Someone whose glucose rises by 80 mg/dl during an 8 hour test and has a TDD of 30 units a day will need a one unit basal increase, so over an 8 hour period, their current basal rate could be raised as much as 0.125 u/hr.

Never assume that changing your basal rates makes them work better. Write down any changes you make or use an alternate basal profile to try new rates. If a new basal worsens your control, return to the earlier settings and discuss your findings with your physician or diabetes educator. Basal rates may need to be adjusted and tested several times to find your optimal rates. Your basal rates may need to be quickly adjusted if you change your weight or activity level, during sick days, if stress levels rise or fall, and if you begin or stop a diet.

Retest to verify after a successful test. Work closely with your physician or nurse educator to get accurate basal rates. As you gain experience, you'll gradually be able to make your own basal adjustments.

Signs your basal rates are too high:

- Your glucose is often low before breakfast when no bolus was given during the night.

- Your glucose often goes low when you skip meals or more than 5 hours since your last bolus.

- Your glucose is often low before meals

- You have frequent lows through the day and your daily basal total makes up more than 55% of your TDD.

Signs your basal rates are too low:

- Your breakfast reading is usually higher than your bedtime reading.

- Your glucose rises between the middle of the night and breakfast.

- Your glucose rises when you skip meals.

- You have frequent highs and your basal makes up less than 45% of your TDD.

Example of A Needed Basal Adjustment

On the first morning after her pump start, Gwenn's breakfast reading was 87 mg/dl (4.8 mmol/L). She was thrilled that her reading was finally in her target range when she woke up. Her pump settings were perfect!

At her clinic visit that day, her doctor pointed out that before Gwenn woke up at 87 mg/dl (4.8 mmol/L), she had been 181 mg/dl (10 mmol/L) at 2 a.m. Her last bolus was given around 6 pm at dinner the night before and she had not taken a correction bolus for the 2 a.m. reading. Even so, her glucose had fallen more than 90 mg/dl (5 mmol/L) by the time she awoke!

Her physician pointed out that basal insulin should keep her glucose flat and not cause an excessive drop like this. Gwenn realized her overnight basal rate needed to be lowered despite her "perfect" reading.

**Optimal basal rates keep your glucose from rising or falling
more than 30 mg/dl (1.7 mmol/L) when you go to sleep or skip a meal
and when your last bolus was taken at least 5 hours
before the start of the test.**

Concealing an illness is like keeping a beach ball under water.

Karen Duffy

Sample Basal Rate Test

Example 11.8 shows an example of Chris' basal test.

11.8 Example: Chris' Overnight Basal Test

Chris' average TDD is 60 units a day with a single basal rate of 1.1 u/hr (44% basal). On this basal test, his bedtime reading of 116 mg/dl (6.4 mmol/L) rose by 11 mg/dl (0.6 mmol/L) at 1:47 a.m. to 127, and on waking his glucose had risen a total of 60 mg/dl (3.3 mmol/L) to 176 mg/dl (1.7 mmol/L).

Basal Test

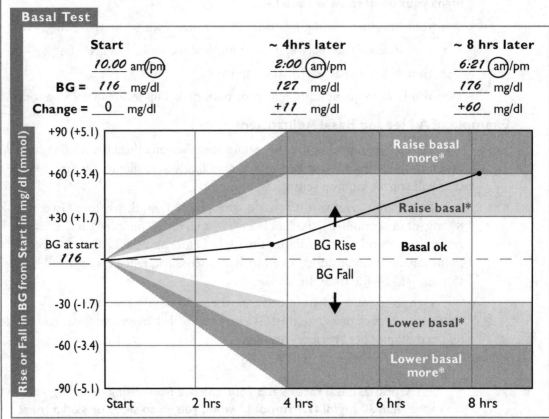

	Start	**~ 4hrs later**	**~ 8 hrs later**
	10.00 am/**pm**	*2:00* **am**/pm	*6:21* **am**/pm
BG =	*116* mg/dl	*127* mg/dl	*176* mg/dl
Change =	*0* mg/dl	*+11* mg/dl	*+60* mg/dl

Chris saw that his glucose was already rising by 2 am and he needed to raise his basal before then. Using Table 11.7, his TDD of 60 units meant he would need as much as 1.5 additional units in his overnight basal to stop the 60 mg/dl (3.3 mmol/L) rise in his glucose. After discussing these results with his doctor, he raised his basal from 1.1 u/hr to 1.20 u/hr between 9 pm and 1 am, and to 1.275 u/hr between 1 am and 6 am, or a total of 1.45 additional units over 9 hours.

A follow up basal test showed that his glucose still rose by 25 mg/dl (1.4 mmol/L). His doctor suggested raising his 9 pm rate to 1.25 u/hr and his 1 am basal to 1.3 u/hr, and these rates finally kept his overnight glucose perfectly flat overnight.   © 2012 Diabetes Services Inc.

Basal Rate for a Dawn Phenomenon or Type 2 Diabetes

The Dawn Phenomenon is strongest during the teen years when large amounts of growth and other hormones are released into the blood during the early morning hours. This causes excess glucose release from the liver and more insulin resistance. The strength of a Dawn Phenomenon varies from person to person and generally disappears by middle age.

Among teens or young adults with Type 1 diabetes, 50 percent to 70 percent need a higher basal rate starting between 1 a.m. and 3 a.m. to control the Dawn Phenomenon. Of these, 20 to 30 percent

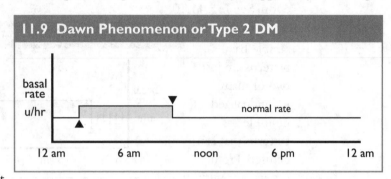

11.9 Dawn Phenomenon or Type 2 DM

may need to increase their basal as much as 20% in the early morning hours to offset a Dawn Phenomenon[89] and keep the breakfast readings in range.[1,14.45]

For someone who averages 1.0 u/hr during waking hours, a 20% increase could be applied as an extra 0.2 u/hr for six to eight hours during the pre-dawn period. For example, a middle of the night basal rate may need to rise to 1.2 u/hr between 2:30 a.m. until 8:30 or 10:30 a.m. after which it returns to the daytime rate of 1.0 u/hr. Remember that when started early a smaller basal rate increase often works as well as a large basal increase at a later time.

In Type 2 diabetes, insulin resistance is often greatest during the early morning hours. This also requires higher basal rates between midnight and 3 a.m. until 10 a.m. or so, for typical sleep hours, but for a different reason. In Type 2, excess fat is released from the abdomen into the blood at night, adding to insulin resistance. This causes the liver to increase glucose production unnecessarily and the person wakes up with a high reading.

Pumps are ideal for managing the Dawn Phenomenon because basal delivery can be increased at the right time to prevent this early morning rise. Be sure to raise the basal rate early for the best effect at least two hours before the glucose begins its rise.

One option for both teens with Type 1 or 2 and others with Type 2 diabetes is to use a medicine developed for Type 2 diabetes called *metformin*. Metformin reduces the excess glucose production by the liver that causes the fasting glucose to rise with a Dawn Phenomenon. Although never approved for use in teens, one meta-analysis of several well-conducted studies using metformin in adults with Type 1 diabetes found that insulin use was reduced by 5.7 to 10.1 units a day, weight was reduced by 3 to 13 lbs, and cholesterol levels were also lowered.[90]

Basal Rate for Night Insulin Sensitivity with a Dawn Phenomenon

Many people are more sensitive to insulin just after midnight, so a decrease in the basal rate may be needed around 8 p.m. to avoid having too much insulin at this time. A lower basal may be needed before bedtime to offset the increased insulin sensitivity after midnight, along with higher basal rates around 2 or 3 am to handle a Dawn Phenomenon. See Fig. 11.10.

These sample basal patterns are just two of many individualized multiple basal patterns that can be used. From experience with

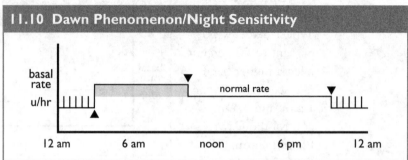

11.10 Dawn Phenomenon/Night Sensitivity

you and many other pumpers, your health care professional will select a basal rate profile that is likely to work for you.

Night Lows

Middle of the night lows at 1 or 2 am can be caused by too much basal insulin or by insulin stacking from carb and correction boluses given during the evening. Never assume that middle of the night lows are always caused by the basal rate. Boluses lower the glucose for about 5 hours after they are given, so the dinner bolus is often working past bedtime. Snack or correction boluses given later in the evening will lower the glucose for another 5 hours, so insulin stacking is a frequent cause for middle of the night lows, especially in pumps that do not subtract excess BOB from carb boluses.

11.11 Common Basal Percentages of TDD	
40-45%	Kids and adults who are sensitive to insulin, physically fit, on a high carb diet, or have residual insulin production in first 5 years after diagnosis.
45-55%	Most people
56% or more	Adults or teens who are on a low carb diet or often miss their carb boluses.

© 2012 Diabetes Services, Inc

If you have 2 am lows, how can you tell if your basal rate is to blame, or if it was your dinner and evening boluses? A great clue comes from adding up how many units of basal insulin you received in the previous 5 hours and comparing this total to how many units of carb and correction bolus insulin were still active during this same period. (This would be a useful tool to add to future pumps to clarify whether your basals or boluses are actually causing highs and lows.) Middle of the night lows are usually caused by the dose that is larger. You can also recheck your basal rates by eating dinner at least 5 hours before bed and not taking any boluses after that. If you go low in the middle of the night on that night, your basal rate is very likely the cause. Otherwise, suspect residual bolus activity.

To prevent night lows caused by bolus stacking, make sure that you:

1. Set your DIA time to at least 4.5 hours so that your bolus calculator will fully measure how much BOB (residual bolus insulin activity) remains,

2. Look to see how much BOB is still active when you check your bedtime glucose.

Temporary Basal Rates

Temporary basal rates are ideal when more or less basal insulin is needed for 30 min. to 24 hours, up to 72 hours. Temp basal rates can be programmed as a percentage of your normal basal rate profile like 85%, 90%, or 120%, or as a set basal rate like 0.75 u/hr. *Percentages usually work better especially if you have more than one basal rate per day.* When this time period ends, the basal rate automatically returns to what it was before the temporary rate began.

A higher temp basal rate might be used during illness or stress, for a brunch or holiday meal that you eat over a period of time, or to cover the conversion of protein to glucose that occurs during the night following a large protein steak or bean soup dinner. A lower temp basal rate is useful during exercise, as well as overnight following a day of increased activity. Like alternate basal profiles, temp basal rates can be used to test higher or lower basal rates to see how they perform before you program them as your regular rates.

With today's pumps, some users find it helps to use a temporary basal rate reduction to offset excess BOB. For example, if someone has 2 units of BOB still active at bedtime and their blood sugar drops 50 mg/dl (2.8 mmol/L) per unit, a bedtime reading of 150 mg/dl (8.3 mmol/L) would likely be followed by a low during the night if nothing were done. Rather than eating a bedtime snack, a temporary basal reduction equal to 1 unit can be used over the next two hours to prevent a low reading.

Alternate Basal Profiles

Alternate basal profiles are 24-hour basal rate profiles stored in pump memory that you can switch between when a different basal profile (weekend, exercise, menses, etc.) is needed. Most pumps allow four alternate basal profiles. If your eating, activity, or stress is different on weekends, consider setting up an alternate basal profile to cover this. If you exercise

> **11.12 Clever Pump Trick - Use Alternate Basals to Test New Basal Rates**
>
> An easy way to test new basal rates after you've been on the pump for awhile is to use an alternate basal profile in your pump. Just create an alternate basal profile with the basal rates you want to try. Switch to this new profile and adjust these rates or their timing until your readings improve. If your readings don't improve, continue to modify them or switch back to the basal rates saved in your original profile.

regularly on Monday, Wednesday, and Friday, you can switch to an alternate basal profile that has lower basal rates before and after the time you exercise on these three days.

Many women manage their varying insulin needs around the time of their period with an alternate basal profile. Some women find they need three different profiles: a standard profile, a higher premenstrual profile, and a lower-than-normal profile for a day or two near the end of their period when insulin sensitivity can increase.

Unlike temporary basal rates, today's alternate basal profiles don't automatically shut off and return the pump to your usual basal profile. You have to remember to do this. It would be safer and more convenient if future pumps allowed you to set how long an alternate basal profile would run so that it automatically switched back to your normal profile at the time desired. In current pumps, it may be better to use a temporary basal profile. If your pump allows a maximum duration of only 24 hours, be sure to set an alert to signal when the temp basal ends so you can reset it as needed.

Basal Rate Tips

- Test and adjust your overnight basal first. This lets you sleep soundly through the night without going low and wake up with good readings.
- Adjust basal rates at least 5 to 8 hours before the high or low reading occurs, or 2 to 3 hours before any fall or rise in your glucose begins.
- Check your glucose often or wear a CGM during basal testing if you suspect you might go low.
- When you adjust your basal rates, adjust by 0.05 or 0.1 units per hour unless frequent high or low readings clearly indicate a larger change is needed.

Never assume your basal rate is correct from a single test. Test at least twice.

Quick Check: Do your basal doses make up 40% to 55% of your TDD?

Summary

Once your basal rates keep your glucose flat while you are sleeping or fasting, you're ready to test and tune your carb and correction boluses by testing your CarbF and CorrF.

If at first you don't succeed, you're about average.

Anon.

Test and Adjust Your Carb Factor

# CHAPTER 4

How accurately you use carb boluses to cover meals affects approximately half your control each day. "How much insulin do I take to cover a bagel, a plate of pasta, or a piece of fruit?" Pump wearers who are most successful at controlling their glucose answer these questions through carb counting.

A carb factor (CarbF) is the number of grams of carbohydrate that one unit of insulin will cover for you. (This is sometimes expressed as the tenths of a unit of insulin needed to cover 10 or 15 grams of carb.) The bolus calculator (BC) in your pump divides the carbs you enter for a meal or snack by your CarbF to recommend an exact carb bolus. Having your carb boluses work requires entry of accurate carb counts and having an accurate CarbF setting in your pump. In the APP study, 92% of pumpers routinely used their pump bolus calculator to give carb boluses.[63]

This chapter shows:

- How to select, test, and adjust your starting CarbF
- How to use combination and extended boluses
- How to time your boluses to avoid post-meal spikes
- How to give a Super Bolus
- More about carb boluses and CarbFs

12.1 Simple Math for Carb Boluses

Though your pump BC calculates this, the math for finding a carb bolus is fairly easy:

Carb Bolus   =   Grams of Carb / CarbF

Example – for 44 grams of carb and a CarbF of 11:

44 grams/11 grams per unit = 4.0 units as your carb bolus

Know your CarbF and this formula to double-check your pump BC recommendations.

© 2012 Diabetes Services, Inc.

141

Even a small change in your CarbF can make a big change in your glucose. Consider someone with good glucose management who weighs 160 lbs. (73 kg) and has a TDD of 40 units. A change in their CarbF from 1 u/10 grams to 1 u/9 grams will lower their glucose by an extra 33 mg/dl (1.8 mmol/L) for meals with 60 grams of carb, and by about 54 mg/dl (3.0 mmol/L) for every meal with 100 grams of carb.

Increments for CarbFs that are smaller than 1 gram per unit are being introduced into new pumps to improve the accuracy of carb boluses. An exact CarbF, like 1 unit for 8.5 grams or 1 unit for 11 grams, can give the bolus doses you actually need. Once your BC recommends a bolus, you can decide whether to take that dose or adjust it for things like increased activity or an illness.

What You Need to Cover Carbs Accurately

- A CarbF that is based on an accurate TDD and your weight
- Accurate carb counting
- Appropriate basal rates that are already tested and adjusted
- An accurate DIA to avoid hidden insulin stacking and track BOB accurately

Once basal rates are accurate, your carb counting or your CarbF become the likely culprits if you have high or low readings after meals.

Select, Test, and Adjust Your Carb Factor

To ensure accurate CarbF testing, be sure to read through all the steps in this section.

Select a Starting Carb Factor

Select a starting CarbF with your health care professional's help from Box 12.2, using *the 2.6 Rule*, or from Tables 9.5 or 12.3, and enter it into your pump as a setting to start your testing. A full range of starting settings for basal rate, CarbF, and CorrF can also be found for your TDD in Table 9.5.

Start with a single CarbF for the entire day. If you need slightly different CarbFs at different times of the day, these adjustments can be made later through testing and experience.

12.2 Calculate Your Own Carb Factor with the 2.6 Rule

In the APP study, the CarbF formula for the better control group was (2.6 x Wt(lb)/TDD).[69] To find your CarbF, multiply your weight by 2.6 and divide this by your TDD:

$$\text{CarbF} \quad = \quad \left(\frac{2.6 \times \text{Wt(lb)}}{\text{TDD}} \right) \quad \text{or} \quad \left(\frac{5.7 \times \text{Wt(kg)}}{\text{TDD}} \right)$$

For example, if a person's weight is 160 lbs. and their 14 day average TDD is 40 units a day, their CorrF would be 2.6 x 160 / 40 = 10.4 grams per unit.

As shown in Box 12.10, most CarbFs range between 1 unit for 3 grams of carb for someone who is less sensitive to insulin, to 1 unit for 20 grams for someone who is more sensitive. Someone who is very resistant to insulin may need a lower CarbF number, while a higher CarbF number may work better for someone who is very sensitive to insulin. Most CarbFs range between 6 and 13 and nearly all range between 2 and 22 grams per unit.

Test Your Carb Factor

A simple way to test your CarbF is to do a backward CarbF test. Make sure no BOB is present and count your carbs accurately. Use your BC to calculate the insulin dose and then see whether you go high or low. Once a carb bolus works for a large carb meal, divide the number of grams of carb in that meal by the carb bolus you gave for them. For instance, this might involve eating 3 or 4 large carb breakfasts over a few days. If you have 100 grams of carb in each breakfast and get great results when you take 9.0 units, your CarbF would be 100 g/9.0 u = 11 g/u.

12.3 Select a Starting Carb Factor for Testing

Find your TDD in the left column and look across that row to where it intersects with your weight. Approximate or round off your CarbF number as needed.

	Carb Factors for Various Weights and TDDs					
Wt = **TDD:**	**100 lb** **(45 kg)**	**120 lb** **(55 kg)**	**140 lb** **(64 kg)**	**160 lb** **(73 kg)**	**180 lb** **(82 kg)**	**200 lb** **(91 kg)**
20 u	13.0	15.6	18.2	20.8	23.4	
25 u	10.4	12.5	14.6	16.6	18.7	20.8
30 u	8.7	10.4	12.1	13.9	15.6	17.3
35 u	7.4	8.9	10.4	11.9	13.4	14.9
40 u	6.5	7.8	9.1	10.4	11.7	13.0
45 u	5.78	6.9	8.1	9.2	10.4	11.6
50 u	5.2	6.2	7.3	8.3	9.4	10.4
60 u	4.3	5.2	6.1	6.9	7.8	8.7
70 u	3.7	4.5	5.2	5.9	6.7	7.4
80 u		3.9	4.6	5.2	5.9	6.5
90 u			4.0	4.6	5.2	5.8
100 u				4.1	4.7	5.2

© 2012 Diabetes Services, Inc.

Be sure to eat enough carbs to test your CarbF as discussed in the Test Your CarbF section in Workspace 12.5. This CarbF then has to be tested at different meals of the day to ensure that the same CarbF works for breakfast, lunch, and dinner.

Testing your CarbF requires a ***clear-out period***, shown in Fig. 12.4, that eliminates any glucose lowering effects from boluses and any glucose raising effect from carbs. Wait at least 5 hours to eliminate previous bolus effects and 3 hours for food digestion.

Count carbs accurately. For your test, eat foods that have the carb count available on a label or in a book, phone app, or software. Weigh or measure foods as needed to get precise a carb count. Plain carb foods without excess fat or protein like cereal or oatmeal with fruit, or a bagel or toast with fruit work best.

To test your CarbF, eat enough carbs to actually challenge it. An easy way to do this is to eat the grams of carb equal to half your weight in pounds or equal to your weight in kilograms. For example, someone who weighs 150 lbs. would eat 75 grams of carb for their test, as would someone who weighed 75 kilograms.

Be sure to bolus 20 minutes before eating. A post-meal rise in your glucose does not matter for this test. How to prevent post-meal spiking is covered below. If your glucose goes above 250 mg/dl (13.9 mmol/L), test more often to make sure it is coming down.

For a successful CarbF test, your glucose will end up within 30 mg/dl (1.7 mmol/L) of your starting glucose 5 hours later as shown by arrow A1 in

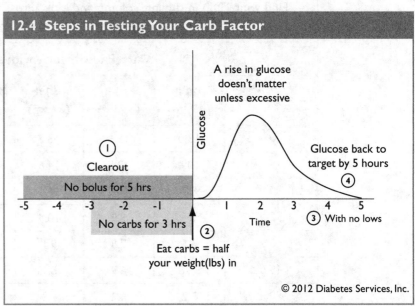

Figure 12.7. If this happens, no adjustment in your CarbF is needed, but test at least 2 or 3 more times and at different meals to verify this CarbF. For the next few days, try to eat a similar number of grams of carb at regular meal times to quickly verify this CarbF.

A CGM trend line, of course, provides a convenient way to test and adjust your CarbF.

An accurate CarbF will bring your glucose to within 30 mg/dl (1.7 mmol/L) of your start about 5 hours later without going low.

1. Start your CarbF test when your glucose is between 80 and 140 mg/dl (4.4-7.8 mmol/L) and it has been at least 5 hours since your last bolus and 3 hours since you ate any carbs.

2. Bolus 20 minutes before eating.

3. Eat grams of carb equal to half your weight in pounds (or equal to your weight in kilograms). Plain carb foods like cereal or oatmeal with fruit, a bagel, or toast and jelly with milk work best.

4. Check your glucose every hour for 5 hours or more often if you may go low (or wear a CGM). If your glucose goes below 70 mg/dl (3.9 mmol/L), stop the test and eat carbs.

5. Record and plot below how your glucose changes during the test.

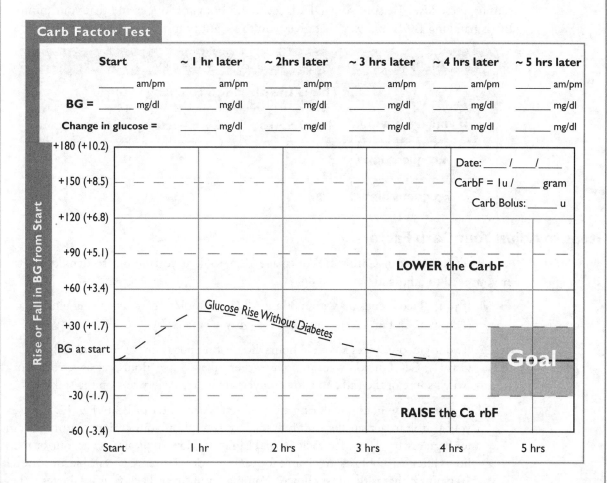

Carb Factor Test

	Start	~ 1 hr later	~ 2hrs later	~ 3 hrs later	~ 4 hrs later	~ 5 hrs later
	_____ am/pm	_____ am/pm	_____ am/pm	_____ am/pm	_____ am/pm	_____ am/pm
BG =	_____ mg/dl	_____ mg/dl	_____ mg/dl	_____ mg/dl	_____ mg/dl	_____ mg/dl
Change in glucose =		_____ mg/dl	_____ mg/dl	_____ mg/dl	_____ mg/dl	_____ mg/dl

Date: _____ / _____ / _____

CarbF = 1u / _____ gram

Carb Bolus: _____ u

LOWER the CarbF

Glucose Rise Without Diabetes

Goal

RAISE the Ca rbF

Rise or Fall in BG from Start

+180 (+10.2)
+150 (+8.5)
+120 (+6.8)
+90 (+5.1)
+60 (+3.4)
+30 (+1.7)
BG at start
_____
-30 (-1.7)
-60 (-3.4)

Start   1 hr   2 hrs   3 hrs   4 hrs   5 hrs

Adjust Your Carb Factor

If your glucose goes low at any point or remains at least 30 mg/dl (1.7 mmol/L) higher than your starting glucose after 5 hours, try the CarbF adjustments suggested below. Always adjust your CarbF in the opposite direction to your glucose problem. For example, if you have high readings before lunch, lower your CarbF number at breakfast to make breakfast boluses larger. If you are having too many lows before lunch, raise your breakfast CarbF number to make breakfast boluses smaller.

For example, if lows often occur after giving carb boluses, increase your CarbF number, usually by one point or less, to make your carb boluses smaller. If you use 1 unit for every 9 grams, try 1 unit for every 9.5 or 10 grams. Check that your daytime basal is not significantly higher than your overnight basal rate, as an excessive morning basal can also cause lows at lunch. Also check your average basal/bolus balance for 7 days or more to make sure that basal rates make up less than 55 or 60% of your TDD. If carb boluses make up more than 50% of your TDD, this is a good indicator that your carb boluses are causing these lows. Be sure your DIA is set to 4.5 hours or longer and that your pump BC is handling BOB in a way that gives you the safest bolus recommendations.

12.6 Which Way Do You Change Your Pump Settings?			
	This is the direction to change your:		
If you are having:	**Basal Rates**	**Carb Factor**	**Corr Factor**
Frequent lows	↓	↑	↑
Frequent highs	↑	↓	↓

Steps to Adjust Your Carb Factor

After testing your CarbF in Workspace 12.5, look at your results to decide whether you need to adjust it:

1. If your glucose ends up within 30 mg/dl (1.7 mmol/L) of your starting glucose (Arrow A1 in Fig. 12.7), your CarbF is fairly accurate. Try it to see how it works.

2. If your glucose spikes a couple hours after eating but is fine at 5 hours (A2), your CarbF is OK, but you want to bolus earlier, take a Super Bolus, eat fewer carbs, or switch some of the carbs to a lower glycemic index variety to stop the spiking.

3. If your glucose goes low during a CarbF test (Arrows B1 or B2 in Fig. 12.7), raise your CarbF to get smaller carb boluses. For example, if your current CarbF is 1 unit for 9 grams, try 1 unit for each 10 or 11 grams. If lows typically occur four or more hours after carb boluses, try 1 unit for each 9.5 or 9.6 grams, if available, or for each 10 grams if that is the next choice. (You may want to recheck your basal rates if they make up more than 55% of your TDD.)

4. If your glucose stays more than 30 mg/dl (1.7 mmol/L) above your starting glucose at 5 hours (C1 or C2), lower your CarbF to get larger carb boluses. (Or recheck your basal rates if they make up less than 45% of your TDD.)

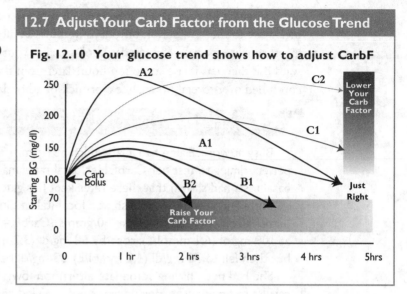

12.7 Adjust Your Carb Factor from the Glucose Trend

Fig. 12.10 Your glucose trend shows how to adjust CarbF

© 2012 Diabetes Services, Inc.

Consider these actions if you have frequent lows or highs after meals:

- Change your CarbF (raise for excess lows, lower for excess highs).
- Improve your carb counting, especially if you frequently go high.
- Check your basal/carb bolus balance. For example, if your basal rates make up more than 55% of your TDD, this may be the source for lows. If basals make up only 45% of your TDD, this would be a likely cause for highs.
- Make sure the DIA time in your pump is longer than 4 hours if you are having low.

Sample Carb Bolus Test

As an example, look at how Elaine tested her CarbF at lunch on the next page.

Combo and Extended Boluses

Low glycemic index foods and carbs mixed with fat or protein digest more slowly. For some of these foods, you may want to stretch out your bolus delivery. Bean dishes, pasta *al dente*, and pizzas are often covered better with a combo or dual wave bolus that slows insulin delivery than with a standard bolus.

For these foods and meals, use either:

- A **combination (combo or dual wave) bolus** that gives part of the bolus right away and the rest over a period of time. For example, 60% of the bolus can be given immediately and the remaining 40% delivered over the next two hours.
- Or an **extended (square wave) bolus** that delivers the entire bolus over a period of time, such as delivering 5 units over an hour and a half. This is the same as a combo bolus with 0% now and 5 units delivered over an hour and a half.

147

A standard meal bolus that is taken 20 minutes before eating will work best for most meals due to the slow action of today's insulins. Combo boluses work well for foods that digest slowly, especially if a standard bolus makes your glucose go low an hour or two afterward but then lets it rise six to ten hours later from the delayed digestion or when a meal is consumed over several hours, like a brunch or a holiday meal. Keep in mind that a standard

12.8 Example: Elaine Tests Her Carb Factor

Busy at work, Elaine had a late lunch at 1 p.m., six hours after her breakfast bolus, perfect timing to test her CarbF. Her basal rates made up half of her TDD and previous basal tests had shown that these rates kept her glucose flat when she was not eating.

For a linguine and clam dish at a local Italian diner, Elaine took the 8 units her pump recommended for these 80 grams (CarbF = 1u/10 grams). Her glucose started at 109 mg/dl (6.1 mmol/L), rose by 58 mg/dl (3.2 mmol/L) to 167 mg/dl an hour later, but then fell to 76 mg/dl (4.2 mmol/L), 33 mg/dl below her start after 4 hours.

She had been having some late afternoon lows, so she faxed her carb bolus test results to her doctor. Her doctor's nurse called back to suggest raising her CarbF to one unit for every 10 grams to one for every 11 grams. This lowered her lunch boluses enough to eliminate most of Elaine's afternoon lows.

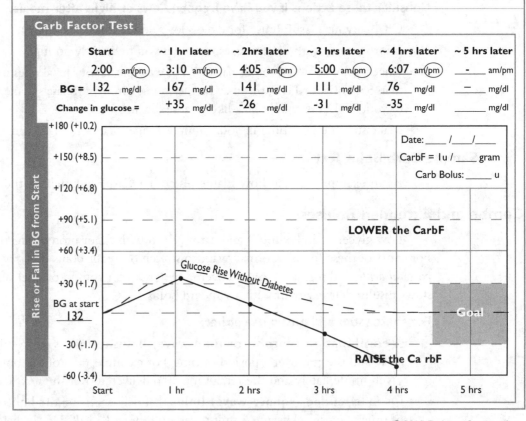

Carb Factor Test

	Start	~ 1 hr later	~ 2hrs later	~ 3 hrs later	~ 4 hrs later	~ 5 hrs later
	2:00 am/**pm**	3:10 am/**pm**	4:05 am/**pm**	5:00 am/**pm**	6:07 am/**pm**	- am/pm
BG =	132 mg/dl	167 mg/dl	141 mg/dl	111 mg/dl	76 mg/dl	— mg/dl
Change in glucose =		+35 mg/dl	-26 mg/dl	-31 mg/dl	-35 mg/dl	_____ mg/dl

Date: ____ /____ /____
CarbF = 1u / ____ gram
Carb Bolus: _____ u

LOWER the CarbF

Goal

RAISE the CarbF

bolus is preferred if certain sauces or toppings, or overcooking make a low GI food like pasta spike the glucose.

Combo boluses are especially helpful for people who have gastroparesis where digestion has been slowed by nerve damage, and when a prescription medication like Symlin® (pramlintide), Precose® (acarbose), or a GLP-1 agonist is used to slow digestion to improve post-meal readings.

Never assume that a combo bolus will actually improve your control. Test your glucose two hours after the bolus was given or wear a CGM to find out. Ideally, your glucose will have risen no more than 40 to 60 mg/dl (2.2 to 3.3 mmol/L) above where it started. Also track your glucose over the next 6 to 8 hours because a delayed bolus will lower your glucose over a longer period of time. Keep a record of the bolus ratio and duration when a particular combo bolus works for a certain food or situation so that you can use it again when you have that meal.

A carb bolus is NOT needed for carbs that are:

- Used to raise a low glucose
- Used to compensate for excess BOB or
- Used to cover exercise or increased activity
- That you may not be able to keep down due to nausea or vomiting

Post-Meal Glucose Goals

In healthy individuals without diabetes, the glucose level after a meal will usually rise no more than 40 mg/dl (2.2 mmol/L) above its start, for example, rising from 90 mg/dl (5.0 mmol/L) to a peak of 130 mg/dl (7.7 mmol/L). How high your glucose rises one to two hours after a meal shows how well the size and timing of your bolus matched these carbs.

In 2001, the American Diabetes Association recommended that post-meal readings in diabetes rise no higher than 180 mg/dl (10 mmol/L) two hours after a meal.[91] In 2002, the European Diabetes Policy Group recommends that they go no higher than 165 mg/dl (8.9 mmol/L) in Type 2 diabetes to prevent diabetes complications like retinopathy and that post-meal readings go no higher than 135 mg/dl (7.5 mmol/L) to prevent heart attacks and strokes in those at risk for cardiovascular disease.[92] From similar evidence, the International Diabetes Federation recommended in 2007 that postprandial glucoses go no higher than 140 mg/dl (7.8 mmol/L) at two hours as long as hypoglycemia can be avoided.[93] In pregnancy, post-meal targets are even tighter, with a goal of going no higher than 120 mg/dl (6.7 mmol/L) after meals and rarely going above 140 mg/dl at any time.

Most foods digest and start to raise your glucose quicker than today's insulins can lower it. This makes glucose spikes after meals a common problem. Most meals start to raise the glucose within 10 minutes of eating and reach their peak glucose 40 to 150 minutes later, with the glucose reaching a peak at 87 minutes for the average meal.[94] *A bolus only begins to lower the glucose about 20 minutes after being taken.*

12.9 The Carb Factor Measures Insulin Sensitivity

Insulin sensitivity (IS) can be measured as the amount of insulin required to move a certain amount of carbs into cells. Your CarbF measures the same thing and is a good measure of your insulin sensitivity (IS).[69] Your personal CarbF can be found by multiplying an average CarbF by your relative IS. The average CarbF in the APP study was 10.8 grams/unit* for the 132 insulin pump wearers who were in excellent control.

This makes finding your relative IS (and CarbF) easy:

1. Find the expected TDD for your weight on the assumption your IS is average:
   Your expected TDD = Wt(lb) x 0.24 u/lb (or Wt(kg) x 0.53 u/kg).[63]

2. Then find your average actual TDD for the last 10 days or more on your pump's history screen or from a recent computer or internet download.

3. Correct your actual TDD to your iTDD in Chapter 10.

4. Divide #1 by #3 to get your relative IS:

$$\text{Your IS} = \frac{\text{Wt(lb)} \times 0.24 \text{ u/lb}}{\text{Your iTDD}}$$

On this relative IS scale, the number 1.0 represents an average sensitivity to insulin. A number larger than 1 suggests greater sensitivity and a number smaller than 1 suggests greater resistance to insulin.

Your CarbF can then be found from this equation:

$$\text{Your CarbF} = 10.8 \times \text{your IS} = \left(10.8 \times \frac{\text{Wt(lbs)} \times 0.24}{\text{TDD}}\right) = \frac{2.6 \times \text{Wt(lb)}}{\text{TDD}}$$

Someone who is more sensitive to insulin will use a CarbF higher than 10.8, while someone who is less sensitive will use a number that is lower, when both people are counting carbs with reasonable accuracy. If you tend to undercount carbs, your CarbF number will be lower to compensate for the undercounting.

Note: Healthcare professionals can use the Pump Settings Tool at www.opensourcediabetes.org to quickly find starting CarbFs, CorrFs, average hourly basal rates, and relative insulin sensitivities.

* The average CarbF in the APP Study was found from an average of over 37,000 meals as the grams of carb divided by the carb bolus taken for each of these meals.

© 2012 Diabetes Services, Inc.

If you're unsure whether carbs or insulin is faster, eat a high carb meal with an exact carb count and cover it with a carb bolus taken just before eating. Check your glucose every 10 to 15 minutes for the first 90 minutes, then every 30 minutes for 4 hours after that (or use a CGM). The slow speed of today's insulins makes it hard to keep your glucose from rising less than the desired 40 to 60 mg/dl (2.2 to 3.3 mmol/L) after a meal.

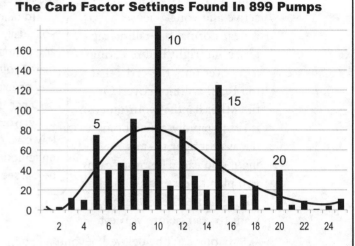
Prevent Post-Meal Spikes

Timing is everything in carb boluses. Although many people find it convenient to take boluses when they begin to eat, ***this is the most common cause for post-meal spiking.*** Today's rapid-acting insulins (Novolog®, Humalog®, and Apidra®) are simply too slow to be effective when taken just before eating a high carb meal. This might work for a meal with fewer carbs, such as less than 1/4 of your weight in pound (or 1/2 your weight in kilograms) as grams of carb, or for a meal with a low glycemic index.

Most meals that have more carbs than this are covered better when the carb bolus taken at least 15 to 20 minutes before eating. A bolus has little effect on the glucose over the first 15 to 20 minutes. Taking a bolus earlier provides a better match for normal digestion and can greatly reduce post-meal spiking. Spiking can occurs when a carb bolus is too small, but many spikes occur because carb digestion more quickly raises the glucose than the bolus can begin to work. About half of a bolus's action is seen during the first 2 to 2.25 hours, with the other half tailing off over the next 3 or more hours. It takes 5 to 6 hours for insulin action from a bolus to stop lowering the glucose. Insulin's long action can cause the glucose to go low 5 or more hours after a bolus is taken.

Today's insulins do not start fast enough and last too long, so they don't always provide optimal carb coverage. For better glucose results, bolus early, adjust bolus timing for your current glucose, and take into account how much BOB is still present.

Using a CGM helps. For example, if you have quite a bit of BOB still active and your glucose is near normal but falling rapidly, bolus right before eating and cover only the carbs that the BOB will not cover. On the other hand, if your glucose is rising rapidly, take a bolus but wait longer to start eating if you can. The more carbs you plan to eat and the higher your glucose, the longer you want to wait before you eat.

Eating can't be delayed beyond a reasonable time once you give a bolus, so be realistic about whether you may get distracted. Bolus early for meals only when you are certain you can eat on time. Keep fruit juice, regular sodas, or other quick carbs handy in case eating gets delayed. When a meal's timing is uncertain at a new restaurant or elsewhere, bolus when you have the food in front of you, or use one of the bolus tricks from Box 12.14. Also consider how many carbs you will eat and the meal's glycemic index.

When your glucose is elevated before a meal, don't send it higher by eating when you're already high. If possible, take a carb plus correction bolus but delay eating until your glucose is closer to your target. A guide for delayed eating is shown in Table 12.15.

Taking boluses right before or even after eating can sometimes be necessary if it isn't clear when a meal will start or when with a child, it is not clear how many carbs will be eaten. Researchers are working to develop faster insulins and microneedle infusion sets to speed insulin uptake. These will help eliminate some of the post-meal spiking and delayed hypoglycemia that is often seen with today's insulins.

Most current pump BCs don't subtract BOB from carb boluses if the BOB exceeds the units needed to lower your glucose. For example, if your glucose target is 100 mg/dl (5.6 mmol/L), your glucose is 102 mg/dl (5.7 mmol/L), and you plan to eat 30 grams of carb (CarbF = 10), most pump BCs recommend that you take 3 units to cover the carbs. This is OK when there is no BOB lowering your glucose, but if you have 3 units of BOB still working from a previous bolus, most pumps recommend that you take 3 more units even though the previous meal's carbs are probably no longer raising the glucose. Carbs in pizza and in some mixed meals digest more slowly, but most carbs are digested within two hours. Here, you may want to override the BC recommendation and calculate your own bolus.

The Super Bolus

One way to reduce post-meal spiking or rapidly lower a high glucose is to give a **_Super Bolus_**.[95, 96] Current pumps do not do this, but you can create your own Super Bolus by using a temp basal reduction to lower your basal rate and then adding the units you took from your basal on top of your usual carb or correction bolus. The larger bolus starts to work more quickly, but avoids having a later low because the basal delivery is reduced by an equal amount. A Super Bolus delivers more insulin quickly for better coverage of high carb or high glycemic index foods, and can also lower a high glucose reading faster.

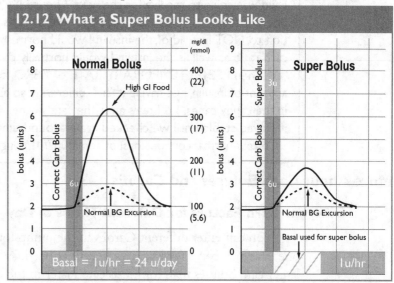

12.12 What a Super Bolus Looks Like

© 2012 Diabetes Services, Inc.

To give a Super Bolus, use a temp basal reduction to lower your basal delivery over the next 2 to 4 hours, and then add the same number of units as were taken out of the future basal delivery into the immediate bolus being given as a carb or correction bolus. An example is shown in Fig. 12.12. Keep in mind that when a Super Bolus is given, the basal insulin that is shifted into a bolus will appear to be extra BOB when it is not. Future pumps could handle this correctly.

Super Boluses help when eating more than 40 grams of carb, especially high GI meals like cereal. For example, instead of someone taking their usual 6 units for breakfast cereal, they can give a Super Bolus instead. If their basal rate is 1.0 unit an hour, a temp basal rate can be given at 20% of normal (80% reduction) over the next 3 hours. The 2.4 units from the basal reduction (0.8 u/hr times 3 hours = 2.4 units) is added to the 6.0 unit meal bolus to give an 8.4 unit bolus (6.0 u + 2.4 u) for the cereal. The cereal gets better bolus coverage with little risk of going low later.

To Reduce Post-meal Spiking:

- Bolus earlier – at least 15 to 20 minutes before eating
- Eat fewer carbs
- Include more fiber, lower glycemic index carbs or carbs mixed with protein or fat
- Use a Super bolus
- Talk with your doctor about pramlintide (Symlin®) or acarbose (Precose®) medications

More About Carb Boluses and CarbFs

Different Carb Factors for Different Times of Day

You can enter different CarbFs in the pump for different times of day. For example, one unit may cover fewer grams of carb at breakfast, so a smaller CarbF is needed to get larger carb boluses than for meals eaten later in the day. Larger breakfast boluses may be needed if more insulin resistance is present in the morning hours due to higher growth hormone, cortisol, and free fatty acid levels in the blood at this time of day. Keep in mind that a basal rate that is too low during the early morning hours also makes you need larger carb boluses at breakfast compared to other meals of the day. A quick way to check whether your morning basal rate is adequate is to delay eating breakfast for 3 or 4 hours one morning. If your glucose rises, then your basal rate is too low.

If your CarbF differ for different meals of the day, the CarbFs are usually within 1 or 2 grams of each other through the day. If your CarbF varies more than this, recheck your basal rates. For instance, if your CarbF for breakfast is 1 u/8 grams but is 1 u/12 grams the rest of the day, your night basal rates may be too low or your daytime basal rates too high.

If you generally eat a bedtime snack, you can program a higher CarbF for the evening hours to get smaller carb boluses at bedtime and reduce the risk for night lows.

Missed Carb Boluses

A carb bolus may be forgotten or started but never completed because of a distraction. Unfortunately, most pumps will not alert you that a carb bolus was never completed. Many current pumps can be set to beep at a certain time of day, such as at 8 am, noon, or 6:30 pm each day, as a reminder to take a meal bolus.

Signs that you may be missing carb boluses include having your TDD vary a lot from day to day or having an unrealistically low average daily carb count on your pump's history screen (See Box 12.11). If you can't remember if a bolus was given or your glucose has risen more than usual after a meal, check your history to see if it was given.

Unusual Food Effects

Some foods affect everyone's glucose badly but others may affect you in particular. You probably have experienced a food that had an unusual effect on your readings. For instance, certain fats, such like those in some chips and fried foods cause insulin resistance and raise your readings higher and longer than their carb count would indicate. Some sugar-free desserts may send your glucose higher than the same product made with sugar.

Research shows that high fat pizza can raise the glucose higher, later and longer than the carb content suggests it should,[97] confirming many people's experience. However, a pizza that is lower in fat, such as a vegetarian pizza or a particular pizza brand may not do this. Experiment. When a meal or dessert causes unusual readings, make a note of it. If it does the same thing a second time, place it on your verboten list, eat less of it, or use a larger bolus or combo bolus as needed to match it. Use a CGM, if available, to really open your eyes to how different foods and bolus types affect your readings.

Avoid Blind Bolusing

Blind bolusing is taking boluses without testing to find your current glucose. People sometimes get busy and think "I don't have time to test so I'll skip it." Blind bolusing does not allow the pump BC to adjust a bolus for BOB to give a more accurate bolus. Always check your glucose or wear a CGM when you bolus.

Delayed eating is the most common cause of severe hypoglycemia.
Don't delay eating if you have hypoglycemia unawareness,
a history of frequent lows, or you may get distracted.

12.15 Clever Pump Trick – How Long to Wait to Eat with a High Glucose

For a high reading before a meal, try taking a combined carb and correction bolus to lower it and delay eating. Be sure to test every 30 minutes (or wear a CGM) until your glucose goes below 150 mg/dl (8.3 mmol/L).

If you can't delay a meal, eat the fat or protein portions first and the carbs last to allow more time for the bolus to start working.

If you have hypoglycemia unawareness, may get distracted, or may forget to eat, always take your bolus and eat right away.

How Long to Delay Eating

A high glucose before a meal rarely falls faster than 3 mg/dl (0.17 mmol/L) per minute. This allows a reasonably safe estimate for how long you might wait to eat after a carb plus correction bolus.

Pre-meal BG	Approx. Wait Time
90-120 mg/dl	10-20 min
150 mg/dl	30 min
180 mg/dl	40 min
210 mg/dl	50 min
240 mg/dl	60 min
270 mg/dl	70 min
300 mg/dl	80 min

© 2012 Diabetes Services, Inc.

Keep Your Circumstances in Mind when You Bolus

Consider your circumstances before you bolus. If you are having pain or are under stress, your usual carb and correction bolus doses may need to be raised, along with a temporary basal increase. If you plan to go running or dancing after a meal, your pump does not know this. If your reading is over 300 mg/dl (16.7 mmol/L) and your urine shows moderate or large ketones, you may need to double or triple your pump's recommended correction bolus, give this dose as an injection, and then replace your reservoir and infusion set. Always keep your current circumstances in mind before you bolus.

Tips on Carb Counting and Coverage

- Most people undercount and guesstimate carbs. Keep your skills current. Review carb counting periodically in Chapter 3.
- Early boluses are the quickest way to improve your readings but don't forget to eat!
- Set and test your CarbF only after you have accurate basal rates.
- If a particular food or drink seems to raise your glucose excessively, try omitting it or have less of it to see if your readings improve.
- Try a combo bolus for foods that make your glucose rise slower or later than usual.
- Make an appointment with your dietitian, diabetes educator, or physician to sort out any food issues. Bring a 3-day diary of food and glucose readings with you.

12.16 A CGM Helps Determine Carb Bolus Timing and Size

After a meal, a glance at your CGM trend line lets you see how the carb bolus matched the meal. This helps tailor boluses to particular meals and quickly identifies foods that may have a low or high glycemic index for you.

The trend line lets you see how combo and extended boluses work for mixed meals and low GI meals. If potato chips or a meat pizza cause your glucose to rise higher than predicted by their carb content, try bolusing earlier or increase the bolus. If the glucose rises longer than expected, try a larger combo bolus to match the meal and extend your bolus longer.

When eating a new meal, your CGM trend line over the next 5 hours shows how it affects your glucose and lets you modify the timing, size, and type of bolus to match. Keep track of boluses that work for specific foods for use next time.

- Use food labels or a carb database in your pump, PDA, or cell phone to improve your carb counts. Use books, measuring cups and spoons, a calculator and a gram scale.
- The **Diabetes Carb and Fat Gram Guide** and **Calorie King's Guide To Calories, Fat, and Carbohydrates** listed in Chapter 3 are handy books for eating out.
- Reduce your pump BC bolus recommendation if you will be active after eating.

12.17 Checklist for Carb Boluses

If your carb boluses usually work, but a high or low reading happens after a particular meal, the problem is usually not your carb factor.

Consider:

- Did you have an accurate carb count?
- Did you eat a high or low glycemic index food?
- Did you eat more fat or protein than usual?
- Did you take your bolus early enough?
- Were you more or less active than usual?

Experience is a dear school, but a fool will learn in no other.

Benjamin Franklin

12.19 How Much Insulin Did You Miss in Your Last Meal Bolus?

If a meal bolus is too small, this is easy to spot because your glucose 4 to 5 hrs later ends up higher than where it started. How much higher your glucose goes shows how many units were missing in that bolus.

To see how many more units you actually needed:

1. Find your TDD on the left.
2. Look across to find the column nearest your glucose 4 or more hours later.
3. The value you find shows about how many more units you needed in that bolus.

Your TDD (u/day)	Your Glucose 4-5 hrs after Your Last Bolus [mg/dl (mmol/L)]						
	160 (8.9)	200 (11.1)	240 (13.3)	280 (15.6)	320 (17.8)	360 (20)	400 (22.2)
20 u	-0.4 u	-0.8 u	-1.3 u	-1.7 u	-2.1 u	-2.5 u	-2.9 u
30 u	-0.6 u	-1.3 u	-1.9 u	-2.5 u	-3.2 u	-3.8 u	-4.4 u
40 u	-0.8 u	-1.7 u	-2.5 u	-3.4 u	-4.2 u	-5.1 u	-5.9 u
50 u	-1.0 u	-2.1 u	-3.2 u	-4.2 u	-5.3 u	-6.3 u	-7.4 u
60 u	-1.3 u	-2.5 u	-3.8 u	-5.1 u	-6.3 u	-7.6 u	-8.8 u
70 u	-1.5 u	-2.9 u	-4.4 u	-5.9 u	-7.4 u	-8.8 u	-10.3 u
80 u	-1.7 u	-3.4 u	-5.1 u	-6.7 u	-8.4 u	-10.1 u	-11.8 u
100 u	-2.1 u	-4.2 u	-6.3 u	-8.4 u	-10.5 u	-12.6 u	-14.7 u

Assumes that your control is generally good and that your basal rates keep your glucose flat when you do not eat.

© 2012 Diabetes Services, Inc.

If you find it hard to laugh at yourself,
I would be happy to do it for you.

Groucho Marx

Test and Adjust Your Correction Factor

An accurate correction factor (CorrF) tells your pump how far your glucose drops on each unit of insulin. Your pump BC can then recommend correction boluses that start to lower your high readings in about 30 to 60 minutes and bring them down to your target 4 to 5 hours later without going low. With a high glucose, any BOB from previous boluses will be subtracted from the correction bolus recommendation.

Everyone needs correction doses, even those in good control. In the APP study, the 132 pumpers with the lowest average glucose averaged 1.9 correction boluses and 4.2 units for their corrections each day, or about 9% of the TDD. This compares to 2.4 correction boluses and 7.0 units a day for the third with the highest average glucose.

This chapter shows how to
- Select a starting CorrF
- Test and adjust your CorrF
- Test your DIA
- Keep correction boluses below 9% of your TDD

13.1 Simple Math for Correction Boluses

The pump uses the same simple math you would to get a correction bolus

Corr. Bolus = (Current BG − Target BG) / CorrF

Example – with a correction target of 100 mg/dl, a glucose of 220 mg/dl, and a CorrF setting of 40 mg/dl:

**220 mg/dl − 100 mg/dl = 120 mg/dl / 40 mg/dl per unit
= 3.0 units as your correction bolus**

Know your CorrF and this formula to check your pump BC recommendations.

© 2012 Diabetes Services, Inc

Both Sides of Corrections Are Important

Correction boluses make up for the deficits or mistakes in your basal rates, carb counting, and carb boluses. They also help in situations where insulin requirements are temporarily increased, such as with stress, pain, a steroid medication, or a failed infusion set (once the bad set has been replaced).

When you test your glucose, you usually need either insulin to lower it or carbs to raise it or offset excess BOB. Your CorrF helps you lower high glucose levels successfully, but it can also help you determine how many grams of carb you need to treat a low glucose or to offset excess BOB. Both sides are critical to bringing your next glucose into your desired target range. Table 10.4 shows how to successfully raise a low glucose.

Select, Test, and Adjust Your Correction Factor

Select Your Correction Factor

Select your starting CorrF with your health care professional's help from Table 13.2 and enter it into your pump. Look for your starting TDD or an improved iTDD in the left column and the CorrF that you want to test in the right column. For a full choice of basal rate, CarbF, and CorrF from your TDD, go to Table 9.5.

13.2 Select Your Correction Factor	
Find your TDD or improved TDD on the left, then a starting CorrF on the right.	
TDD or iTDD	CorrF 1 u lowers BG by:
	1960 Rule (110 Rule)
15 u	131 (7.26)
20 u	98.0 (5.44)
25 u	78.4 (4.36)
30 u	65.3 (3.63)
35 u	56.0 (3.11)
40 u	49.0 (2.72)
45 u	43.6 (2.42)
50 u	39.2 (2.18)
55 u	35.6 (1.98)
60 u	32.7 (1.81)
70 u	28.0 (1.56)
80 u	24.5 (1.36)
90 u	21.8 (1.21)
100 u	19.6 (1.09)

¹ CorrF = 1960/TDD (mg/dl) or 109/TDD (mmol/L) – how far 1u lowers your BG in mg/dl (or mmol/L).

Larger CorrF numbers give smaller correction boluses. People who are in better control and those who use less insulin per day need larger CorrF numbers. Someone whose average TDD is 25 units a day will find their glucose falls about 80 mg/dl (4.2 mmol/L) per unit, while for someone who uses 100 units of insulin per day, their glucose will fall only 20 mg/dl (1.1 mmol/L) per unit. Correction boluses for the second person will be about four times as large as the first person's to lower the same high glucose. *Larger CorrF numbers like 2200 or 2400 work better for those whose glucose levels are often normal or who have frequent lows* because smaller correction doses are needed to cover the smaller deficits (or excesses) that exist in their basal rates and carb boluses.

On the other hand, *if your average glucose or A1c is routinely elevated, smaller CorrF rule numbers like 1800 or 1500 work better* because larger correction doses are needed to cover the larger deficits in basal rates or carb boluses.

13.3 Calculate Your Own Correction Factor

In the APP study, the average CorrF Rule Number (an average of each individual's CarbF times their average TDD) in the best control third was 1960 mg/dl (109 mmol/L).[63] Your starting CorrF can be found from this average CorrF Rule Number. Simply divide 1960 by your average TDD in a calculator to find your CorrF:

$$\textbf{CorrF} = \frac{\textbf{1960 mg/dl}}{\textbf{TDD}} \quad \text{or} \quad \frac{\textbf{109 mmol/L}}{\textbf{TDD}}$$

For example, if a person's 14 day average TDD is 47.3 units a day, their CorrF would be 1960/47.3 = 41.4 or 41 mg/dl per unit (2.3 mmol/L per unit).

1960 can be replaced by 2000 for easy mental math, or by a 110 Rule for those who measure glucose in millimoles per liter. Use a smaller number CorrF Rule Number like 1800 or 1500 to calculate a CorrF if your readings are mostly high, or a larger number like 2200 or 2400 for mostly normal readings or frequent lows.

Know your CorrF to double-check the pump's correction bolus before taking it.

© 2012 Diabetes Services, Inc

Start with a single correction factor for the entire day. If you need slightly different CorrFs at different times of the day, these adjustments can be made later through testing and experience.

To find your CorrF, you will first need:

1. Accurate basal rates

2. Accurate CorrF

3. Accurate glucose readings

4. A single correction target or narrow correction target range in your pump

5. An accurate DIA

Test Your Correction Factor

Your CorrF is tested in Workspace 13.5. Similar to testing basal rates, some fasting is required. As shown in Fig. 13.4, the test is started when your glucose is above 250 mg/dl (12.9 mmol/L), you have not eaten in the last 3 hours nor given a bolus in the last 5 hours, and you can wait to eat for another 5 hours – small amounts of protein (nuts, cheese, boiled egg, etc.) are OK. Set your Correction Target to 100 mg/dl (5.6 mmol/L) in your pump. Once the correction bolus is given, reset to your usual target.

A successful CorrF test will bring a high glucose down to a value between 70 and 130 mg/dl (3.9-7.2 mmol/L) 5 hours later without going low. If your glucose goes below 70 mg/dl (3.9 mmol/L), stop the test and eat. Once a CorrF works

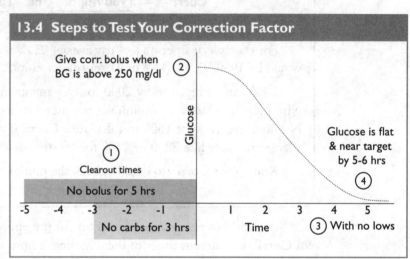

13.4 Steps to Test Your Correction Factor

Give corr. bolus when BG is above 250 mg/dl ②

① Clearout times

No bolus for 5 hrs

No carbs for 3 hrs

Glucose

Time

Glucose is flat & near target by 5-6 hrs ④

③ With no lows

© 2012 Diabetes Services, Inc

well, repeat the test to verify it. Adjust and retest your CorrF until it consistently does this. See Example 13.7 as a guide.

A good time to check your CorrF is when a bedtime reading is above 250 mg/dl (13.9 mmol/L) and it has been at least 5 hours since your last bolus. Be sure to set an alarm that load enough to wake you up at regular intervals to check your glucose. A CGM with its alarms provides extra security. Another good time to test your CorrF is a high reading at lunch or dinner if your glucose was relatively normal 5 hours earlier, no bolus has been taken since then, and you can wait to eat for another 5 hours.

A high breakfast reading is not always a good time for CorrF testing. If your glucose was already high at bedtime and stays high overnight, your liver will be making excess amounts of glucose because your insulin level was low all night. (The liver reads your insulin level, not your glucose. The low insulin level tells the liver to make extra glucose to raise your "low" glucose.) Here, your correction bolus has to be larger than normal to overcome the extra insulin resistance created by several hours of high readings and to turn off the liver's excess glucose production. This makes the CorrF number appear to be lower than it would be if your overnight basal rate or dinner carb bolus had been adequate. Test your CorrF at another time if your glucose has been constantly high for more than about 5 hours. A CGM helps evaluate these situations.

13.5 Test Your Correction Factor

An accurate CorrF will bring your high glucose down to between 70 and 130 mg/dl (3.9 to 6.8 mmol/L) in 5 to 6 hours without going low.

1) Start your test when:

    a. Your glucose is over 250 mg/dl (13.9 mmol/L)

    b. You have not eaten in the last 3 hours nor given a bolus in the last 5 hours

    c. You can wait to eat for another 5 hours – small amounts of protein are OK

2) Set your Correction Target to 100 mg/dl (5.6 mmol/L) for the test. Reset to your normal target after you give this correction bolus.

3) Take the correction bolus that your pump BC recommends.

4) Check your glucose hourly or wear a CGM. Check more often if glucose is dropping quickly.

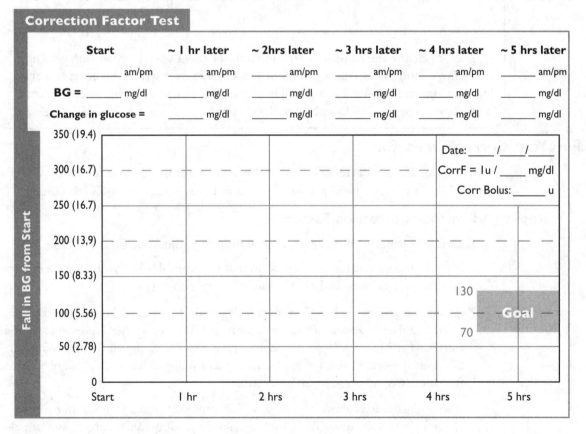

Correction Factor Test

	Start	~ 1 hr later	~ 2hrs later	~ 3 hrs later	~ 4 hrs later	~ 5 hrs later
	_____ am/pm	_____ am/pm	_____ am/pm	_____ am/pm	_____ am/pm	_____ am/pm
BG =	_____ mg/dl	_____ mg/dl	_____ mg/dl	_____ mg/dl	_____ mg/dl	_____ mg/dl
Change in glucose =		_____ mg/dl	_____ mg/dl	_____ mg/dl	_____ mg/dl	_____ mg/dl

Date: _____ / _____ / _____

CorrF = 1u / _____ mg/dl

Corr Bolus: _____ u

13.6 Correction Bolus Testing with a CGM

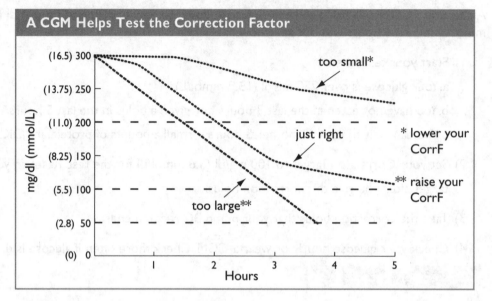

A CGM Helps Test the Correction Factor

too small*

just right

* lower your CorrF

** raise your CorrF

too large**

© 2013 Diabetes Services, Inc.

A CGM clearly shows how correction boluses affect your glucose with readings every five minutes or so during the 5 or more hours over which the bolus is working. Readings and a trend line are visible as the glucose comes down, and the trend line lets you see pending lows before they happen.

Adjust Your Correction Factor

If you need larger correction boluses from your pump, you will lower the CorrF number. Likewise, if you need smaller correction boluses, raise your CorrF number.

Steps to Adjust Your Correction Factor

Your results from Workspace 13.5 show how to adjust your CorrF:

1. If your glucose ends up within 30 mg/dl (1.7 mmol/L) of your pump's correction target, celebrate and check one more time to verify.

2. If your glucose goes below 70 mg/dl (3.9 mmol/L) within 5 hours, raise your CorrF number by about 10% to make correction boluses smaller. For example if your CorrF is 1 u:20 mg/dl (1 u:1.1 mmol/L) raise it to 1 u:22 mg/dl (1 u:1.2 mmol/L), or if 1 u:80 mg/dl (1 u:4.4 mmol/L) raise it to 1 u:88 mg/dl (1 u:4.9 mmol/L), etc. Retest the CorrF to verify this new setting.

3. If your glucose stays above 130 mg/dl (7.2 mmol/L) after 5 hours, lower your CorrF by 5 to 10%, using Table 13.8 to make correction boluses larger. For example, to get a 10% increase in the size of your correction boluses, if your CorrF is 1 u:20 mg/dl (1 u:1.1 mmol/L) lower it to 1 u:18 mg/dl (1 u:1.0 mmol/L), or if it is 1 u:80 mg/dl (1 u:4.4 mmol/L) lower it to 1 u:72 mg/dl (1 u:4.0 mmol/L), etc. If your

reading stays above 200 mg/dl (11 mmol/L) at 5 hours, a smaller CorrF may be needed. Retest to verify that the new setting works.

4. Once a CorrF appears correct, repeat the test to verify it.

Box 13.7 shows an example of how Elaine tested and adjusted her CorrF.

13.7 Example: Elaine Tests Her Correction Factor

Elaine had tested her basal rates recently so she knew they kept her glucose flat when she was not eating. For a Tuesday lunch, she had a pasta dish at a nearby restaurant but underestimated how many carbs she ate. At 5 p.m. when she had a chance to check, her reading was 328 mg/dl (18 mmol/L). It had been 5 hours since her last bolus, so she decided to skip dinner and test her CorrF.

Her CorrF is 1 unit for every 50 mg/dl (2.8 mmol/L) above her target of 100 mg/dl (5.6 mmol/L), so she bolused 4.6 units to lower her glucose by 228 mg/dl (12.7 mmol/L). [228/50 = 4.6 units]

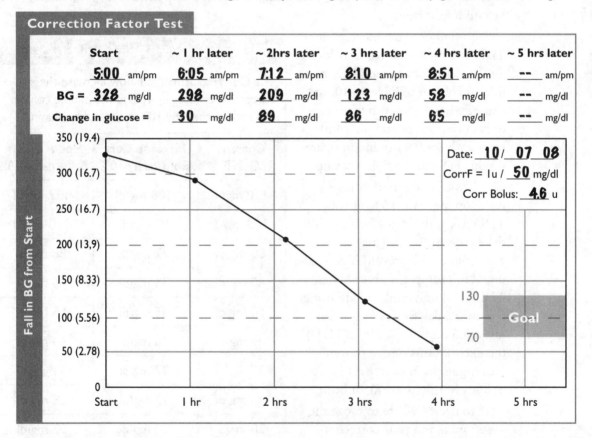

Correction Factor Test

	Start	~ 1 hr later	~ 2hrs later	~ 3 hrs later	~ 4 hrs later	~ 5 hrs later
	5:00 am/pm	**6:05** am/pm	**7:12** am/pm	**8:10** am/pm	**8:51** am/pm	-- am/pm
BG =	**328** mg/dl	**298** mg/dl	**209** mg/dl	**123** mg/dl	**58** mg/dl	-- mg/dl
Change in glucose =		**30** mg/dl	**89** mg/dl	**86** mg/dl	**65** mg/dl	-- mg/dl

Date: **10** / **07** **08**
CorrF = 1u / **50** mg/dl
Corr Bolus: **4.6** u

Elaine checked her glucose each hour but went low to 64 mg/dl (3.6 mmol/L) less than 4 hours later. After treating the low, she raised her CorrF to 1 unit for each 55 mg/dl (3.1 mmol/L) and planned to retest on another day.

© 2013 Diabetes Services, Inc.

If high readings are often followed by lows, your CorrF number will likely need to be increased, your DIA time lengthened to 4.5 hours or longer, or your basal rate lowered. Be sure to recheck your basal rates if they make up more than 55% of your TDD.

Keep Corrections Below 9% of the TDD

Correction boluses are needed on most days by most pumpers, but when correction boluses become large and frequent, this indicates there is a deficit in either your basal rates or your carb boluses. Frequent highs mean your basal rates are too low, your CarbF is too high, carb boluses are being missed or taken too late, or carb counts are being undercounted. Always address the real control issue.

With good glucose control, correction boluses usually make up less than 9% of the TDD, or 0.09 times your TDD.[69] Some pumps provide the average percentage of the TDD that comes from correction boluses on a history screen, while others provide this after downloading or uploading your pump. See your pump manual for how to access this helpful information.

To find out how much of your TDD you use for corrections, look for your current average TDD in the left column of Table 13.10, and compare how your current average daily correction bolus total compares with the 9% maximum figure for this TDD in the right column.

If your correction boluses make up more than 9% of your TDD, ask your doctor how to shift the excess into your basal rates or carb boluses and prevent high readings. For example, if your average TDD is 40 units and you are using 5.6 units a day for correction boluses (3.6 units is 9% of this TDD), the extra 2 units can be moved into higher basal rates, larger carb boluses (smaller CarbF), or both.

To decide where to move the excess insulin in your correction boluses, check your basal/carb bolus balance. A typical balance, shown in Table 8.14, would be 40 to 55% basal and 36 to 51% carb boluses

13.8 Sample CorrF Adjustments

The CorrF adjustments below increase the size of correction boluses by 10% in the middle column and reduce them by 10% in the right column.

Current CorrF	Increase Corr Boluses by 10%	Reduce Corr Boluses by 10%
120 mg/dl	108 mg/dl	132 mg/dl
100 mg/dl	90 mg/dl	110 mg/dl
80 mg/dl	72 mg/dl	88 mg/dl
60 mg/dl	54 mg/dl	66 mg/dl
50 mg/dl	45 mg/dl	55 mg/dl
40 mg/dl	36 mg/dl	44 mg/dl
30 mg/dl	27 mg/dl	33 mg/dl
25 mg/dl	22 mg/dl	28 mg/dl
20 mg/dl	18 mg/dl	22 mg/dl
15 mg/dl	14 mg/dl	16 mg/dl
10 mg/dl	9 mg/dl	11 mg/dl

13.9 Test Your DIA Time

Once your basal rates keep your glucose flat when you are not eating and your CorrF is accurate from testing, you can test your DIA time to see how fast your insulin really works. Your DIA time and your CorrF can both be tested anytime your glucose is above 250 mg/dl (13.9 mmol/L) and it has been 5 or more hours since your last bolus and 3 or more hours since you last ate. Give the recommended correction bolus and check your glucose every 30 to 60 minutes (or watch it on a CGM) over the next 5 to 6 hours to see how long it takes for the high reading to return to target. Your DIA time is revealed when your glucose stops falling and becomes a flat line *without going low*. If your glucose goes low before 5 or 6 hours. Your correction bolus was too large

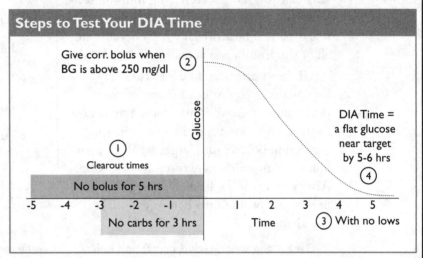

or your basal rate was too high. For a successful test, your glucose will reach 70 to 130 mg/dl (3.9 to 7.2 mmol/L) and not fall any further over the next 60 minutes. The time at which your glucose starts to stay flat is the DIA time to enter in your pump.

For example, if your pump DIA time is set to 3 hours, you should reach a glucose of 70 to 130 mg/dl (4.4 to 6.7 mmol/L) within 3 hours and not have your glucose fall any further over the next 90 minutes. If your glucose continues to fall after 3 hours, your DIA time is longer than 3 hours. Keep in mind that although insulin action has largely trailed off about 4 hours after a bolus, the glucose usually continues to fall at a slower rate from the trailing action of the bolus insulin. Your DIA includes this time. Repeat a successful test to verify it.   © 2013 Diabetes Services, Inc.

with the rest for corrections. If your basal rate total per day is less than what you give for carb boluses, you probably want to shift the excess in your correction boluses into higher basal rates. If the basal and carb bolus totals are similar, add half of the excess correction insulin to each.

If your readings are often higher at a particular time of day, add some or all of the excess in your correction boluses to the carb bolus or to the basal rates that are delivered before you typically go high. For example, if your readings usually rise after dinner and remain high at bedtime, raise your basal rate from the early or mid afternoon through the mid evening hours, or select a lower CarbF that starts in the afternoon to get larger carb boluses for dinner.

When calculating an average for your correction boluses, do not include those given for unusual circumstances. For instance, if you have been having infusion set problems, your correction boluses during this time will be artificially high because not all of this insulin was actually delivered.

Likewise, if your TDD is artificially high because you've needed lots of correction boluses to lower highs caused by overtreating lows, don't add the excess in your correction boluses into larger basals or carb boluses. This will only worsen the situation. **Always stop lows first.** Discuss with your health care professional before you make any changes.

13.10 Keep Corr. Boluses below 9%	
If Your TDD is:	Corr. Boluses Should Average No More Than:
10 u	0.9 u/day
20 u	1.8 u/day
30 u	2.7 u/day
40 u	3.6 u/day
50 u	4.5 u/day
60 u	5.4 u/day
70 u	6.3 u/day
80 u	7.2 u/day
90 u	8.4 u/day
100 u	9.0 u/day

Over a one week period, correction boluses generally make up 9% or less of your TDD. When correction boluses average more than 9%, move any excess above 9% into basal rates or carb boluses.

More about Correction Boluses

Don't assume everything is fine if your BC says that you don't need a correction bolus for a particular glucose. Instead, check out how much excess BOB is present. When your BOB happens to be larger than the correction bolus for your glucose, you may need to eat carbs to compensate for this excess BOB. To find the number of carb grams you need, check your BOB and multiply any units above what you need to correct your glucose by your CarbF (See Box 10.4 for details.).

If you gave a correction bolus 3 or more hours ago but your glucose is still as high or higher than when you gave the bolus, suspect that you have a delivery problem. Check for ketones and carefully consider whether you need to replace your infusion set.

Be Patient when Bringing Down Highs – Don't Overtreat

About 70% of the glucose-lowering impact from today's insulins is seen in the first 3 and half hours, but the remaining insulin activity will continue to taper off over another 2 to 3 hours. Be patient when you bring down high glucose readings. Don't take repeated correction boluses without considering how much BOB you have. If you desire a faster reduction in the glucose, carb and correction boluses can be combined as described later in this chapter, or a Super Bolus can be given, as shown in Fig. 12.12.

Don't stack insulin. If you had a high reading before a meal and are still high a couple of hours later, the remaining BOB from the combined carb and correction bolus taken earlier may be adequate. For example, if your reading was 225 mg/dl (12.5 mmol/L) before the meal and is now 250 mg/dl (12.9 mmol/L) 2 hours later, your reading will likely come down from your earlier combined bolus. A good rule of thumb is that if your glucose does not rise more than 40 mg/dl (2.2 mmol/L) about 2 hours after a meal for which you gave a combined carb and correction bolus, no additional correction bolus is likely needed.

> ### 13.11 Get Regular A1c Tests
>
> Have your A1c level tested every three to six months to evaluate your overall control. The A1c test provides an average of the last several weeks' glucose readings.[40] It reflects your control over the last 4 to 6 weeks and provides a good guide for whether you need to increase or occasionally decrease your TDD.

Not Every High Reading Is the Same – Circumstances Matter

The correction bolus you need to lower a high reading can be affected by more than just the glucose value. The bolus recommendation for a glucose of 360 mg/dl (20 mmol/L) will need to be adjusted at times for the circumstances that surround this high reading. For example, if you have a mid-morning reading of 360 mg/dl (20 mmol/L) and started with a normal reading before breakfast but forgot to take your bolus, taking the correction bolus recommended by your pump BC will be appropriate. The carbs eaten 2 hours earlier have typically already digested, so a carb bolus would not be taken for these missed carbs.

On the other hand, correction boluses need to be much larger than what your pump BC recommends if you are in ketoacidosis, have a bacterial infection, your infusion set got detached, you've started a steroid medication, or you just had a severe low that released lots of stress hormones and you overate. If your infusion set came out several hours ago and your blood or urine shows moderate or large ketone levels, you'll need a much larger bolus than your pump recommends, sometimes as much as 1 unit for every 2 lbs (1 kg) of body weight with large ketones. Ketoacidosis creates lots of resistance to insulin, plus you did not get any basal insulin for several hours.

But a correction bolus may not be needed at all if you simply had jelly on your finger when you checked your glucose. For any unexpected high reading, always start by washing your hands and rechecking your glucose.

What if Correction Boluses Often Don't Work?

If correction boluses don't consistently return you to your target 4 to 5 hours later, one or more of your BC settings is likely incorrect. The real source for frequent highs will be basal rates that are too low or a CarbF number that is too high. If your average meter

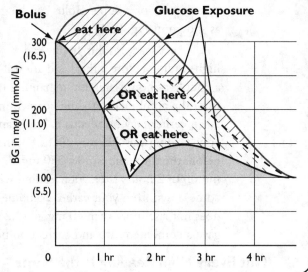

13.12 Delay Eating when High to Reduce Glucose Exposure

Rather than driving an already high glucose higher by eating a meal right away, delay eating when possible until your glucose gets closer to your target glucose.

Do not delay eating too long to avoid going low.

Do not try this if you might forget to eat or you have hypoglycemia unawareness.

glucose is above 160 mg/dl (8.9 mmol/L) or a recent A1c was above 7.5%, and correction boluses don't bring high readings down to your target:

- Check your basal/carb bolus balance. One or both is not providing enough insulin – usually the one that is smaller, or both if there is an equal balance.

- If correction boluses sometimes work for highs and other times do not, consider other factors like erratic delivery from your infusion sets (try a different brand and anchor the infusion line with tape), or episodes of stress or pain.

How to Combine a Carb and Correction Bolus

When your glucose is high before a meal, you want to take a carb plus correction bolus but avoid sending your glucose higher by eating right away.

Options to consider include:

1. Take a carb bolus plus correction bolus, but delay eating if possible when your glucose is above 150 mg/dl (8.3 mmol/L) before a meal. Enter your glucose reading and how many carbs you will eat into your pump, and take your BC recommendation. Wait to eat if you can until your glucose is below 150 mg/dl (8.3 mmol/L). (See Table 12.15 for estimated wait times.) Make sure you eat at the planned time and set an alarm to avoid any delay. Recheck your glucose within an hour to determine how the combined bolus is working or watch the trend line on your CGM.

2. If you can't wait to eat, take a correction bolus and eat a low carb meal with a smaller carb bolus.

3. Take your carb plus correction bolus and then eat any protein or low GI carbs first followed by any high GI carbs.

4. Give a Super Bolus that takes some basal insulin and delivers it immediately with the bolus. (See Fig. 12.12.)

Tips on Correction Doses

- An accurate CorrF lowers a high reading to within 30 mg/dl (1.7 mmol/L) of your target glucose within 5 hours without causing a low.

- If high readings often fail to come down to your glucose target after correction boluses, lower your CorrF by 10% (See Table 13.8.) to make correction boluses larger.

- If high glucose readings often go low after correction boluses, raise your CorrF by 10% or so (See Table 13.8.) to make correction boluses smaller.

- If you use more than one CorrF for different times during the day and they vary quite a bit, retest your basal rates to make sure they have been correctly set.

- To prevent night lows after treating high readings near bedtime, use a larger CorrF starting about 4 hours before bedtime to lessen this risk.

- If you have occasional unexplained highs, consider a problem with your infusion sets, a loose connection at the hub, bad insulin, an infection, or excess stress or pain.

- Anytime you have two unexplained high readings in a row, use a new bottle of insulin and change out your entire infusion set and reservoir from a new bottle before you correct the second high reading.

171

- When you lose weight or increase activity, your CarbF and CorrF will need to rise and your basal rates fall to get less insulin, and vice versa.
- When the TDD is too low, correction boluses start to make up a larger percentage of the TDD as they replace missing basal and carb bolus insulin. If your correction boluses make up more than 9% of your TDD, distribute the excess from your correction boluses into a higher basal rate or a lower CarbF (or both) to prevent the highs.

Don't treat lows with too many carbs or highs with too much insulin.

Experience teaches you to recognize a mistake when you've made it again.

Anon.

Pattern Management Secrets

Once you find your appropriate TDD and derive pump settings from it for better overall glucose control, pattern management becomes easier for making the fine adjustments needed in basal rates, bolus factors, and food choices. *A glucose pattern is any consistent repetition of high or low glucose readings at the same time of day.*

This chapter shows

- How to find and fix unwanted glucose patterns
- Common patterns and their solutions

Glucose monitoring is the first step to good control, but simply testing your glucose is not enough.[99] In the APP Study, pump users with the highest average glucose checked their glucose 4.0 times a day, nearly as often as those with the lowest average glucose who checked 4.7 times a day.[69] Your glucose will not improve until you or your doctor use your glucose results to make insulin and lifestyle adjustments.

Find Patterns

To find patterns, know where to look. Patterns may show up everyday, only on some days, or only in relation to a particular food or event. At least a week's worth of records are needed to spot most patterns. Regular meter testing and recording or wearing a CGM and downloading the data often reveals patterns. This analysis is critical to making the decisions that let you adjust your pumps settings and lifestyle. Check your meter or CGM records at regular intervals to get a clear picture of your patterns and to keep glucose readings in a desired range.

Your glucose patterns can only be seen when you carefully look at all your readings in front of you. A written record or device download of your readings is the easiest way to identify high and low patterns, and take steps to determine their cause.

How to Find and Fix Your Patterns

1. Select a glucose goal range or ranges that improve current readings. Select different ranges for before meals, after meals, at bedtime, and in the middle of the night.

2. Check your glucose at least 5 to 7 times a day or wear a CGM.

3. Record or download your readings. The last 30 days help you find long-term patterns, while the last 7 to 14 days let you see recent dose or lifestyle changes.

14.1 The Path to Better Control

- Monitor glucoses frequently (or wear a CGM), match boluses to your carbs and current glucose, bolus for every meal and snack (unless there's a good reason not to do so), and don't overtreat lows with carbs or highs with insulin.

- Stop frequent lows first. Lower your TDD by 5% for frequent, mild lows or by 10% for frequent, severe lows.

- Find an improved TDD (iTDD) from your A1c or average glucose (Table 10.3).

- Get new pump settings from this iTDD (Table 9.5).

- Adjust these starting settings with testing and pattern analysis (Chapters 11-14).

- Keep your average basal rate and carb bolus totals balanced, and compare your insulin use with that of pump wearers in excellent control (Workspace 8.14).

- Keep correction boluses at or below 9% of your TDD (Chapter 13).

- If control issues arise, double check your current pump settings against the optimal values for your TDD (Table 9.5).

- Use a DIA time of 4.5 hours or longer to minimize insulin stacking.

Use doses that give you good control, no matter what best practices may be.

© 2013 Diabetes Services,.Inc.

4. Mark all readings above or below your goals. Make your lows and highs easy to spot by highlighting each with a different color or shape. Record EVERY low you have, whether a meter reading was done or not, to review with your doctor.

5. Use *Smart Charts* in Fig. 5.6 or the *Enhanced Logbook* in Fig. 5.7 to count how many readings are below, within, and above your goal range at each time of day.

6. Over time, try to get 5 out of 7 of each week's readings into your glucose goal range at each time of day.

To find out why glucoses are too high or too low, log events in your meter or CGM so you remember what caused them. For context, add notes about missed insulin, certain foods, illness, menses, stress and exercise on the computer download.

Bring a record of your readings, food, exercise, stress, and basal/bolus doses to all clinic visits, so your physician or diabetes educator can help you eliminate unwanted patterns. You'll get better advice if you take the initiative and have your records ready to analyze. If you don't do this, he/she won't be able to see your glucose patterns and make the insulin adjustments you need. Of course, don't guesstimate or make up any readings.

If you can't download meter, CGM, and pump data, hit your meter's recall button and write down each glucose and the time and date it was checked for at least the last 14 days into Table 14.13 at the end of this chapter. Then transfer these meter readings to a copy of the *Enhanced Logbook* in Fig. 5.7 or to a standard logbook so you can see at what time of day you have control issues. Add any details you remember about particular highs and lows.

Review your readings each week. Change one basal rate or bolus setting at a time until an unwanted pattern improves. Usually, you want to wait 3 to 4 days after a bolus adjustment and 5 to 7 days after a basal adjustment to see if this change corrects the unwanted pattern before you make another adjustment. Particular events like exercise or a particular food may cause unusual readings, so pay attention to these using *Smart Charts*, a phone app, etc.

> ### 14.2 Good Control Is Possible if You:
> - Are motivated
> - Are educated in diabetes management
> - Have appropriate pump settings
> - Receive good feedback through glucose monitoring
>
> From Dr. Robert Tattersall: **Workshop On Home Monitoring of Blood Glucose**, Nottingham Univ., 1980.

When glucoses are out of range, look for patterns that happen most of the time, such as three out of four or five days. You may also see a single occurrence out of range. Circle the highs on the printouts of the reports in one color and the lows in another. Lows are eliminated first because they have more immediate danger.

Fix Your Patterns

Analyze data in order of importance: overnight glucose patterns first, then pre-meal readings, and finally post-meal readings. Look for when the greatest number of glucoses is out of your target range, look for reasons, and make changes to bring them back in.

Things that Make Your Glucose Go High and Low:

1. When boluses are being missed for meals or snacks, this shows up as unusually high glucose spikes after a meal. Here, the high glucose will come down about 4 to 5 hours after a correction bolus is given. If the high reading does not come down, suspect an infusion set or other problem.

2. Certain foods, illness, menses or stress can all cause high readings. For example, if you spike every time you eat a food or on days you are stressed, your records will gradually show the connection. Glucoses often vary around a woman's menses. Putting comments into a logbook or applet lets you connect these occasional causes for highs.

3. Watch for lows-to-highs where a low glucose is followed shortly later by a high reading. These can be easily eliminated by not over-treating lows. Highs-to-lows can be corrected with a higher CorrF number or a longer DIA time.

4. Track your exercise and activity. Low glucose levels can occur during, immediately after, and several hours later. Later lows may show up that evening, during the night, and even the next day with more vigorous activity.

14.3 Questions to Ask when You Cannot See a Pattern

If you're on a roller coaster, put your thinking cap on and answer these questions. Deal with issues checked "yes" or "unsure" to get more consistent readings.

Are you:	Yes	No	Unsure
skipping meal boluses?	☐	☐	☐
taking boluses just before or after eating?	☐	☐	☐
not counting or measuring your carbs accurately?	☐	☐	☐
having frequent or severe low blood glucoses?	☐	☐	☐
having excess lows due to fear of complications?	☐	☐	☐
excessively afraid of having a low?	☐	☐	☐
skipping meals?	☐	☐	☐
not exercising?	☐	☐	☐
changing insulin doses a lot from day to day?	☐	☐	☐
not changing infusion set often enough?	☐	☐	☐
exercising at different times, intensities, or durations?	☐	☐	☐
sleeping at irregular hours?	☐	☐	☐
under stress?	☐	☐	☐
experiencing pain?	☐	☐	☐
ill, have an infection, or have other significant change?	☐	☐	☐

5. Patterns caused by incorrect pump settings often create consistent patterns of highs or lows at a particular time of day, or on pie charts as larger slices of highs or lows at that time of day. Adjust your basals or CarbF about 5 to 6 hours before the highs or lows occur.

Consider changes to your insulin doses, timing, food choices, lifestyle or behavior. For example, if your breakfast carbs vary from 30 grams to 90 grams but you always take a 5 unit bolus to cover them, it is easy to see why your lunch readings would be erratic. You might want to have a consistent number of carbs for breakfast or start to base your breakfast bolus on the actual grams of carb you eat. Try a temp basal increase for short-term issues like illness, stress or menses.

Common Glucose Patterns

It takes experience and trial and error to see and correct unwanted glucose patterns. It helps to use software and to write down readings outside your goals. Get your doctor or nurse educator's help if you can't seem to find patterns. Ask a family member or friend whose judgment you respect to review them with you for suggestions. Keep at it. Over time, your ability to see and correct patterns will improve.

Find any pattern of frequent lows and correct these first. Then identify other patterns that best match yours in the pages that follow. Make one of the suggested changes to improve or eliminate that pattern. Discuss with your doctor or nurse educator if you have any questions.

No Pattern

If there really is no pattern among your highs and lows, this is often caused by the wrong TDD or pump setting errors. The first thing to do is to double-check how you are currently using your insulin and how your current pump settings compare to the optimal settings for your TDD in Workspace 8.14. This often brings up ideas for basal or bolus changes to try.

If you think something else is involved, see Workspace 14.3 for some possibilities.

Frequent Lows

Stop frequent lows first because they can be dangerous. Stopping lows tends to reduce many rebound highs caused by stress hormone release and overtreatment.

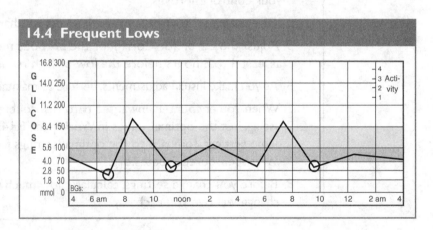

Lows that happen at about the same time each day can be eliminated with appropriate basal or bolus adjustments. Select a limit for how low your glucose can go with your physician for your age and any history of hypoglycemic seizures or hypoglycemia unawareness.

Frequent lows at varied times of day strongly suggests you need a lower TDD. Decrease your TDD by 5% for frequent mild and moderate lows, such as going below 70 or 65 mg/dl (3.9 or 3.6 mmol/L) nearly every day. Decrease your TDD by 10% for frequent moderate and severe lows, such as going below 50 mg/dl (2.8 mmol/L) every 2 or 3 days, as shown in Table 10.2. Review specific pump setting adjustments with your physician. It is sometimes better to find new pump settings directly from Table 9.5 using a smaller TDD.

14.5 Adjustment Tips

Always address the source of glucose problems. For instance, high readings before the evening meal can be caused by a basal rate that is too low from mid-morning through the afternoon, by a lunch CarbF that is too high, by not counting all of the carbs eaten at lunch, by eating white rice for lunch, or by missed boluses at lunch or in the afternoon.

To get rid of lows, basal rates go down, while the CarbF or CorrF goes up. To get rid of highs, the basal rates go up, while the CarbF or CorrF goes down. Develop a plan but always ask your doctor for advice if you are unsure about what to do.

Rules for Making Insulin Adjustments

1. Make one dose change at a time.

2. Start with the smallest change that seems likely to help. If your readings are relatively steady and close to your target range, a small change in your basal rates or boluses should be sufficient. CarbFs are usually changed by one point or less, CorrFs by three to ten points, and basal rates by 0.025 to 0.1 u/hr for a few hours. Frequent or severe lows or highs may require larger changes.

3. Adjust basal rates every 7 days and adjust bolus factors every 4 days until your control improves.

4. Give changes 3 to 7 days to work unless you have lows after the change.

5. Adjust the CarbF (or CorrF) for the previous meal or adjust your basal rates at least 4 to 8 hours before the low or high reading you want to avoid happens.

6. As you make insulin adjustments, be sure to maintain your basal/carb bolus balance.

7. When you encounter unwanted patterns, double-check your current insulin use against the optimal values in Workspace 8.14. Also check how your current pump settings compare to the optimal settings for your TDD in Table 9.5 or at www.opensourcediabetes.org.

8. Before you change settings, calculate how much more or less insulin that change will give you each day.

© 2013 Diabetes Services, Inc.

Frequent Breakfast Lows

Frequent breakfast lows, as well as frequent lows that occur within a 3 hour period before breakfast, are usually caused by an overnight basal rate that is too high. If these lows are occasional and mild, a small basal reduction should eliminate them, while for frequent and stronger lows a larger reduction will be needed. See Table 11.7 for suggestions on how much the basal change will lower your insulin dose. Be sure to check some middle of the night readings or wear a CGM to find out when these lows begin. Most people do not wake up when they first go low and may already have been low for several hours without knowing it. A *basal test* is the best way to reset the basal rates.

Frequent Highs and Lows

Frequent highs and frequent lows usually indicate that the TDD is too high. Try lowering your TDD as described above for frequent lows. One exception to this is when lows are being caused by a short DIA (hidden insulin stacking) or by excessive correction boluses caused by a CorrF number that is too low or when correction boluses are being raised above the BC's recommended dose,

Frequent Highs

Frequent highs at different times of day are a common problem in diabetes and a sure sign that you need to raise your TDD, unless instead you need to stop

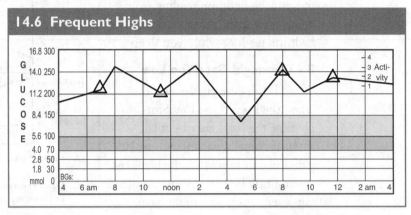

14.6 Frequent Highs

indulging on so many sugared sodas and sweets. If the average glucose in your meter is above your glucose goal, review your diet and whether you are covering all the carbs you eat with adequate boluses. Be sure your carb counts are accurate and take a carb bolus for every meal and snack. Identify whether it is your lifestyle or insulin doses or both that need to change.

Check your basal/carb bolus balance. Increase your basal rates or carb boluses (lower CarbF) depending on which is lower. Increase both if they are about equal. For each 6 mg/dl drop desired in the average glucose, add 1% to the TDD. For example, if your current average meter glucose is 220 mg/dl with few lows, and you want to lower it to 160 mg/dl, you would increase your TDD by 10% for a 60 mg/dl drop in average glucose.

Breakfast Highs

The breakfast glucose is the most important one of the day to control. If it is high, it directly affects your A1c because it has likely been high for at least a several hours during the night and often remains high into the late morning or early afternoon hours. When your readings stay flat overnight and you wake up with a normal reading, the rest of the day is easier to control. If other unwanted patterns appear, they become easier to fix.

Fig. 14.7 shows patterns that lead to high breakfast readings and their causes.

A – Already High at Bedtime

Always fix the bedtime high first if that's the cause for high breakfast readings. Find where your daytime glucose is highest and increase insulin doses there. If you have been giving full correction boluses for bedtime highs, but the glucose did not come down during the night, the bedtime CorrF may be too weak and needs to be lowered or the overnight basal is too low and need to be raised. If you are concerned about night lows and have not been giving full correction boluses at bedtime, reconsider this, keeping in mind that it is often easier to prevent the bedtime reading from being high than it is to fix a high bedtime reading while you sleep.

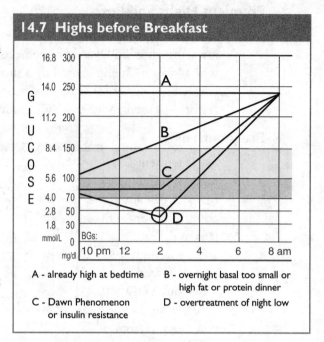

B – Overnight Basal Too Low

The glucose rises overnight when the basal is too low. Simply raise the basal rates by small amounts, usually starting at 8 to 10 p.m. Keep in mind that the breakfast reading may be OK on some mornings even with a low night basal if correction boluses are given at bedtime or during the night. Do a night basal test if you are not sure of the basal.

C – Dawn Phenomenon/Insulin Resistance

In someone without diabetes, a low insulin level reflects the fact that the glucose is also low. The liver does not read glucose levels but does read the insulin level and will respond when insulin is low by making and releasing glucose into the blood. Unfortunately, when the insulin level is low in someone with diabetes, the liver makes glucose even though the glucose is already high.

Once the liver starts producing extra glucose, whether due to a Dawn Phenomenon in Type 1 diabetes or a rise in insulin resistance during the early hours in Type 2 diabetes, larger than normal correction boluses are needed to lower the high breakfast reading.

Make sure your night basal rates are correctly set to stop the liver from releasing glucose during the night. With a Dawn Phenomenon in teens and young adults, the basal rates may need to be raised at 1 or 2 am. Insulin resistance with Type 2 diabetes or the presence of abdominal obesity in Type 1 diabetes often requires a similar rise in basal rates to stop excess glucose production and release by the liver. The earlier the basal is raised, the smaller this increase needs to be. Metformin, a medicine that specifically blocks excess glucose production by the liver is helpful in these situations. Talk with your doctor if you think you might benefit from metformin.

D – Over-treatment of Night Lows

Occasional morning highs will be seen if someone awakes during the night with a low glucose and overeats. This pattern is easy to spot because the night low is usually followed by a breakfast high. Other breakfast readings are normal or at least lower.

Find the letter below that best describes when your glucose goes high or low, then look at that letter below that has suggested fixes.

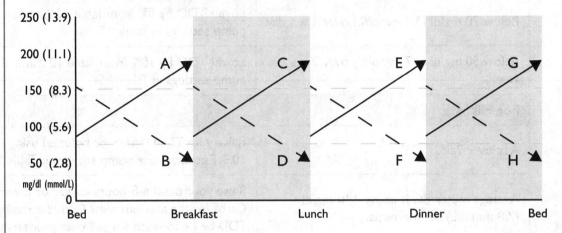

A) Raise your overnight basal rate if your reading usually rises overnight. Raise it 2 hrs before the glucose begins to rise. (Go to G or H if your bedtime glucose is usually high or low.)

B) Lower your overnight basal rate(s) if your reading usually falls overnight. Decrease it about 2 hours before the fall begins.

C) Lower your breakfast CarbF OR raise your basal from before breakfast through mid morning.

D) Raise your breakfast CarbF OR lower your basal from before breakfast through mid morning.

E) Lower your lunch CarbF OR raise your basal from before lunch through mid afternoon.

F) Raise your lunch CarbF OR lower your basal from before lunch through mid afternoon.

G) Lower your dinner CarbF OR raise your basal from before dinner through mid evening. Consider whether after-dinner snacks may be causing the rise.

H) Raise your dinner CarbF OR lower your basal from before dinner through mid evening.

For regular patterns of lows or highs, add up the total bolus units that were active in the previous 6 hours and compare this to the total basal insulin delivered during these 6 hours (6 x your hourly basal rate). To prevent lows, you will usually want to lower the one that is larger. To prevent highs, you will usually raise the one that is smaller.

For example, Leonard took 8 units for lunch and his basal rate was 1.0 u/hr through the morning and afternoon, or 6 units over 6 hours. For lows near dinner, he could lower his 8 unit lunch bolus, while for pre-dinner highs, he might raise his basal rate around 10 am.

14.9 Fixes to Try for Glucose Patterns You Don't Want

For Lows	What to Do:
Below 70 mg/dl (3.8 mmol/L) over 1 x a day.	Lower TDD by 5% from Table 10.2 and check pump settings in Table 9.5.
Below 50 mg/dl (2.7 mmol/L) over 2 x a week.	Lower TDD by 10% from Table 10.2 and check pump settings in Table 9.5.
For Highs	
A1c over 7.5%.	Raise your TDD (basals or boluses) using Table 10.3. Recheck your pump settings in Table 9.5.
Average meter BG is above 140 mg/dl (7.8 mmol/L) before meals.	Raise your basal 4-8 hours earlier or lower your CarbF for the previous meal. Consider raising your TDD by 1% for each 6 mg/dl over your target.
Average meter BG is above 150 mg/dl (8.3 mmol/L) with few lows	Raise your TDD using Table 10.3 and recheck pump settings in Table 9.5.
BG often rise more than 80 mg/dl (4.4 mmol/L) after meals and still high at 4 hrs.	Bolus earlier, lower your CarbF number, eat different or fewer carbs, add lower GI foods.
Correction boluses average over 9% of TDD.	Shift excess over 9% into basals or carb boluses.
Unexplained highs.	Check infusion set and site. Consider bad insulin.
For Readings that Vary	
BG readings vary but have no pattern	Lower TDD, recount carbs, check infusion site, make lifestyle consistent, take bolus for every bite.
Regular highs or lows at a particular time of day, such as high readings before breakfast	Adjust basal rates or CarbF from Table 9.5 and review fixes in Table 14.8.
High or low readings after a particular food like pizza or cereal	Recheck carb count, adjust carb bolus for that food, or try different type of bolus (combo, etc.).
High or low readings after eating out	Recheck carb count, adjust bolus next time

To lower TDD, check basal/carb-bolus balance and reduce the larger one, or both if equal.
To raise TDD, check basal/carb-bolus balance and increase the smaller one, or both if equal.

Make a record of all night lows, not just the ones for which you do a fingerstick, so your doctor knows why the high breakfast readings are happening.

Lows or Highs at About the Same Time of Day

When lows or highs often happen at about the same time before lunch, before dinner, or at bedtime, look for that pattern in Table 14.8 and try one of the fixes that is suggested. Look for the time of day when your glucose has its largest fall or rise out of your goal range and work on that pattern first. For example, if your glucose rises about 60 mg/dl (3.3 mmol/L) between breakfast and lunch, and another 40 mg/dl (2.2 mmol/L) between lunch and dinner, fix the after breakfast rise first.

Lows to Highs

If your glucose rises above 150 mg/dl (8.3 mmol/L) only an hour or two after a low, eating too many carbs is the likely cause. The fear, confusion, and extreme hunger that accompany a low can make emptying the refrigerator seem quite sane. Overeating, however, only makes the glucose go sky-high for hours afterward. Stress hormone release, indicated by sweating and shaking, tends to raise the glucose over a several hours, but by itself will not cause a rapid rise from 36 to 329 mg/dl (2.0 to 18.3 mmol/L) over a two hour period as shown in Fig. 14.10.

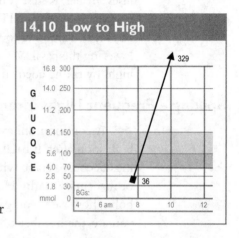

Be patient any time you treat a low. Fast carbs take 20 to 30 minutes to raise the glucose. Release of fight or flight hormones during a low makes you ravenous much longer than this. Use glucose tablets or fast-acting carbs for lows to bring your brain back quickly. Even in the panic of a low, it is harder to overdose on glucose tabs than it is on cookies or candy bars. One gram of carbohydrate raises the glucose by three to five points for most adults, so only 10 to 20 grams of quick carbohydrate is typically needed to stop most lows.

Once your thinking has sufficiently cleared, check your BOB and eat enough slower carbs to cover this active insulin. More than 15 to 20 grams is usually needed when you have residual BOB, or if a recent increase in activity caused the low.

If you overeat for a low, count how many grams of carb you actually ate. Enter these carbs and your low glucose into your pump BC to calculate the bolus you need to cover the extra carbs. Taking a bolus may seem strange when you are low, but it's exactly what is needed to cover the excess carbs and prevent a high reading later. Check your glucose a couple of hours later to ensure your bolus was correct.

Do not skip your bolus for the next meal after a low! It does nothing for the previous low. It just makes your next reading high and puts you on a roller coaster. Instead, look at what caused the low and fix that.

Highs to Lows

If you often plummet from a high to a low glucose within 4 or 5 hours after giving correction boluses, as shown in the Fig 14.11, your correction boluses are too large.

Make sure your DIA is set to at least 4.5 hours to eliminate hidden insulin stacking and don't give larger correction boluses than your pump BC recommends. If this doesn't work, raise your CorrF to make your correction boluses smaller. Retest your basal rates if they make up over 55% of your TDD in case an excessive basal is contributing to the lows and consider lowering the basal. Make sure to avoid post-meal highs by taking adequate carb boluses.

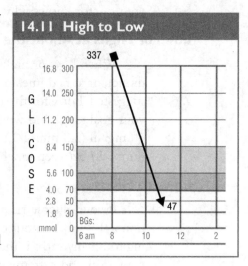

Spiking – Frequent Highs after Meals

A common, annoying pattern is to have a normal glucose before eating and go high soon after. If basal testing has verified your basal rates are accurate but your readings become erratic when you eat, the problem likely arises from inaccurate carb counts or inaccurate CarbF. How high your glucose rises after eating depends on the size of the bolus, how early you gave it before you ate, the number of carbs, your activity level after the meal, the food's glycemic index, and whether you missed a carb bolus. Compare the glucose patterns in Fig. 14.12 for help in identifying these.

A – Missed Carb Bolus

Line A in Fig. 14.12 shows a typical pattern when a carb bolus is not taken for a meal. Forgetting to take a bolus is hopefully rare, but if you sometimes forget boluses, set a time alarm in the pump to remind you or wear a wristwatch with alarms to remind you to bolus for meals.

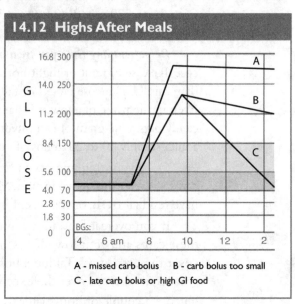

A - missed carb bolus   B - carb bolus too small
C - late carb bolus or high GI food

If you are unsure whether a bolus was actually given for a recent meal or snack, check your pump history to confirm.

B – Carb Bolus Too Small

Line B shows a pattern when the carb bolus for a meal is too small for the number of carbs eaten. This happens when carbs are not counted or inaccurately counted, when portions are not measured, when snacks are not fully covered, when there is hesitation to cover carbs due to a fear of hypoglycemia, or when the CarbF number is too large. Even if you usually count carbs accurately at home, you may misjudge carb boluses for meals that are eaten out. Casseroles and combination food are difficult to count also.

Learn carb counting. The time spent on this will benefit you day after day. If you already practice carb counting, double-check your counts periodically. Review Chapter 3 to be sure you have a good understanding of this excellent tool. Learning to quantify the effect that foods have on your glucose becomes invaluable to your control over time.

Skimping on the insulin you need only generates unwanted highs. When a reading goes high after a meal, many people think, "I shouldn't have eaten so much." This assessment may be accurate and if it is, eating less can be a good choice. But if the carbs eaten were not excessive or you will eat the same thing again, a wise decision may be: "Next time I'll bolus enough insulin to cover those carbs!" Make sure you are getting adequate carb boluses to stop any post-meal highs, usually at least 40% of your TDD.

Retest your CarbF to ensure that your carb boluses are matched to the carbs in your meals. If a CarbF number is too high, it can work for small carb meals but leads to highs when a large amount of carbs is eaten. You may want to eat the same meals with known carb counts until you find a CarbF that works.

Many restaurants have nutritional information available to guide your bolus doses. Pay attention to meals that consistently cause high readings so you can choose a larger bolus to match the carbs when you later reorder the same meal. You may want to create a personal list of restaurant meals with their accompanying insulin doses to make post-meal readings more reliable. With this list in your pocket or purse, you can eat out with far more enjoyment. Mark meals where a mismatch occurs so you can better match your bolus next time. Table 12.19 provides a way to estimate how much insulin you missed in your last carbs bolus when your reading is still high about 4 hours later.

C – Late Bolus or High GI Food

Bolusing early to better match today's relatively slow insulins to your faster digestion is one of the best-kept secrets to control. If your glucose spikes between meals but is usually back to normal before the next meal, bolus earlier, switch some high glycemic index foods to low GI ones, or talk with your doctor about different medications that stop post-meal spiking.

To reduce problems caused by inaccurate carb counts or poor bolus timing, check your glucose before, two hours and four hours after meals. Record your readings for a week or two to find out whether high and low readings relate to particular meals.

Summary

Don't avoid checking or reviewing your readings because you fear a reminder of how bad things are. Trust in your own ability to tackle any glucose problem you are having. Readings outside your target range present a learning opportunity. Pretend your readings belong to someone else or consider improved readings as a game to play. Share your records with friends, family members, your accountant, your math teacher – anyone who can help you spot your patterns and make needed changes.

For control problems, check your pump's history to see how the percentages of your basal rates, carb boluses, and correction boluses compare to the optimal percentages for each found in Workspace 8.14. Also compare your CarbF and CorrF settings against the optimal settings for your TDD in Table 9.5. Discuss your current TDD and basal/bolus balance with your physician if you have any questions

Easy street is a blind alley.

Anon.

14.13 Download Your Meter's Memory

Write down each glucose test, its time, and your 14 day avg. BG from your meter. Transfer to a logbook to find patterns.

14 day avg. = _____ mg/dl(mmol/L)   # tests = _____

Date	Time	Glucose
___/___/___	_____ am/pm	_____ mg/dl (mmol/L)
___/___/___	_____ am/pm	_____ mg/dl (mmol/L)
___/___/___	_____ am/pm	_____ mg/dl (mmol/L)
___/___/___	_____ am/pm	_____ mg/dl (mmol/L)
___/___/___	_____ am/pm	_____ mg/dl (mmol/L)
___/___/___	_____ am/pm	_____ mg/dl (mmol/L)
___/___/___	_____ am/pm	_____ mg/dl (mmol/L)
___/___/___	_____ am/pm	_____ mg/dl (mmol/L)
___/___/___	_____ am/pm	_____ mg/dl (mmol/L)
___/___/___	_____ am/pm	_____ mg/dl (mmol/L)
___/___/___	_____ am/pm	_____ mg/dl (mmol/L)
___/___/___	_____ am/pm	_____ mg/dl (mmol/L)
___/___/___	_____ am/pm	_____ mg/dl (mmol/L)
___/___/___	_____ am/pm	_____ mg/dl (mmol/L)
___/___/___	_____ am/pm	_____ mg/dl (mmol/L)
___/___/___	_____ am/pm	_____ mg/dl (mmol/L)
___/___/___	_____ am/pm	_____ mg/dl (mmol/L)
___/___/___	_____ am/pm	_____ mg/dl (mmol/L)
___/___/___	_____ am/pm	_____ mg/dl (mmol/L)

Unexplained Highs? — Check for a Pump Problem

15

When unexpected high glucoses occur, most pumpers automatically blame themselves for eating too many carbs. Although excess carbs can certainly cause highs, keep in mind that your pump may be the real source for these high readings.

Pump problems can originate from an insulin leak at the infusion site, infusion line, hub connection, or between the O-rings in the reservoir. It may also come from a pump programming error or defective insulin. A pump and any part of the insulin delivery system can fail and result in a high glucose. In these situations, immediate attention must be directed at finding and solving the real cause for the high readings.

If you've been told you have "poor absorption," "scarring," or that you have "bad sites," you may want to look for is a more reliable infusion set. Set problems are a frequent source for unexplained highs that often last 10 to 36 hours on a pump downloads but disappear when the set is changed. Giving another bolus from the pump will not correct the problem. Always give an injection from a new bottle of insulin or a pen to get the glucose under control before you start your detective work.

In this chapter, we will troubleshoot

- Clogs
- Leaks
- Tunneling of insulin

Is a Pump Problem Causing Highs?

The first sign of a pump problem is usually an unexplained high glucose that goes up gradually or quickly, depending on how much insulin is being lost. The rise usually begins a couple of hours after delivery is interrupted. A complete interruption of delivery causes ketone levels to rise at 0.2 mmol/L or more per hour. After 3 hours or so, blood ketone levels may rise above normal levels of 0.5 mmol/L, as shown in Table 16.6, and moderate blood ketone levels (1.5 mmol/L or higher) can be seen after 5 to 8 hours.

187

If your glucose is unexpectedly high on two consecutive glucose tests, check for ketones as described in the next chapter. If ketone levels are moderate or large, either your insulin is not being delivered or you have a serious medical problem underway. With an insulin delivery problem, both basal and bolus insulin delivery has been interrupted, so a larger correction bolus than that recommended by your BC will be needed. Take an injection to lower your reading before you start to troubleshoot the pump.

When an unexpected high glucose occurs, keep site problems, mechanical problems, and bad insulin in mind as possible causes. Pumps have audible alarms designed to alert you if there is a clog or blockage.

However, other problems like a displaced infusion set or bad insulin **will not sound an alarm**. If bad insulin is causing high readings, open a new bottle to fill the reservoir. Box 15.5 describes how to detect bad insulin in the insulin bottle.

Steps to Troubleshoot Unexplained Highs

Pump problems need to be corrected quickly. Be familiar with your pump to check and correct problems efficiently. When the first unexplained high glucose occurs, give a correction bolus. If a second unexplained high occurs, check the blood (or urine) for ketones. *If ketones are moderate or large, give an injection by syringe.* This injection will need to larger than that recommended by your pump to also replace the missing basal insulin and to overcome the insulin resistance found in the ketotic state. See Table 16.6 for suggested doses.

Check at the infusion site and work back to the pump for delivery problems:

1. Check whether the infusion set is displaced or loose

2. Feel around the site for a lump caused by bleeding under the skin or an infection

3. Look for blood in the line (a good sign of bleeding under the skin)

4. Check for air in the infusion line

5. Look for damage to the infusion line, then run the entire line between your fingers and smell them for an insulin leak (Box 15.2)

6. Check that the hub is firmly attached to the reservoir (smell for an insulin leak)

7. Look for a leak between the O-rings in the reservoir if they are visible

8. Consider bad insulin (Box 15.5)

After the injection is given, replace the reservoir and insert a new infusion set right away at a new site, using a new bottle of insulin.

Clogs and Blockages

A clog or blockage in the infusion line rarely occurs. Some causes are easily seen, while others take time to solve. A complete clog or a partial blockage often occurs when a Teflon infusion set gets kinked, bad insulin is used, or there are defects in plastic within the infusion line. If you see a speck or particle in your insulin vial, your insulin is likely to clog and won't work well in your pump. (See Box 15.5.)

Novolog® (aspart) and Humalog® (lispro) may be *slightly* less likely form a clog than Apidra® (glulisine). Under stress conditions, 24 insulin pumps randomly switched between the three insulins, a low basal of 0.1 u/hr was run at 93° F (34° C) with 3 boluses of 2.0 units given 3 times a day in each pump. Over 5 days of stress testing, 9.2% of the lines occluded with Novolog®, 15.7% with Humalog®, and 40.9% with Apidra® insulin.[100]

Insulin can interact with any defect or change in the interior of an infusion line and cause a clog. Foreign materials like betadine or alcohol that contact the reservoir or infusion line can cause a clog or blockage. Hand lotions, hair sprays, or solvents on your hands, skin, clothing, or in the air may penetrate the infusion tubing and cause this problem.

Insulin is a protein, just like an egg white, that needs to be kept away from heat and sunlight. If your tubing comes in contact with very hot water, such as in a steaming shower or hot tub, heat may coagulate the insulin. It is wise to disconnect and take the pump and tubing away before coming in contact with very hot water to avoid this problem.

Pumps have sensors that detect clogs so an alarm should sound once a unit or two is not delivered. A medium or large bolus will trigger an occlusion alarm quickly but if only basal insulin is being delivered, it will take longer for pressure to build in the line and trigger an alarm. With a low basal rate, this delay could be several hours. The glucose may already be high by the time the alarm sounds.

Most common sign of a clog or blockage: an alarm or a high glucose.

15.1 Clogs and Blockages

Problem	Causes	Solutions
Clogs occur when insulin comes out of solution and crystallizes, usually near the end of the infusion line or in the Teflon cannula.	This may be caused by a bad lot of infusion sets, a kinked Teflon cannula, bad insulin, heat or sunlight on the line, or when hair spray, hand lotion, or solvent contacts the infusion line.	Remove the Teflon catheter or metal needle and give a 5 unit bolus. If insulin comes out easily, a clog is not the cause of the high. If no insulin comes out, a clog is present. Fill a new reservoir with insulin from a new bottle, and replace the infusion set.

Will Pump Alarm? Only after a Complete Clog or Blockage Occurs

Leaks

If insulin leaks from your reservoir or infusion set, it will usually evaporate quickly and be difficult to see or feel unless you use a large bolus. *Unfortunately, your pump cannot warn you that you have a leak.*

Insulin has a distinctive smell, as described in Box 15.2. A good way to detect a leak is to run your fingers along the line from the hum to infusion set. Then smell your fingers for insulin. If your sense of smell is weak, ask someone else to do this. A leak between the O-rings at the back of some reservoirs cannot be smelled but can often be seen (see Fig. 7.5). The infusion set can detach partially or completely and leak insulin. A partial detachment is usually difficult to see. Fortunately, leaks tend to be rare when the user's setup technique is good.

> ### 15.2 The Smell of Insulin
>
> Insulin has a distinctive smell derived from m-creosol and phenol that help stabilize the insulin molecule and also act as anti-bacterial agents. The odor is often described as smelling like creosote, railroad ties, or Band Aids. If you smell an odor like this, look for an insulin leak.

Most common sign of a leak: a high glucose.

How to Check for Clogs or Leaks

After two unexplained high glucoses in a row, check for ketones, and give an injection if needed. Then remove the Teflon catheter or metal needle and follow these steps:

- To check for clogs, give 5 units as a "fill tubing" after removing the infusion set. (This does not create any BOB as a bolus would.) If insulin appears immediately at the tip, there is no clog. If no insulin appears at the tip, the infusion set is clogged and the 5 units should trigger a high-pressure alarm.
- If there is no clog, check the infusion line, hub, or O-rings for leaks. Look and smell for insulin at the hub, along the infusion line, and between the O-rings.
- If neither a clog nor leak is present, replace the infusion set and consider other causes.

Tunneling of Insulin

Another cause for unexplained highs is *tunneling*. Insulin that is infused beneath the skin leaks back to the skin surface along a path around the cannula. When you slide the needle of an infusion set through the skin, the surrounding tissue becomes mildly inflamed and swollen. As time passes, the tissues around the Teflon or metal needle heal.

This healing process may allow a small path to form along the length of the Teflon tubing under the skin. If the set is moved during a game of golf or tennis, or an unanchored infusion line is tugged, insulin delivered at the infusion tip may leak back to the surface of the skin. Control will be impossible with this infusion set and it must be changed.

Tunneling is more common with Teflon infusion sets that go straight in and have a shorter length than slanted Teflon sets. Straight-in sets also cover their entry point, so any leakage of insulin back to the skin surface cannot be seen. When tunneling occurs with

15.3 Leaks and Detached Sets

Problem	Causes	Solutions
Infusion Site		
Infusion set partially or completely detaches.	Set gets loose from sweat or tugs, infusion line not taped down, problem during insertion.	Replace the infusion set. Use good technique and tape the line down. Switch to a different brand of set if problem continues.
O-Rings		
Seal between the O-rings and reservoir wall is bad and lets insulin leak backward.	When reservoirs sit in a pharmacy, O-ring lubricant pools at the bottom of the reservoir.	Use a new reservoir and relubricate the O-rings (Box 7.5) before drawing up insulin. Take care inserting reservoir into the pump.
Hub		
Insulin leak starts when infusion line hub is not tight in the reservoir, or overtightened, cracking the hub.	Occurs when tightentened with a weak or excessive grip, or when not paying attention to twisting the hub.	Look for fluid around the hub. Check for the smell of insulin and a crack in the hub. If hub feels loose, retighten it using small pliers if needed.
Line		
A break in the line has occurred.	Infusion line can be damaged by pets, sharp objects, or rarely as a manufacturing defect.	Feel and look for damage along the infusion line. After giving a bolus, check for any insulin along the line. Replace the infusion set.
Will Pump Alarm? Not Yet.		

slanted Teflon sets, a drop of insulin will occasionally be visible around the set's entry point after a large bolus. Tunneling also can happen with metal needles but is rare.

If your infusion set causes unexplained highs, switch to a different type or brand.

Most common sign of tunneling: a high glucose.

Don't Leave an Infusion Set in Too Long

Another cause of high glucoses is leaving your infusion set in too long. When an infusion set is left in longer than three days, it may loosen and allow tunneling to occur

15.4 Tunneling		
Information	**Causes**	**Solutions**
Glucose rises if insulin leaks from the end of a cannula or metal needle back to the skin. More common in 90 degree Teflon cannulas when no tape is used to anchor the infusion line, especially after activities like golf or tennis.	Bumps or movement of the infusion set loosens contact between Teflon cannula and surrounding tissues, opening a path for insulin to escape to the skin.	Use insertion sets no longer than 3 to 4 days. Always anchor infusion lines with 1" tape. Replace infusion set and anchor it.
Will Pump Alarm? No		

around it, or it may cause irritation or infection that will drive up the glucose. Check for redness of the skin at the site. Change your set and see whether the glucose comes down. You may need an antibiotic if an infection has occurred. It is best to change your sets every two to three days and avoid the problem entirely.

Running Out of Insulin

Running out of insulin can also cause high glucose readings. Today's reservoirs hold 176, 200, 300 or 315 units of insulin. Many pumpers forget how quickly this insulin disappears. The following tips help in managing your insulin supply:

- Keep a bottle of rapid insulin and a syringe or an insulin pen available at all times in case you run out of insulin in your pump.
- Set the low reservoir alarm on your pump to alert when about half of your usual TDD is left in the pump. For instance, if your TDD is 50 units a day, set your alarm for about 25 units. When you hear the alarm, start planning how to deal with it.
- Fill your reservoir and change your infusion set on a regular schedule. Choose a convenient time to change your set and site every second or third day, and have your pump remind you to do it at that time. **Be careful not to do this near bedtime since you will not know if a problem develops during the next eight hours.**
- If you don't have enough in your reservoir to last until your next scheduled change, you can use the insulin in your pump for your basal delivery, and temporarily inject with a syringe or insulin pen for boluses. Make sure there is enough insulin left in your reservoir to provide the basal insulin you need.
- Some pumps have a hidden reserve that remains available for basal delivery. When the pump reaches "zero insulin left," 10 units or so are left that can be used only for basal insulin delivery. This is often enough to get you to the next scheduled infusion set change, but not every pump model has this!

- If you run out of insulin and have no other insulin available, remember there are 10 to 20 units in your infusion line that can be accessed in an ***extreme emergency***. To do this, separate the line from your pump, hold the hub low with the opening up and raise the rest of the line high to fill the hub with insulin. Remove insulin as needed from the filled hub with a syringe for injection.

Contact the Manufacturer

If you suspect a problem with the pump itself, call your manufacturer. (The phone number can be found on the back of the pump or controller.) The customer service representative will help you check your pump. If a problem is found, they will send you a replacement and packaging to use to return your current pump. It is wise to have a vial of long-lasting insulin on hand and know how to use it if you have to rely on injections for a day or two. See Box 15.6 for how to replace your pump with injections.

Summary

If your glucose goes high without a clear reason, carefully consider whether extra carbs, a missed bolus (check your pump history), or too little basal or bolus insulin could be the cause. Consider other causes, such as an infection, or bad insulin. Check your pump and infusion site for mechanical causes.

Anytime your glucose readings are over 250 mg/dl (12.9 mmol/L) twice in a row without a clear reason, take an injection of rapid insulin and test your glucose often until you are sure you have corrected the problem. Check for ketones and call your

15.6 My Pump Stopped Working – What Do I Do?

A pump can stop working or you can run out of reservoirs or infusion sets. When something goes wrong, you will need to switch back to injections for awhile.

Always keep a record handy of your current basal rates, TDD, CarbF, and CorrF in case there's a pump failure. Keep on hand a bottle or insulin pen with a long-acting insulin, like Lantus® or Levemir®, to replace your basal insulin delivery. NPH® insulin is available at a local pharmacy without a prescription and can replace your basal insulin if your total basal per day is split into 3 equal injections of NPH® through the day.

To Switch Back to Injections, Replace Your Basal and Bolus Delivery:

1. For basal delivery (about half your daily insulin), take the same number of units of Lantus® or Levemir® at bedtime as your current basal total for the day following your pump crash. (See #2 for temporary basal replacement if it will be several hours till bedtime.) If you know only your approximate TDD, take half of this amount as Lantus® or Levemir®.

2. Basal insulin can also be replaced temporarily with more frequent injections of the same rapid insulin you use in your pump. To do this, give an injection of your rapid insulin every 4 hours that is equal to 4 times your hourly basal rate.

3. For boluses, use rapid insulin and your CarbF and CorrF to mentally calculate the boluses you need.

4. To keep track of BOB from recent injections, calculate that 20% or 25% of the last bolus will be used each hour.

5. Check your glucose frequently to be sure these doses are working until you can get your pump replaced and go back on it.   © 2012 Diabetes Services, Inc.

physician/health care team immediately if your ketones are moderate or high. Replace your reservoir, insulin, and infusion set before relying on your pump again.

Keep all possible causes for an unexplained high in mind. It is important to differentiate between whether a high glucose is due to a problem unrelated to insulin delivery or whether you have a delivery problem with your site, infusion set, reservoir, or pump.

An insulin pump enhances control when it is working properly, but it is a mechanical system that can also fail to function. Common pump problems are usually encountered in the first six months of use. It is important to know how to troubleshoot clogs, leaks, dislodged infusion sets, and tunneling of insulin to correct the problem quickly and minimize its severity. Fortunately, pump and infusion set problems decrease in frequency as the pumper's experience grows.

Irony is just honesty with the volume cranked up.

George Saunders

Keys to Treating Ketoacidosis

CHAPTER 16

When you have little insulin in the blood, your glucose readings will rise and may become a serious medical problem. Ketosis begins when the body mobilizes and breaks down excessive amounts of fat for fuel because it cannot use glucose with the low insulin level. Glucose and fat levels both rise as less glucose enters cells and more fat is mobilized to make up the difference. *Diabetic ketoacidosis (DKA) begins as the blood becomes more and more acidic as ketone levels rise.*

This chapter covers severe highs, ketosis, and DKA

- Causes
- Symptoms and detection
- Treatment and prevention

In 2007, among all people with diabetes, the Center for Disease Control reported 123,000 hospitalizations for DKA at a total cost of $2.4 billion. Ketoacidosis is often seen when Type 1 diabetes is first diagnosed. DKA occurs when too little insulin is available to the body. This can happen from a severe infection, other serious illness, with use of steroid medications like prednisone, when insulin doses are missed, or when insulin has lost potency.

Ketoacidosis is more common in pump wearers if their glucose levels are routinely elevated, when boluses are often missed, when infusion sets or patch pumps often get detached or leak, or when empty reservoir alarms are ignored. Hospitalization for ketoacidosis in Type 1 diabetes occurs about once for every 30 years of insulin use but it is more common in children.

In children and adolescents, ketoacidosis can occur during normal growth spurts if basal rates and boluses are not sufficiently raised to meet the increased need for insulin. Hormone changes during puberty require large increases in basal and bolus doses. Avoiding DKA in children is especially important as this appears to lower a child's IQ by a small amount each time an episode occurs.[101]

The risk of ketoacidosis is lower in Type 2 diabetes, but the larger number of people who have Type 2 makes the actual number of cases of ketoacidosis greater with Type 2 diabetes. DKA carries a much higher death rate of 5% to 10% in older people with Type 2 diabetes because of age and because the DKA is often triggered by a severe illness like pneumonia, a heart attack, or a stroke.[102]

195

Ketosis can begin 3 to 6 hours after an infusion set or patch pump leaks, clogs, pulls out, or fails, and be quickly followed by DKA. If an infusion set gets displaced near bedtime, the rising glucose is unlikely to be detected for several hours. Tiredness may cause a person to go to bed without testing if the glucose is very high. Giving a correction bolus will not

> ### 16.1 Causes of Severe Highs and Ketoacidosis
> - Onset of Type 1 diabetes
> - Severe infection
> - Heart attack, stroke, or serious illness
> - Insulin doses that are skipped or too low
> - Nondelivery from infusion set or pump failure
> - Growth spurts in kids and adolescents
> - Use of prednisone or other steroid
> - Severe stress

help if there's an insulin delivery problem. Treatment will be delayed further if you go to work or school without the supplies needed to correct your high reading.

When insulin levels fall after an infusion set failure or for other reasons, the use of fat for fuel increases. Burning fat sounds good but when done to excess, ketone levels rise and cause the blood to turn acidic, and acidity leads to nausea and vomiting. The vomiting, along with high glucose levels, can rapidly lead to dehydration where the kidneys can no longer get rid of excess glucose and ketones. Once vomiting begins, death may occur if IV re-hydration is not started within a few hours in a hospital or ER. The rapid replacement of fluids and insulin are both critical to survival.

Symptoms

Symptoms of ketoacidosis are nearly identical to those caused by a flu or food poisoning. Ketoacidosis caused by an infusion site problem or bad insulin can be mistaken for a viral or other illness. Symptoms of DKA and the flu are very similar. NEVER assume your symptoms are just caused by the flu. Always test your glucose (and ketones when it is above 250 mg/dl) before going to bed when you are unusually tired.

The major difference a viral illness and DKA is that the ketoacidosis can kill you. If you feel ill or tired, check your glucose, then check your ketone level. Recheck ketones every 4 hours over the first 12 hours and then once a day during the course of any illness. Be especially careful to check for ketones at the first sign of nausea. If you take a bolus for a high reading with no ketones at bedtime, set an alarm and test two hours later to ensure that your glucose is coming down.

If you find moderate or large levels of ketones in your urine or blood, this suggests the "illness" may be due to failed insulin delivery. The presence of ketones will require larger than normal correction boluses by injection or by pump once the delivery problem is resolved. Call your doctor immediately if your urine or meter test shows moderate or large ketones. *Go directly to an emergency room any time you start to vomit and can no longer keep fluids down.*

Know how to recognize and treat ketoacidosis. Early symptoms include tiredness, excessive thirst, frequent urination, dry skin, a fruity odor to the breath, abdominal pain, and nausea, basically the same symptoms that many people experienced if they had very high glucoses at diagnosis. Advanced symptoms include vomiting, shortness of breath, rapid breathing, and unconsciousness. Early symptoms may be confused with the flu or food poisoning. Because they may be due to ketone poisoning, they should never be ignored. As soon as a person begins to vomit or has difficulty breathing, immediate treatment in an emergency room is required to prevent coma or death.

Detection

If ketones are present, they can be detected in the blood with a ketone meter about 2 to 4 hours before they can be detected in the urine with ketone test strips. Ketones can be detected in the blood with the same lancing device used for glucose meters and an Abbott Precision Xtra™ or Nova Max™ Plus ketone meter, or in the urine with Bayer Ketostix® or foil-wrapped Ketodiastix® urine test strips. These can be found at any pharmacy.

Keep blood or urine ketone strips on hand, store them in a dry area, and replace them as soon as they are outdated. Most people will only occasionally use ketone test strips, so it is better to buy ones that are individually wrapped. Ketone meters use a special strip that is individually wrapped in foil for freshness. These are advantageous for pump wearers, parents of children with diabetes, and anyone prone to ketoacidosis. A blood ketone level above 0.5 mmol/L suggests excess ketones are present, while a level of 1.5 mmol/L suggests ketoacidosis may happen quickly. A level of 3.0 mmol/L or higher demands immediate medical attention. A urine test that shows large ketones is roughly equivalent to 3.0 mmol/L or higher but takes a longer time to appear in the urine.

16.2 Ketoacidosis

Early Symptoms

- any unexplained high glucose reading
- nausea
- vague flu-like symptoms
- increased thirst and dry mouth
- excessive urination
- increased hunger
- excess tiredness or weakness
- confusion
- an acetone or fruity odor of the breath
- abdominal pain

Late Signs

- vomiting
- severe abdominal pain
- rapid breathing
- shortness of breath
- unconsciousness

Call your physician or go to an emergency room immediately anytime a blood ketone level of 3.0 or higher or large amounts of ketones in urine or blood, and any late sign is present.

16.3 Steps to Treat Ketoacidosis on a Pump

Always check for ketones if you have nausea, an unexplained high glucose, or a reading above 300 mg/dl (16.7 mmol/L). If you have moderate or large ketone levels, your pump is not delivering insulin or you have a very serious illness. Follow the directions below for normal to small, or moderate to ketone levels.

If Ketones Are Normal or Small:*	If Ketones Are Moderate or Large:**
1. Give a correction bolus with the pump.	1. **Stay hydrated.** Drink 8 to 12 ounces of non-caloric fluid every 30 min. even if you do not feel thirsty until control is regained. Use water, water with a pinch of Nu-Salt™ to restore potassium levels, or diluted Gatorade.
2. Drink 8 to 12 ounces of water or non-caloric fluid every 30-60 min. until control is regained.	2. *Give insulin by injection from Table 16.6 until your glucose is below 200 mg/dl (11.1 mmol/L).* More insulin will be needed with ketones, if basal insulin has been missed, or you have an illness or fever.
3. Check your glucose at least every 2 hours when a reading is above 250 mg/dl (13.9 mmol/L).	3. *Call your doctor if your glucose is over 250 mg/dl (14 mmol/L) and moderate or large ketones are present.*
4. In 2 hours, if your glucose has not fallen and ketones are again small, change the infusion set and site, and follow the procedure to the right.	4. *If vomiting begins when ketones are large, immediately call your doctor or go to an ER* for IV hydration and treatment. Medical treatment is required. Call 911 if no one is available to drive you.
5. If the glucose is about the same or lower, recheck in another one to two hours and enter this reading into your pump to determine if an another correction bolus is needed.	5. Replace the pump insulin cartridge and entire infusion set at a new site, using a new bottle of insulin. Check your pump settings
6. If your reading stays high or ketones appear, call your physician and follow the procedure to the right.	6. Once your glucose is less than 200 mg/dl (11.1 mmol/L), **drink fluids with carbs**, like Gatorade, to avoid having a low glucose and to speed up the fall in ketones.

* Urine ketones are normal or small; blood ketones are less than 0.6 to 1.2 mmol/L
** Urine ketones are moderate or large; blood ketones are above 1.2 or 3.0 mmol/L

Thanks to Geri Wood, RN, BSN, CDE and John Stanchfield, MD, of Salt Lake City for their helpful suggestions.

If no blood ketones are present, an insulin delivery problem is less likely and a high reading should respond to a correction bolus. If a urine ketone test is negative, repeat the test 2 hours later because ketones appear later in the urine than blood. Keep in mind that ketones may not form but your glucose can remain unusually high if an infusion set is only partially delivering insulin.

If ketones are present, however, a pump delivery problem is likely.

Remove the set and inspect the infusion site, line, hub, and pump for the source of the problem. If a lump is felt under the infusion site, squeeze it to see if blood or pus is present. Look for any kinks in the Teflon catheter. Replace everything and use a new bottle of insulin. A larger than normal correction bolus will be needed to replace the basal insulin that has also not been delivered for several hours and to overcome the insulin resistance caused by DKA. Give special attention to increasing fluid intake to feel better and call your physician immediately if blood ketones are over 0.6 mmol/L in the blood or a urine test shows moderate or large levels of ketones.

Is your glucose high for no reason? Wash your hands and retest.
Your finger might just have something on it!

Prevention and Treatment

Infections and other illnesses can cause ketoacidosis and ketoacidosis can easily be confused with the flu. Frequent monitoring of glucose and ketone levels is critical during any illness to prevent unrecognized ketoacidosis from complicating an already serious situation. When feeling ill, you may be tempted to stop checking your glucose and fail to recognize how serious the situation has become.

If you feel especially tired, never go to sleep without checking your glucose and ketones. Do not go to sleep with a high glucose level without checking ketones, your infusion site and pump delivery. If you suspect an insulin delivery problem, use an injection to bring the glucose down and change the entire pump setup. Check your insulin's expiration date and do not use vials that have been opened for more than a month or were left in a car on a hot day. Open a new insulin vial if you have any doubts about your insulin.

With any sudden, unexplained rise in glucose, suspect an infusion set or pump problem. Pump failure can cause ketoacidosis within a few hours. If moderate or large amounts of ketones are present, more injected insulin than normal will be needed to lower the glucose. Change your reservoir and infusion site immediately, and set an alarm to awaken you in two hours to monitor your progress.

Some episodes of ketoacidosis occur after several weeks or months of inattention to testing or to its results. Basal and bolus doses may have gradually become inadequate due to growth, weight gain, or stress. When monitoring is not done or high glucose readings are ignored for weeks, a missed insulin dose or the start of an infection can quickly cascade into ketoacidosis.

When an infection or illness causes glucose levels to go high, the underlying problem must be dealt with to lower the glucose. Medications like prednisone and cortisone can cause very high glucoses. Very large increases in basal and bolus doses may be needed to deal with infection, a serious illness, or some medications. Call your doctor right away to discuss how to treat any underlying problem and how much to increase your doses.

An unexpected high glucose or the presence of ketones while on a pump should raise a red flag. If there is not a clear reason, such as illness or infection, the cause may come from the pump itself, from bad insulin, an infusion set that has come loose; or a leak from a hub or an infusion line. Other causes include incorrect basal or bolus settings, forgetting or neglecting to take boluses, or pain or depression that cause personal care to be neglected.

Ketoacidosis can be debilitating, painful, expensive, dangerous, or deadly. Take care to avoid it. If it occurs, treat it quickly with extra insulin and fluid intake. Discuss any problems you have regarding high readings, the presence of ketones, or personal issues regarding diabetes with your physician so you can resolve them quickly and avoid problems.

For high glucoses and ketones, drink water, inject insulin to ensure delivery, and call 911 or go to the ER as soon as vomiting begins. Unless caused by an obvious error such as bolusing and neglecting to eat, emergencies usually require an immediate change in TDD, basal rates, or boluses, as well as a review of the lifestyle factors that contributed to the crisis. After an emergency occurs, do not fall back into the old routine that created the problem. Determine what you need to change to avoid repeating it in the future.

16.6 Approximate Correction Insulin Requirements Based on Blood Ketone Levels (Illness or DKA)

Blood Ketone Level	What It Means	BG = 100-180 mg/dl (5.5-10.0 mmol/L)	BG = 180-250 mg/dl (10.0-14.0 mmol/L)	BG = 250-400 mg/dl (14.0-22 mmol/L)	BG > 400 mg/dl (> 22 mmol/L)
0.5 mmol/L or less	Normal ketones	Give usual correction bolus from pump.	Extra fluid. Give usual correction bolus from pump.	Extra fluid. Give usual correction bolus from pump.	Extra fluid. Give usual correction bolus from pump.
0.6 to 1.5 mmol/L	Ketones are building up. Check infusion set and pump.	Extra carbs and fluid. Give usual bolus doses if infusion set is OK. Recheck in 2-3 hours.	Extra carbs and fluid. Give extra 5% of TDD or I u for every 80 lbs (40 kgs). Recheck in 2-3 hours.	Extra fluid. Give extra 10% of TDD or I u for every 40 lbs (20 kgs). Recheck in 2-3 hours.	Extra fluid. Give extra 15% of TDD or I u for every 25 lbs (12 kgs). Recheck in 2-3 hours.
1.5 to 2.9 mmol/L	Ketoacidosis (DKA) is developing – contact doctor. Check pump, replace infusion set & reservoir.	Extra carbs and fluid. **Inject** extra 5% of TDD or I u for every 80 lbs (40 kgs). Recheck in 2-3 hours.	Extra carbs and fluid. **Inject** extra 10% of TDD or I u for every 40 lbs (20 kgs). Recheck in 2-3 hours.	Extra fluid. **Inject** extra 15% of TDD or I u for every 25 lbs (12 kgs).	Extra fluid. **Inject** extra 20% of TDD or I u for every 20 lbs (10 kgs).
At about 3 mmol/L	Severe DKA – call doctor or have someone take you to ER, esp. if vomiting starts. Check pump, replace infusion set & reservoir.	Extra carbs and fluid. **Inject** extra 5% of TDD or I u for every 80 lbs (40 kgs). Repeat every 2-3 hours until ketones come down.	Extra carbs and fluid. **Inject** extra 15% of TDD or I u for every 25 lbs (12 kgs). Repeat every 2-3 hours until ketones come down.	Extra fluid. **Inject** 20% of TDD or I u for every 20 lbs (10 kgs). Repeat every 2-3 hours until ketones come down.	Extra fluid. **Inject** 25% of TDD or I u for every 15 lbs (7 kgs). Repeat every 2-3 hours until ketones come down.

The doses above are correction bolus or injection doses only. (See Table 16.7 for percentage of TDD.) More or less may be needed. *Basal or long-acting insulin must also be given! Do not stop basal delivery even if you are not eating.*
Do not go to sleep if you are alone and ketones are 1.5 mmol/L or higher. Call someone to stay with you.
Check your glucose and ketones every 2 hours if your last glucose was above 300 mg/dl (16.7 mmol/L). In pregnancy, do this when above 150 mg/dl.

Modified from recommendations by the International Society for Pediatric and Adolescent Diabetes[104]

16.7 Correction Doses as a Percentage of Your TDD (total daily dose)					
Total Daily Dose	**5%**	**10%**	**15%**	**20%**	**25%**
20 u	1 u	2 u	3 u	4 u	5 u
30 u	1.5 u	3 u	4.5 u	6 u	7.5 u
40 u	2 u	4 u	6 u	8 u	10 u
50 u	2.5 u	5 u	7.5 u	10 u	12.5 u
60 u	3 u	6 u	9 u	12 u	15 u
70 u	3.5 u	7 u	10.5 u	14 u	17.5 u
80 u	4 u	8 u	12 u	16 u	20 u
100 u	5 u	10 u	15 u	20 u	25 u

For use in Table 16.6 with an illness or diabetic ketoacidosis. These correction doses, as a percentage of your average TDD, should be given by injection if blood ketones are 1.5 mmol/L or higher. Your average TDD includes both your usual basal and bolus doses.

Let your doctor help you find new ways to maintain better control. It is rare for someone who has erratic readings to leave the office of an experienced pump specialist on the same basal rates and boluses they came in with. An open mind combined with open discussion with others will speed your progress.

**During even mild episodes of ketosis, staying hydrated is VITAL.
Drink lots of fluids.**

**As soon as your glucose falls below 250 mg/dl (14 mmol/L),
start eating or drinking some carbs to speed up the fall in blood ketone levels.**

*I have such an extensive collection of seashells that I must display them
on all the beaches of the world.*

Anon

Other Things that May Impact Your Control

When glucose readings have a pattern and go high or low at the same time each day, this is usually easy to track down and correct with basal, bolus, or diet adjustments. But when readings are erratic without an obvious pattern, how do you correct them?

In this chapter, we cover things that contribute to erratic readings:

- Fear of lows
- Erratic schedule
- Menses
- An illness
- Stress
- Pain
- Steroid medications
- Over-the-counter products
- Thyroid disease
- Celiac disease
- Gastroparesis

Lifestyle factors like infrequent monitoring, skipping meal boluses, taking boluses late, overeating, and poor food choices often lead to erratic readings. Pain, stress, or too many lows also increase the likelihood for wacky readings. Erratic readings almost always indicate that the amounts or timing of your basal and bolus doses needs to change.

A little detective work and patience generally uncovers the sources for out-of-control readings. Most lifestyle issues and the pump settings that affect your readings are usually under your control. You may already be aware of things you have been thinking of changing. Before you look for other causes, be sure to recalculate your iTDD using Table 10.1 or Table 10.3, and check your current pump settings against those derived from your iTDD in Table 9.5. Answer the questions in Table 14.3 to assess what may be affecting your readings.

Fear of Lows

An excessive fear of lows can lead to high readings if basal rates and boluses are underdosed to avoid having them occur. One pumper got into the habit of skipping carb and correction boluses to ensure he had no lows, so for a few years, his A1c hovered around 9%. After he had a hemorrhage in one eye that required laser treatment, he started to check his glucose regularly and use his pump's bolus calculator to avoid insulin stacking. With some work on his fear of lows and a few changes in his management, he eventually brought his A1c down into the upper 6% range with no serious hypoglycemia.

The risk of having lows rises as glucose readings are brought into a range that would otherwise allow you to live a long and healthy life. For those who fear lows, acknowledge your fear but don't let it make decisions for you. Rather than base your dose decisions on fear, use clear judgments to match your doses to your real needs. This is the best way to prevent lows and highs. Counseling focused on behavior change and wearing a CGM can be extremely helpful. See Chapters 19 and 20 for more information on lows.

Erratic Schedule

Eating and exercising at irregular times and an erratic work or school schedule challenges management skills and creates ups and downs in your readings. Living a more consistent lifestyle helps you find pump doses more quickly that work for you. If regulating your lifestyle is not possible, take extra glucose readings and adjust your basal and bolus doses to match your lifestyle. Realize that your learning curve may be a bit steeper. Wear a CGM if at all possible. Try to eat a similar number of carbs for breakfast, lunch, and dinner.

Menses

Women often find that their readings rise a few days before their menstrual period begins. On average, the TDD needs to rise by 3 units a day to offset these hormonal changes.[103] Keeping your glucose better controlled with extra insulin tends to lessen premenstrual symptoms. To do this, increase basal rates and bolus doses during these few days to avoid high readings as determined by trial and error. For women who have regular periods, the required insulin adjustments are often consistent from month to month, while for others with irregular periods dose adjustments can vary from month to month.

Set up an alternate basal profile for this time of the month or use a temp basal increase, especially if your pump allows a longer duration for this change, such as 72 hours or more. The advantage of using a temp basal rather than an alternate basal profile is that the pump automatically returns to your usual basal, rather than having to manually switch back to your usual basal profile.

Prior to your period, the need for extra insulin may show up gradually but often returns to normal quickly once your period begins. Reduce basal and bolus doses just as quickly when this occurs. Some women find that they need a lower than normal basal rate for a couple of days after their period starts. Figure out your own pattern and be prepared to make these adjustments to stay in good control.

An Illness

Bacterial infections like pneumonia, strep throat, an impacted wisdom tooth, a bladder infection, or a sinus infection, especially with a high fever, can double or triple your TDD. An infection causes insulin resistance from the release of stress hormones and inflammatory substances like tumor necrosis factor and cytokines. Higher basal rates and larger bolus doses are needed to counteract these changes. Once an antibiotic is started, the increased need for basal and bolus doses gradually returns to normal over a few days as the excess insulin resistance disappears.

Viral illnesses like a cold or flu usually have less effect on glucose levels and can often be managed by giving additional correction boluses as needed. Raising the basal rates may or may not be needed. Viral illnesses that last longer, like hepatitis and mononucleosis and those associated with a high fever are more likely to require an increase in both basal rates and boluses.

Illnesses that cause vomiting or diarrhea may keep you from eating. Omit carb boluses, but continue basal delivery and use correction boluses as needed for high readings. Always check your glucose and for ketones for any nausea or vomiting and drink plenty of non-caloric liquids for any illness with diarrhea or vomiting if the glucose is 150 mg/dl (8.3 mmol/L) or higher. Drink fruit juice or sip clear sodas regularly if the glucose is 150 mg/dl or less. Dehydration can be very serious if you don't drink enough to compensate for fever, diarrhea, or vomiting.

If a low glucose occurs when the stomach is unsettled, a half can of regular clear soda with one teaspoon salt often works well. During an illness, small doses of glucagon can also be given to prevent hypoglycemia. For children, mix all the saline in the kit with the glucagon powder. Then use a standard U-100 insulin syringe to give the glucagon. For children, give 1 unit of glucagon for each year of age, i.e. 10 units for a 10-year-old child.[104] An adult can be given one unit for every 10 lbs of weight, such as 15 units for a 150 lb (60 114 kg) adult to prevent a low glucose.

Frequent glucose checks guide your insulin adjustments toward better control so that your body heals sooner. Ask a health care professional for guidance any time you become ill and are unsure how to bring your readings under control. Check your glucose often or have someone else test it during any illness.

Stress

Sudden stress, such as that caused by a car accident, is easy to spot and deal with. Chronic stress from a relative's or friend's extended illness or death, problems at work, or difficulties in a relationship can have a dramatic impact on control but be less obvious and especially hard to measure.

How different you feel when you go on vacation is often a good indicator of the amount of stress you are under in your day-to-day life, especially when your glucose suddenly becomes easier to control. Listen to family and friends. They often recognize your stress before you do, and can alert you to making changes or seeking treatment earlier.

In someone who does not have diabetes, the extra glucose released with stress is matched by an equal increase in insulin to produce the energy needed for fight or flight. In diabetes, when glucose release is not matched with enough insulin, the high glucose levels magnify emotional reactions and cause more stress hormones to be released. This can cause additional depression and irritability that impairs the ability to deal with the stress at hand. The challenge of caring for your own diabetes can add to stress and frustration as readings jump in unexpected ways and improvements are slow in coming.

Controlling your readings during stress becomes difficult not only because glucose-raising hormones are released but also because the order of daily life often gets disrupted. Stressful events can lead to lost sleep, decreased activity, and increased eating of comfort foods high in sugar and fat. These also cause you to need more insulin.

Intermittent stress with its unpredictable timing is best treated with correction boluses, as the need arises. If you anticipate a limited period of stress, such as a day of tension-filled business meetings, or finals at school, check your glucose more often and take correction boluses as needed. Use a temporary basal increase if past experience tells you this will be needed. For longer periods of stress, such as when a family member is in the hospital, consider raising both your meal boluses and using a higher alternate basal profile to improve your control. Maintaining or increasing exercise during a period of stress, although sometimes difficult to do, lessens the need for extra insulin and helps you better mange stress.

Pain

Pain is often not recognized as a major player in glucose control, but the more pain you have, the more insulin you need. When the body hurts, inflammatory substances like tumor necrosis factor and cytokines are released, causing pain but also making the body more resistant to insulin. Basal and bolus doses have to be increased to counteract pain, whether caused by an accident, joint pain, or an illness.

Chronic pain creates a constant need for higher insulin doses. Work to eliminate or reduce pain with appropriate medical care. Talk with your physician about strategies and medication that reduce pain. Discuss how to adjust your basals and boluses for episodes when pain may be constant and for periods when it becomes more pronounced. Be sure to reduce any increase in basal or bolus doses once the pain is minimized.

Steroid Medications

Steroids like prednisone are often prescribed for poison ivy, allergic reactions to medications, or illnesses like lupus, asthma, and arthritis. Always let the doctor know that you have diabetes and always ask if another medication might work. When a steroid tablet or injection is used to curb a systemic allergic reaction or inflammation, insulin need can rise dramatically, often up to twice your usual total daily dose. This rise is followed by a gradual reduction in doses over several days, depending on how long the steroid affects you. Newer steroids that are injected directly into a joint for injury or pain remain active for longer periods and insulin requirements can be higher for one to three weeks, depending on how much impact it has beyond the joint capsule.

Steroids increase insulin need as soon as they are started and for a few days afterward as their effect gradually wears off. Check your readings often during a short course of oral steroids. Raise your basal and bolus doses quickly in response to the rapid rise in glucose when a steroid is begun, and lower doses as the steroid medication is being tapered off. Insulin needs are often back to normal 3 to 5 days after the last steroid dose is taken.

Any time you require oral, injected, or even nasal spray steroid medications used for inflamed sinuses, notify your diabetes team for guidance on the basal and bolus adjustments that you will need.

Over-The-Counter Products

Certain over-the-counter products can raise or lower your glucose dramatically. Ephedra, a form of "speed," often leads to unexpected high readings. The FDA removed ephedra from sale as a weight loss product after several deaths were reported, but ephedra may be sold under other names, such as ma huang, Brigham tea, squaw tea, joint-pine, jointfir, Mormon-tea, yellow horse, horsetail, sea grape, and others.

Chinese herbal products for diabetes often contain unregulated chlorpropamide, an old prescription medication called Diabenese that increases beta cell production of insulin. This diabetes medication is no longer prescribed because it can lead to severe hypoglycemia in people with Type 2 diabetes. Be careful when you take over-the-counter products and watch for any unexpected readings if you decide to try any new energy drink, supplement, or herbal product.

Thyroid Disease

Thyroid disease is more common in people with diabetes. In Type 1 diabetes, another autoimmune disorder, called Hashimoto's thyroiditis sometimes causes an initial excess release of thyroid hormone followed by a gradual decline. Type 2 diabetes and thyroid disease are associated because they both become more common as people age. Thyroid disease affects one of every 10 women over the age of 65.

In early stages of thyroid disease, thyroid hormone release may become excessive before it gradually falls below normal, or over- and under-delivery may alternate for a while. Glucose levels tend to climb slightly when the thyroid is overactive and fall as the thyroid becomes underactive. It takes time to identify the thyroid as the source for a glucose control problem as the transition into thyroid disease often takes place over weeks or months.

If your glucose control seems to have changed and you have thyroid symptoms such as nervousness, tiredness, sleeping difficulties, constipation, or are feeling hotter or colder than usual, have your thyroid checked. An overactive thyroid may increase your need for insulin, while an underactive thyroid typically lowers your insulin need.

If you have a low thyroid level and are placed on thyroid medications, you may need to raise your basal rates and boluses slightly, especially if these were lowered while your thyroid function was low. If your thyroid is overactive and you receive radioactive iodine or medication or undergo surgery to reduce the excess thyroid production, you may need to lower your basal and bolus doses slightly once the treatment takes effect. Rely on your health care team for advice during these transition periods.

Celiac Disease

Celiac disease is an autoimmune disorder that affects people of all ages, nearly one in every hundred people in the United States. People with Type 1 diabetes, another autoimmune disease, are more likely to develop celiac disease.

Celiac disease is an abnormal response of the immune system to gluten, an ingredient that is present in all wheat foods, several other grains, and in many food additives. Any food can be contaminated with gluten if it is processed in the same equipment used to process gluten-containing grains, or exposed to gluten on surfaces or utensils used at home or in restaurants.

Celiac is a lifelong disease that cannot be outgrown or cured. It can, however, be managed through strict diet changes. In the past, over 90% of those who had it remained undiagnosed and untreated. In recent years, a growing awareness has made an accurate diagnosis more likely. People are generally diagnosed in their 40's through 60's, about nine years on average after developing the disease.

Celiac symptoms vary from vague or "silent" to severe. They overlap those of other diseases like irritable bowel syndrome, ulcerative colitis, diverticulosis, chronic fatigue syndrome, intestinal infections, and depression, so this often delays an accurate diagnosis. Symptoms and complications are wide ranging. They include intestinal problems, such as bloating, cramping, stomach pain, diarrhea, absorption problems leading to vitamin deficiencies, bone loss, osteoarthritis, anemia, "failure to thrive" in children, inflammatory reactions, irritability, headaches, joint pain, itchy skin, and even an increase in some malignancies. If left undiagnosed and untreated, celiac can lead to peripheral neuropathies (numb or tingling hands or feet), tooth enamel defects, an underactive spleen, and infertility.

Celiac disease can be diagnosed through blood tests that look for four different antibodies, especially a positive anti-gliadin antibody, or by endoscopy and intestinal biopsy that detect telltale intestinal changes. Blood tests are easy to use and noninvasive, so they are usually done first to see if there is reason to proceed with a biopsy.

Endoscopy and intestinal biopsy require fasting and an anesthetic, and can be uncomfortable. The presence of a positive anti-gliadin antibody on the screening test, plus a positive biopsy is considered the gold standard for diagnosing celiac disease. Alternatively, a positive biopsy, followed by improvements in symptoms when a gluten-free diet is followed, also provides a certain diagnosis.

A certain diagnosis is important because treatment requires a strict diet that avoids all foods with gluten or gluten contamination for a lifespan. People who are unsure of the diagnosis will have a hard time following the stringent diet. If the diet isn't maintained, celiac disease can be debilitating and lead to serious health problems like those listed above. Intestinal damage can occur if a gluten-free diet is not strictly followed. An initial visit and regular follow-up with a dietitian who is familiar with celiac disease is especially helpful.

Gastroparesis

Gastroparesis is a partial paralysis of the intestine's normal peristaltic or wavelike motion caused when high glucose levels damage the nerves that control this motion. Symptoms that suggest gastroparesis include mild stomach pain, feeling full immediately or for prolonged periods after eating, excessive gas, bloating, nausea, and vomiting.

Gastroparesis is a form of *autonomic neuropathy* and is often accompanied by other damage to the autonomic nerves, such as loss of constriction of the pupils to light, loss of variability in the heart rate, and the inability of the blood vessels to constrict when going from lying in bed to standing. Symptoms that suggest autonomic neuropathy include light-headedness when first standing up, a heart rate that does not rise appropriately when exercising, sweating after eating, and impotence in men.

Fortunately, when simple tests for autonomic neuropathy are positive, they suggest that gastroparesis may also be present. One test involves checking the blood pressure after lying down quietly for a few minutes, and then rechecking it right after standing up. A positive test occurs if there is a drop of more than 20 points in the upper (systolic) blood pressure number or more than 10 points in the lower (diastolic) blood pressure number upon standing.

Autonomic neuropathy can also be detected by how the heart rate varies after deep breathing or how the blood pressure varies while wearing a Holter monitor for 24 hours at home. Gastroparesis shares many symptoms with celiac disease, an autoimmune disease that can be seen in Type 1 diabetes. Clinical testing can help differentiate these.

Gastroparesis often slows the absorption of food after a meal. This can cause lows in an hour or two after a meal bolus as the bolus starts to act before the food is absorbed. This is followed by a climb in the glucose over the next six to eight hours as the delayed absorption continues and the meal bolus is gone.

Combo or extended boluses from a pump that spread bolus activity over time better match the slower carb digestion seen with gastroparesis. How long to delay or spread out carb boluses has to be determined from experience. A CGM provides a much clearer picture of how digestion issues may impact the glucose after a meal.

Gastroparesis symptoms are often reduced by regular intake of acidophilus capsules, yogurt with live culture, and by eating small meals that contain lower glycemic index foods with a more consistent rate of digestion. Several prescription medications (Reglan, erythromycin, Motilium, and anti-emetics) are available to treat gastroparesis and stabilize digestion. Consult your physician if you believe you have gastroparesis.

Praise does wonders for the sense of hearing.

Anon.

Stop Glucose Spikes and Variable Readings

If you are not yet confident about how to change your pump settings, discuss any control issues with an endocrinologist or diabetes health professional who is experienced with pumps to get back on track quickly. Do not keep doing the same things you've always done and expect different results and don't spend weeks or months with unstable readings. When you seek help, solutions come your way.

Ways to Reduce Excess Glucose Exposure and Variability

Glucose variability involves excessive up and down swings in your glucose. Glucose variability can make you feel bad and may also increase the risk of complications. One way to measure variability is with the *standard deviation (SD)* of your glucose readings. A good goal for SD, available in most software downloads from meters or pumps, is to keep it less than 40% of your average glucose. For example, if the average glucose on your meter is 150 mg/dl, you would like your SD to be 60 mg/dl or less (150 x 0.4 = 60). A lab test, called the 1,5-anhydroglucitol or GlycoMark test, can be taken to measure glucose variability. A higher number on this test means your glucose is more stable.

Glucose variability is higher when:

• You have frequent highs because your TDD is too low

• You have frequent lows because your TDD is too high.

• Your pump settings are incorrect and cause both highs and lows.

• Lifestyle issues like missing boluses, bolusing late, not testing, or inaccurate carb counts magnify the variability.

High glucose readings and excess glucose variability are both unhealthy. The suggestions below help reduce excess glucose exposure, measured by an A1c or the average glucose on your meter, and excess glucose variability, measured by your standard deviation or GlycoMark.

Post-meal Spiking

People vary a great deal in how likely they are to have variable glucoses, but going too high after meals is a common complaint. It is also a major contributor to glucose variability and high A1cs. After-meal spikes that rise above 150 mg/dl (8.3 mmol/L) should be avoided whenever possible to lessen both glucose exposure and variability.

Causes

Carb breakdown starts very quickly after eating begins. Many foods will largely be digested and enter the bloodstream within 45 to 60 minutes, unless gastroparesis (see page 209) is present. Today's rapid insulins can't start working this quickly, so when boluses are taken just before eating, the glucose spikes. To offset the rapidity of carb digestion, it helps to take carb boluses at least 15 to 20 minutes before eating.

To make matters worse, people with Type 1 diabetes lack amylin that slows digestion (See Symlin below.) and many people with Type 1 and Type 2 diabetes release larger amounts of glucagon than normal when they eat, raising post-meal glucose levels even higher (See GLP-1 Agonists below.)

Solutions

Learn the glycemic index of the foods you eat and choose those with a ranking below 60 as often as you can. Take your carb bolus earlier than usual, such as 30 minutes for foods that have a high glycemic index, or eat those foods later in the meal. This may not completely solve the problem but will help reduce spiking.

Many breakfast foods like cold cereals, instant oatmeal, yogurt with fruit syrup, and toasted cheese sandwiches are high glycemic index foods that may cause post-meal readings to spike even when the carb bolus is correctly sized. Try a breakfast of old-fashioned oatmeal that does not raise your glucose as fast or as high as most cold cereals.

Tips to Prevent Spiking:

- One of the best-kept secrets is to take carb boluses early, at least 15 to 20 minutes before eating when possible. Don't delay eating and keep quick carbs available.
- Set a reminder in your pump or a watch so you won't forget to take boluses.
- Replace foods that spike your glucose with ones that have a lower glycemic index. For breakfast, try old-fashioned oatmeal, a high-fiber cereal topped with strawberries, or plain yogurt with fresh fruit sliced into it.
- If you plan to eat a high glycemic index food (white bread, white rice, etc.), be sure to take the carb bolus at least 20 minutes before the meal.
- Review carb counting so that you can avoid a mismatch between the carbs you eat and the bolus you take to cover them.
- Add extra fiber like psyllium (sugar-free Metamucil) or guar gum to a meal to reduce its glycemic index. A tablespoon or two of psyllium added to cold cereals can dramatically lower post-meal readings.

- Get 30 to 45 minutes of exercise shortly after the meal. (If you have heart disease, get your doctor's approval before you start.)
- Discuss with your doctor one of the prescription medications below that slow digestion and minimize post-meal spikes.

With post-meal spiking, check your average basal/bolus balance. If your basal insulin is less than 50% of your TDD, raise your basal rates during the day. Having a higher basal insulin level in the blood prior to eating also helps reduce post-meal spiking.

Medications That Lower Post-meal Spiking

Precose® and Glyset®

Alpha-glucosidase inhibitors, also called *starch blockers*, are older medications that help control glucose levels by slowing down the digestion of complex carbs. This reduces the glucose spikes seen after meals, sometimes lowers the fasting glucose, and tends to lessen delayed hypoglycemia once bolus and basal doses are appropriately reduced.

Precose® (acarbose) and Glyset® (miglitol) are taken before each meal. They work by inhibiting enzymes in the intestine that break down carbohydrates. This slows the digestion of carbohydrates in the small intestine and slows the rise in the glucose after a meal.

The way that starch blockers work also causes their side effects. They tend to be very safe drugs that have almost no entry into the bloodstream. Digestive side effects can occur when digestion is inhibited too greatly, including abdominal bloating, gas, and diarrhea.

To minimize or prevent intestinal side effects, start these medications at minimal doses and gradually increase them as tolerance improves in a week or so. Half of the smallest tablet can be taken before one meal a day, with doses gradually extended to all meals and doses then gradually increased. Side effects tend to decrease over time, allowing doses to be increased until post meal readings are controlled. These medications are not advised for those with digestion or intestinal issues.

A low glucose reading when using one of these medications is best treated with glucose tablets or a glucose gel. Starch-blockers delay the digestion of table sugar, fruit, and fruit juice so they do not raise a low glucose as quickly.

When dosed well, Precose and Glyset greatly improve post-meal control and have a very good safety profile.

Symlin®

As antibodies destroy the beta cells in early stages of Type 1 diabetes, the body loses insulin production, but it also loses production of a second beta cell hormone called *amylin*. Insulin, discovered in 1922, is critical to survival. Amylin, less critical and discovered 65 years later, also plays an important role in glucose regulation.

In a person without diabetes, insulin and amylin are released in small amounts all the time, with levels rising sharply at mealtime. Like insulin, amylin production is also lost when beta cells are destroyed. In Type 2 diabetes, its production parallels that of insulin, rising during early stages of the disease, then falling over time.

A modified form of amylin, called Symlin®, is available by prescription. Symlin® decreases glucagon secretion, decreases appetite, and delays gastric emptying. Less hunger is experienced after meals, enabling many people who are overweight to lose significant amounts of weight, yet normal weight individuals lose none. Symlin® can dramatically lower post-meal glucose levels and reduce glucose variability in anyone whose insulin production is limited. These benefits occur from a slowing of digestion and also a lowering of the excessive post meal glucagon release that raises glucose levels in Type 1 diabetes.

If started at full doses, Symlin® can cause severe hypoglycemia in about 30% of users when it is first reintroduced to the body. To lessen this risk, Symlin® can be started at lower starting doses, while carb boluses are reduced by 30% to 50% on the same day that Symlin® is started. Glucose levels may at first go higher until the full Symlin® dose is reached. Once a treatment dose is reached, carb boluses can be appropriately adjusted. The delay in food digestion caused by Symlin® often requires the use of combo or dual wave boluses (some now, the rest over time).

Basal rates may also need to be lowered, especially if current basal doses make up more then 50% of the TDD. If weight loss occurs, both carb boluses and basal rates will need to be lowered gradually as weight comes down.

The manufacturer recommends starting with 15 micrograms before each meal and increasing to 30 micrograms, then 45 micrograms, and finally 60 micrograms if no nausea is encountered for three days. Excess doses are easy to spot by a feeling of fullness or nausea after the dose is given. Vomiting and diarrhea may also occur. If side effects occur, lower the dose by 15 micrograms for a few days and try increasing the dose again after there is no fullness or nausea for at least three days. Doses can be increased every three days as long as nausea or other side effects are not present.

Lower doses of Symlin® are often sufficient to normalize after-meal readings, while maximum doses of Symlin® may assist weight loss. If the goal is to reduce post-meal spiking and glucose variability, the dose is gradually increased until most post-meal readings rise less than 40 to 60 mg/dl (2.2 to 3.3 mmol/L) above where they started. For weight loss, larger doses may be used.

A good balance between Symlin® and insulin doses keeps rises in post-meal readings minimal while causing few lows. In many Type 1s, an injection of only 15 or 30 micrograms taken two or three times a day before meals is needed to do this. Symlin® is usually taken just before meals that contain at least 250 calories or 30 grams of carbohydrate. If a dose is missed, wait until the next meal to take the regular scheduled dose.

With larger doses of Symlin®, the full glucose rise from the slowed digestion may not occur until several hours later. For example, a large carb intake for dinner may not be seen as a higher glucose until breakfast the following morning. To prevent morning highs, an extended bolus over a few hours or a temp basal increase overnight may be needed after a larger carb intake in the evening.

Symlin® and the GLP-1 agonists discussed below delay the digestion of all foods. If a low occurs, use glucose tablets if available. If your glucose is low before a meal, raise it before you take Symlin®. Be patient, as the rise in glucose will be slower. Likewise, high readings can take longer to bring down while food absorption is still ongoing.

Foods that formerly spiked the glucose may require a combo or dual wave bolus once Symlin® slows the entry of glucose into the blood stream. Using Symlin® may cause problems by slowing carbs that already digest slowly, such as *al dente* pasta, causing lows early and highs later unless the bolus is stretched out.

GLP-1 Agonists

GLP-1 agonists that are currently available include Byetta® (injected twice a day), Victoza® (injected once a day), and Bydureon® (injected once a week). Others are being developed. They are approved by the FDA for use with other diabetes medications, as well as with some long-acting insulins. Research studies suggest that GLP-1s also benefit people with Type 1 diabetes. Like Symlin®, hypoglycemia can occur if insulin doses are not reduced (about 20%) when they are started. Combo boluses are often used to balance the delay in food absorption. GLP-1 agonists may help weight loss.

GLP-1 agonists stimulate insulin production and restore first phase insulin secretion in Type 2 but not Type 1 diabetes. They decrease the excess release of glucagon that is seen after meals in both types of diabetes, and this also decreases post-meal glucose readings and improves control. They have multiple sites of action in the body. Research studies suggest that about one third of people lose more weight, about one third lose some weight, and about one third lose none. Carefully discuss any off-label use of a GLP-1 with your doctor. Pump adjustments are similar to those with Symlin®.

Summary

Post-meal glucose control plays a major role in your overall glucose stability and A1c results. You have many options to use in this area of self-management. Wearing a CGM helps to quickly spot problem areas and to find solutions. It can also speed up finding appropriate basal and bolus doses and their timing when Symlin® or a GLP-1 agonist is used to delay food digestion. If you have hypoglycemia unawareness, a longer digestion time along with appropriate insulin dose reductions can help, but this requires the use of a CGM that will reliably alert you if you go low. None of the medications above is recommended for people with gastroparesis where digestion times vary.

216

Keys to Treating Hypoglycemia

Even with good management, the most conscientious person cannot prevent all lows. In the APP Study, the 396 pump wearers had an average of 1.4 readings a month below 50 mg/dl (2.8 mmol/L), while the group of pumpers with the lowest average glucose (144 mg/dl or 8.0 mmol/L) averaged 3.6 per month. Yet, for unclear reasons, 38% of the best control group had less than one glucose below 50 mg/dl per month on their meter.

Although some lows may be inevitable as you bring high glucose levels down, neither frequent nor severe lows are necessary. For safety and accuracy, anyone who is fearful of lows, has hypoglycemia unawareness, lives alone, or has a job where hypoglycemia is a danger could benefit from a CGM that can detect lows early when symptoms are minimal. The CGM alarms and trend line give advanced warning of lows or highs before your glucose reaches an extreme. Hypoglycemia is less common and less severe when someone wears a CGM, especially if they look at it frequently and gain experience in how to test and adjust their basal and bolus doses.

This chapter reviews hypoglycemia
- Symptoms
- Causes and prevention
- Treatment
- Treatment of severe hypoglycemia
- What you can do and how others can help
- Prevention tips

Unlike organs that can switch from using glucose to fat or protein for fuel when the glucose is low, the brain and nervous system depend on glucose for their major fuel. When the brain lacks glucose, thought and coordination become impaired and behavior changes. Mild lows may be annoying or embarrassing but a severe one can be frightening or dangerous. Prevention and early treatment avoids these issues while minimizing stress hormone release that cause the glucose to spike afterward. Frequent lows impair short-term memory, especially for names and words, although avoiding lows can largely reverse this.

Hypoglycemia is usually defined as a glucose of 65 mg/dl (3.6 mmol/L) or less. Symptoms vary greatly from person to person, though. Someone who routinely has readings between 180 and 360 mg/dl (10 to 20 mmol/L) will often experience hypoglycemia symptoms

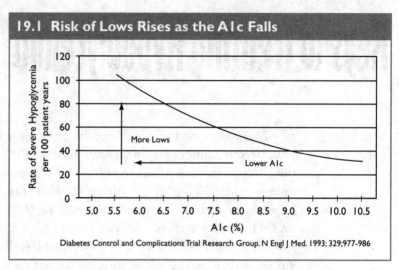

19.1 Risk of Lows Rises as the A1c Falls

Rate of Severe Hypoglycemia per 100 patient years

More Lows

Lower A1c

A1c (%)

Diabetes Control and Complications Trial Research Group. N Engl J Med. 1993; 329;977-986

at 100 mg/dl (5.6 mmol/L). On the other hand, someone who has frequent lows may have little or no symptoms at 45 mg/dl (2.5 mmol/L).

Most lows are mild and cause no damage, but don't think of them as harmless. Treat all lows quickly. Realize that you are not destined to have severe lows simply because you use insulin. It also does no good to use insulin poorly because you have an obsessive fear of lows. This only complicates your goal of good control.

Hypoglycemia can be managed by adjusting insulin doses appropriately, testing glucoses frequently, wearing a CGM, keeping quick carbs on hand, and being willing to consume carbs if anyone asks if you are feeling alright. Wear an ID bracelet or pendant and carry a card in your wallet that shows you have diabetes. This will alert others if you happen to become low and are unable to take care of yourself.

19.2 Hypo Symptoms and When They Occur	
From Stress Hormones	**From Low Brain Glucose**
About 65 mg/dl (3.6 mmol/L)	**Below 55 mg/dl (3.1 mmol/L)**
• Sweating	• Confusion
• Shaking	• Poor concentration
• Irritability	• Mental slowness
• Stubbornness	• Blurred vision
• Fast heart rate	• Sudden tiredness
• Hunger	• Headache
• Feeling amped up or nervous	• Frequent sighing
• Resisting help	• Inability to form words
• Tingling of the lips or fingers	• Silliness
• Nausea	• Yawning
• Vomiting	• Seizure
	• Coma

19.3 How to Prevent Lows

- Test often or wear a CGM.
- Eat every meal or snack for which you've taken a bolus .
- Count carbs and bolus for the carb count and your current glucose.
- Use your experience to adjust your boluses, basals, or carbs. For example, if lows often occur in the afternoon, add an afternoon snack or, even better, increase your carb factor to lower your bolus at lunch or lower your basal rate before and after lunch.
- Check your BOB and eat carbs if BOB is excessive.
- Test before and after exercise, as well as during longer periods of exercise. Strenuous activity can lower your glucose for the next 36 hours.
- Always check your glucose before driving and during long drives. Eat carbs before driving and keep glucose tabs or quick carbs in sight anytime you drive. Being drunk and hypoglycemia are hard to tell apart. If you go low while driving, you may be considered drunk and not get assistance to raise your glucose.
- Be careful with alcohol. More than one to two drinks reduces the normal creation of glucose by the liver and makes lows likely during sleep.

Reduce Your Boluses and Basals

- If lows are frequent or severe.
- As soon as you start a diet or a new exercise program.
- Before, during and after exercise, especially if it is moderate or strenuous, lasts 40 minutes or longer, and is an activity you are not trained for.
- When stress levels drop, such as when you start a vacation.

Reduce Your Carb Bolus (Raise Your CarbF)

- If your lows often occur within one to three hours after carb boluses.
- Anytime daily activity (shopping, cleaning house, etc.) is increased.

Reduce Your Correction Bolus (Raise Your CorrF)

- If your lows often occur after you bolus to correct high readings.

Always discuss frequent or severe lows with your health care team.

19.4 How to Prevent Night Lows

Lows often occur at night because the body is most sensitive to insulin between midnight and 3 a.m. for normal sleep hours. In a person without diabetes, insulin levels are reduced automatically so that a low never happens. An insulin pump can be set to mimic this action with a lower basal rate starting 4 to 8 hours before 2 a.m.

If you suspect night lows, check at 2 a.m. for a few nights or wear a CGM. If your glucose does go low at night, reduce your basal rate starting at 9 p.m. or earlier until your nighttime glucose drops no more than 30 mg/dl (1.6 mmol/L) overnight.

Other Causes and Solutions:

- Covering a high bedtime reading with a correction bolus that is too large is a common cause of night lows. For bedtime highs, take less than your pump's recommended bolus. You can also set your correction factor to a larger number or raise your target glucose about 5 hours before bedtime.

- A short DIA hides BOB remaining at bedtime. Set DIA to 4.5 hrs or longer.

- Extra exercise or activity lowers the glucose for up to 24 to 36 hours afterward. After increased activity, reduce the dinner carb bolus and use an overnight temp basal rate reduction to perhaps 80% to 90% of normal. Eat extra carbs at bedtime. Check your glucose in the middle of the night and upon waking. Keep notes to follow next time.

- Always check your glucose and consider your BOB before you go to sleep. Compensate for any excess BOB with grams equal to BOB times your CarbF.

Lower Your Risk

1. Lower your basal rate, starting 2 to 4 hours before going to sleep.
2. Raise your CarbF and CorrF 5 hrs before bed to reduce BOB at bedtime.
3. Set your DIA to 4.5 hours or longer.
4. Raise your glucose target for the late afternoon and after to raise your bedtime glucose.
5. Use a temp basal reduction after extra exercise.

Symptoms

Hypoglycemia symptoms vary from person to person and from event to event, depending on how often lows occur and how low the glucose goes. Certain symptoms are caused by release of stress hormones, while others are caused when too little glucose reaches the brain and nervous system.

Symptoms usually start when readings fall below 65 to 55 mg/dl (3.6 to 3.1 mmol/L), although some people feel symptomatic at 90 mg/dl (5 mmol/L) and others will drop to 40 mg/dl (2.2 mmol/L) before they have symptoms.

The glucose at which you start to get hypoglycemia symptoms depends on:

1. Your current control – frequent lows reduce warning signs.

2. The level of your stress hormone reserves – frequent lows delay warning.

3. How fast your glucose drops – a more gradual drop gives less warning.

During a low, you may shake, sweat, and feel disoriented, or you may feel rather normal. Symptoms become harder to recognize during exercise, while concentrating, during focused involvement, while drinking alcohol, and when driving. Symptoms may be harder to recognize on a pump because the glucose often falls more gradually, but the slower fall also allows more time to recognize and respond to the low.

Even if you feel normal during a low, those around you will often notice changes in your behavior, personality or capability. Always be willing to check your glucose and treat yourself right away if a family member, friend, or coworker mentions this. Always check any time you suspect a low or anyone around you suggests you are low. Do this immediately and willingly no matter what you are involved in. Refusing to check is common since irritability and stubbornness occur early during a low. Cooperation minimizes embarrassment and will shorten your low.

> **19.5 Good Control Starts with Stopping LOWS!**
>
> Anytime you begin to have frequent lows, reduce your TDD to an iTDD, usually by up to 5 or 10 percent. Use this lower TDD to calculate new basal rates and new bolus factors for a safer pattern that has fewer lows and fewer highs following these lows. See Chapter 10 and Table 10.2.

Nighttime Symptoms

Over half of all lows occur during sleep. Night lows are a major cause of hypoglycemia unawareness because sleep masks the early signs of a low. The symptoms listed below are specific for night lows. If you wake up with any of these, check your glucose immediately or eat quick carbs (See Box 19.6.) and then check. Always keep fast-acting carbs close to your bed within easy reach.

Symptoms at night:

- Nightmares
- Waking up alert with difficulty going back to sleep
- Waking with a fast heart rate (check your pulse for this)
- Waking up with night clothes, sheets, or a pillow damp with sweat
- Waking up with a feeling that something isn't right

Symptoms the next morning that suggest a low during the night:

- Waking up "foggy-headed" or with a headache
- Having an unusually high reading after breakfast or before lunch caused by stress hormones that gradually release glucose from the liver

- A temporary loss of memory for words or names
- Feeling worn out

Wearing a CGM that alarms when you are low or checking your glucose in the middle of the night does wonders to identify and correct night lows. If you have night lows, review causes and adjust your carb intake, doses, or exercise to prevent them. Check more often from bedtime to breakfast until they are no longer a problem.

Causes and Prevention

Lows have many causes but frequent or severe lows mean that too much insulin is being given, especially when lows occur within one to three hours after a bolus, when more than 15 grams of glucose is required to bring the reading back to normal, or when lows occur during sleep or before breakfast. If one of these is happening, call your physician or health care team immediately to discuss how to lower your doses.

Causes of Lows

Lows are more likely

1. When too much insulin is taken
2. When a meal bolus is taken but the meal is missed, delayed, or interrupted
3. Under WAG conditions when carbs are estimated, not accurately counted
4. When a correction bolus is increased to bring a glucose down faster
5. When the DIA is too short and hides BOB
6. When boluses are given without checking the glucose (blind bolusing) or without checking how much BOB is present
7. After several boluses have been stacked over a short period of time
8. After drinking alcohol
9. During and after exercise, especially at night after an exercise for which you are not trained
10. On vacation (more activity and less stress with irregular eating)

Be alert for changes in your daily routine (travel, vacation, weight loss, stress, etc.) that may cause lows. People who exercise strenuously or for prolonged periods benefit

19.7 Check Short Term Basal versus Bolus Insulin

Many things can cause a low. When a low glucose happens, you want to find out if your basal or your bolus insulin caused the problem. To "measure" the relative effect of each, add up all the active bolus insulin at work during the previous 5 hours and compare this to the amount of basal insulin you received during this time. Be suspicious of the insulin dose (basal or bolus) that was larger during these 5 hours.

from frequent basal and bolus adjustments that match these changes in activity. More activity, less insulin. Less activity, more insulin. Alternate basal profiles can be set up to easily switch basal profiles for activity, menses, weekends, or vacations.

Each time you check your glucose, look to see how much BOB you have and consider whether the BOB may send your glucose low later. For instance, if your reading is 120 mg/dl (6.7 mmol/L) two hours after a bolus, you may need to eat some carbs to prevent a low. Know where to find the current BOB or remaining bolus insulin activity in your pump. See Box 19.9 to determine how many carbs you need to eat for a low.

19.8 How Much 1 Gram of Carbs May Raise Your BG	
If your weight is:	**1 gram will raise you about:**
50 lbs (23 kg)	8 mg/dl (0.44 mmol/L)
75 lbs (34 kg)	7 mg/dl (0.39 mmol/L)
90 lbs (41 kg)	6 mg/dl (0.33 mmol/L)
120 lbs (55 kg)	5 mg/dl (0.28 mmol/L)
160 lbs (73 kg)	4 mg/dl (0.22 mmol/L)
200 lbs (91 kg)	3 mg/dl (0.17 mmol/L)

Box 19.3 lists some important steps to prevent lows. The chance of having a followup low after an initial one is very high. After having an initial low, one research study found that there was a 46 percent chance for another low in the next 24 hours, 24 percent on the second day, and 12 percent on the third day after the original low.[105] Awareness of the extra risk that follows a first low can prevent a second one. Stress hormone release during the first low glucose reduces the body's stores for the next two to three days so the symptoms normally caused by stress hormone release during the second low tend to be milder and harder to recognize.

After a low happens, take steps to keep your readings higher for the next 24 to 36 hours, such as raising your correction target and using a temp basal reduction to lessen your risk for a second low. Alternatively, you may want to lower carb boluses somewhat or eat 10 to 15 grams of carb a few times that you do not cover with a bolus for 24 to 36 hours after the first low.

19.9 Treat Hypoglycemia with the Right Number of Carbs

1. Eat 15 grams of quick carbs immediately. (See Box 19.6.)

2. Then check how much BOB remains and eat additional grams of carbs = BOB times your CarbF. Include some slow acting carbohydrates and/or protein to keep you stable until your next meal. Cheese and crackers, bread with peanut butter, half an apple with cheese, a cup of milk, or other carb/protein combinations are good choices after eating the quick carbs.

3. Test your glucose 20 minutes later to make sure it has risen. Some pumps can be set up to remind you to do this.

4. After a moderate to severe low, thinking and coordination may not return to normal as quickly as you glucose reading does. Wait 30 to 45 minutes after the glucose rises above 80 mg/dl (4.4 mmol/L) before you drive a car or operate machinery.

Bolus on Board Tipping

When low, how many units of BOB you have left can tell you how many grams of carb you need to treat the low. Into your bolus calculator, simply enter the low glucose and keep increasing the number of carb grams. When your BOB equals your combined carb plus correction bolus, that number of grams of carb in your pump should be the number you need to treat the low glucose.

No more "15 grams" for all lows. Many bolus calculators do NOT give the correct bolus recommendation in this situation, but if your pump settings are correct you can quickly estimate for how many carbs you will need for each low you have. Bolus Tipping is particularly helpful for bedtime and middle of the night lows.

You Will Need More than 15-20 Grams of Quick Carbs When:

- BOB is present.
- A carb bolus was taken for a meal but you forgot to eat (Lots of BOB).
- Following several boluses when BOB and insulin stacking are excessive.
- You have been more physically active.

Treatment

Treat lows with quick carb products that are easy to keep on hand, but that your family and friends won't consume before you do, and that you will eat or drink when you are low. The quick carbs listed in Box 19.6 relieve symptoms quickly. In 10 to 20 minutes, you'll feel better and your brain, muscles and other organs will thank you for rapidly resupplying the glucose they need. Quick treatment minimizes the release of stress hormones, so that a high is less likely to follow the low. Quick treatment also preserves internal stores of stress hormones and makes it more likely that symptoms will signal the next low.

Glucose is the best treatment for lows. It may be called glucose or dextrose (a glucose-glucose molecule) on the ingredient list. Glucose can be found in glucose tablets, in certain candies like Sweet Tarts, and at a lower concentration in sports drinks like Gatorade. Box 19.6 lists a variety of quick carbs containing 15 grams of fast carbs that will raise the blood glucose 45 to 75 mg/dl (2.5 to 4.2 mmol/L) in most adults. One rule of thumb is 15/20: take 15 grams of carb and retest in 20 minutes (Even glucose takes a while to work.).

Table sugar or sucrose found in soft drinks and most candies is different from glucose or "blood sugar." Table sugar contains one glucose molecule and one fructose molecule. After it breaks down in the stomach, only half of these carbs are available as fast-acting glucose. Fruit juices provide mental relief, but take longer to treat serious hypoglycemia, as do regular candy and desserts. Foods with the highest glycemic index numbers (See Table 3.13.) will raise your glucose the fastest.

Treat lows quickly with quick carbs.
Eat more than 15 grams if you've been active or have BOB.

Treat but Don't Overtreat

The urge to overtreat lows is natural. Release of stress hormones during a low causes panic that may lead to an overdose of orange juice, chocolates, or the entire contents of your refrigerator. This makes your goal of stable readings hard to achieve. If you often rebound and go high after lows, over-treatment is the likely cause, although stress hormone release can also contribute to a rise. Lessen stress hormone release by treating lows quickly. Avoid letting panic take over if you want to avoid gaining excess weight from over-treatment. If your lows are frequent or severe, reduce your boluses or basals so you do not lose this battle.

> ### 19.10 Clever Pump Trick –
> ### What to Do when You Overeat for a Low
>
> If you overeat during a low, count how many carbs you ate as soon as your thinking clears. Enter the carb count into your pump along with the low glucose reading. From the carb bolus required, subtract the "correction" bolus that is usually expressed as a negative number of units and any BOB that is present. This total gives an appropriate bolus to cover your excess carb intake. Check your glucose again in 15 minutes to ensure it has risen. Recheck 2 hours later to to see if an additional bolus or additional carbs may be needed.

Be prepared for lows. Have quick carbs at your bedside, in your pocket or purse, at your desk, in the glove compartment or on the seat beside you, and where you exercise. Know how much you need to bring you out of a low. Stay calm and let your fast acting carbs reduce the panicked appetite that can lead you to overeat.

You may not be able to think clearly during a low, so you and your family and friends must know ahead of time how much glucose you need and where to find it. Fifteen grams of glucose raises the blood glucose about 60 mg/dl (3.3 mmol/L) for most adults (see Box 19.8). Retest 20 minutes after treatment to ensure the low has been corrected.

After quick carbs have been consumed, an additional complex carb and protein snack, like old-fashioned peanut butter and crackers, can help keep your glucose from falling later. Nutrition bars like a PowerBar or an Extend Bar contain raw cornstarch or other complex carbs and protein so they break down slowly. These can be a good choice as a nighttime snack to prevent night lows.

Once you are alert after the low, be sure to factor in any recent activity and any BOB that is still active. If a low happens 4 to 5 hours after your last bolus, only 10 to 20 grams of carbs is likely needed. But if a low happens only two or three hours after a bolus, more carbs will be needed to offset the BOB. If you have been more active than usual or missed a meal for which you bolused for, you will also need more carbs to treat a low.

Always check your current BOB when a test is done to determine how many carbs are needed if you are low or whether additional carbs may be needed to offset any BOB that is still working.

15 grams of quick carbs typically raises the glucose 45 to 75 mg/dl (2.5 to 4.5 mmol/L).

Tips for Treating Hypoglycemia

- Carry quick carbs like glucose tablets at all times. Know how much to eat. Don't use chocolate – it tastes great but it's too slow for lows and too easy to overeat.

- Have 15 grams of glucose tabs and check your glucose as soon as possible.

- Wait 15 to 20 minutes for quick carbs to work and retest to ensure your glucose has risen. Retreat if necessary.

- Assume the primary responsibility for handling your lows, but always be willing to accept help and advice from others.

- Do you feel normal? Does the world look so? Do others think you are acting strangely? Test immediately if in doubt.

- Let your family, friends, and those you are with know about your diabetes and what they can do to help if you become confused or weak suddenly.

- Tell family and friends when you vary your regimen or lifestyle in ways that make lows more likely. Share what is happening with your glucose control so that others will be prepared to help you if you need it.

- Test more often or wear a CGM anytime you change your insulin doses, food choices, activity, or when traveling or on vacation.

- Be very careful anytime lows become frequent, especially night lows.

- If you ever become unconscious or too incoherent to treat a low, discuss this with your physician immediately. A change in insulin doses will likely be needed.

- Work with an endocrinologist who understands and specializes in insulin delivery to improve your control and reduce your risk for lows.

Many people find that arm exercises like lifting, raking, shoveling, or pulling drop the glucose faster than exercises involving the legs.

Treatment of Severe Hypoglycemia

Severe hypoglycemia occurs when a person can no longer handle a low on his or her own. This can be dangerous if it happens while driving, when a person is alone, or if it results in loss of consciousness or convulsions. A Danish study found severe hypoglycemia occurred in 40 percent of people with Type 1 diabetes with an episode about once every 9 months and unconsciousness happening every two and a half years.[106]

Many problems associated with hypoglycemia arise because the brain depends on glucose to operate. As glucose levels fall, the person's ability to think, reason, and solve problems quickly becomes impaired. During a low glucose, a person's actions may range from anger and hostility to becoming lethargic or incoherent, depending on how fast and how far their glucose falls.

Ordinarily, the body releases stress hormones that eventually help raise the glucose, but they can make it difficult to treat the person who desperately needs help. Irritation and anger can be triggered by release of stress hormones, especially when others are asking questions and the person cannot think clearly enough to answer. It is important for those assisting this person to stay calm, recognize that hypoglycemia is underway, not react to the person's irrational actions, and treat the low quickly with fast carbs or glucagon. If irrational thought, anger, irritability, silliness, running away, or an insistence that "I feel fine" occurs, a low glucose level is almost certainly the cause.

What You Can Do

Keep glucagon handy at all times. Glucagon quickly raises the glucose by releasing stored glucose from the liver and can bring someone out of unconsciousness or a seizure in a few minutes. Glucagon kits are available by prescription and should be kept at home by everyone on insulin. *Be sure that a family member or a friend has been trained in how and when to inject glucagon.* A Certified Diabetes Educator, trained nurse, or pharmacist should train anyone who is likely to be present during a severe low glucose in how to inject glucagon.

A glucagon kit contains a syringe with saline and a small vial of dry glucagon powder that must be freshly mixed prior to injection. To prepare glucagon, inject the saline into the glass vial and shake the vial to dissolve the glucagon. The glucagon can be drawn up into the syringe contained in the kit or into a U-100 insulin syringe for more accurate dosing. The glucagon is then injected straight into muscle areas in the upper arm, leg or buttock.

Know how much glucagon to give. The glucagon vial contains 1 mg. of glucagon, which is generally enough for a 200 lb (90 kg) adult. Half this dose is usually all that someone who weighs 100 lbs (45 kgs) will need. For children, dosing is much easier if you put the full 1 milliliter of saline into the glucagon powder, mix, and then use a 30, 50, or 100 unit U-100 insulin syringe to give units of glucagon equal to half their body weight in lbs (or equal to body weight in kg). For example, a child who weighs 60 lbs (27 kg) would get 30 units and one who weighs 90 lbs (41 kg) would get 45 units.[104]

For easy access and fast action during an emergency, keep an appropriately sized insulin syringe inside or attached to your glucagon kit with written instructions on the dose that is needed. After the glucagon is given, the person's awareness should improve within 15 to 20 minutes.

Glucagon can be stored at room temperature or in the refrigerator. Check the expiration date periodically to ensure potency.

Using out-of-date glucagon is always better than not giving glucagon.

Don't Go Low when Driving

Driving a car can be hypnotic or trancelike. With attention focused on the road, you may not notice that your ability to think, make decisions, and interact with others has changed. If the glucose level drops slowly during a longer drive, a low becomes hard to recognize, especially if you are alone or your passenger is sleeping.

Always test and check your BOB before you put the key in the ignition. Have glucose tablets or quick carbohydrate easily accessible in your vehicle. On long drives, wear a CGM or keep it on the dashboard, or test at least every two hours. This is great for family harmony on vacation tips. Always test immediately if someone else in your vehicle requests that you do so, especially if you have hypoglycemia unawareness. Pull over and test your glucose if you have any doubts. The risk of injury or death to yourself and others is very high if you drive while low.

If you're involved in an accident due to a low glucose level, an automatic suspension of your license is likely. Be honest with state licensing to avoid loss of insurance coverage.

Tips for Those Helping Someone Who Is Low

If the person is somewhat responsive and able to swallow, safely encourage them to consume a sugared beverage, glucose gel, or a tube of cake icing. Anytime someone with severe hypoglycemia cannot eat or drink, an injection of glucagon is the best treatment.

Glucagon can be handy when someone resists treatment due to hypoglycemia unawareness, though help from others may be needed to hold them down, or when nausea does not allow carbs to be eaten.

If someone with diabetes is found unconscious, always assume this is caused by a low glucose and treat with glucagon. Never put something in the mouth of an unresponsive person. Get a glucose reading after giving the glucagon. If they do not respond to glucagon, call 911. This may also be necessary if the person having the low glucose is too irate or irrational to accept help, or they are stronger than those trying to help. In an emergency, stay calm and keep your emotions under control. Tell the emergency operator right away that the person has diabetes, is on insulin, and appears to be having a severe low glucose. Give instructions, if needed, on how to get to your location. Let the paramedics who are well trained do a glucose test, give carbohydrates, inject glucagon, or start IV glucose.

What to do if a person resists help:

- Control your emotions. If the person you are helping is stubborn, acts silly or becomes angry, do not take it personally. Recognize that their mental function is impaired. Do not embarrass them. Prepare yourself ahead of time to deal with the variety of hypoglycemia attitudes you may encounter.

- Take charge of the situation. Use a gentle but firm tone. A non-confrontational stance, such as sitting or standing beside the person helps.

- Say, "Here, have this piece of candy," or try "This tastes great. Here, try some." If the person refuses to be persuaded, be kind but firm and say, "You'll feel better after you drink (or eat) this."

- Avoid direct questions like "Are you low?" or "Do you need to test?" A person unable to think is likely to say "NO" and become defensive.

- Do not let the person drive a car, run machinery, or become involved in other dangerous activities that require coordination and thinking. Hiding car keys or disabling a car by pulling the spark plug cable off may be necessary.

- Ask others for help or call 911 if you cannot treat the person yourself. Keep embarrassment to a minimum and cooperation to a maximum.

It's not what we don't know that hurts,
it's what we know that ain't so.

Will Rogers

Avoid Hypoglycemia Unawareness

The symptoms of shaking and sweating caused by the release of stress hormones let most people know their glucose is too low. However, stress hormone levels can become depleted after a series of frequent lows, and this may result in a loss of these warning signs. *Loss of symptoms often leads to hypoglycemia unawareness.*

When hypoglycemia unawareness occurs, a person's thinking becomes sufficiently impaired that they no longer recognize they are low. Even if a meter reading shows a low, they may not be capable of understanding the situation and treating it. If their hypoglycemia is not recognized and treated by someone else, bizarre behavior, a car accident, *grand mal* seizures, or even death may follow.

A 2005 report by the U.S. Department of Transportation reviewed 15 research studies and found that, on average, 25% of those with Type 1 diabetes have hypo unawareness.[107] A study that evaluated tight glucose control in Type 2 diabetes by the Veterans Administration showed that severe lows were about 20 times more common in Type 1 diabetes than in Type 2 primarily because fewer Type 2s are completely dependent on insulin.[108]

The lower a person's average A1c or glucose level, the higher their risk for hypo unawareness. In the Diabetes Control and Complications Trial, hypo unawareness was three times more common in the intensively controlled group compared to the conventionally controlled group.[109] The presence of hypo unawareness indicates that the TDD and one or more pump settings are excessive. Insulin doses must be lowered and glucose targets raised sufficiently to stop both frequent and severe lows.

Causes

The primary cause of unawareness is depletion of the body's supplies of stress hormones from frequent lows. These can occur during the day, but are more frequently seen after long periods of nighttime hypoglycemia that go unrecognized. In the DCCT trial, about 55% of lows occurred during sleep, and typically people wake up for less than half of their night lows. When night lows go unrecognized, hypo unawareness becomes likely.[110]

231

Dr. Thiemo Veneman and his research team in the Netherlands studied the effect of lowering the glucose level of 10 people who did not have diabetes on two occasions.[111] While the participants slept in a hospital, the researchers used insulin to lower their glucose level below 45 mg/dl (2.5 mmol/L) for two hours in the middle of the night. As occurs during most nighttime lows, they did not wake up.

Five people were put through a nighttime low on the first visit and the other five on the second visit. On waking in the morning, all were given insulin to lower their glucose to see when they would recognize the symptoms of a low glucose. After sleeping through a night low, even people without diabetes had more trouble recognizing a low the next day.

> ## 20.1 Risk Factors for Hypo Unawareness:
> - Too much bolus or basal insulin
> - After physical activity that you don't normally do
> - Following a recent low or frequent lows, especially at night
> - A rapid fall in glucose
> - A prior low glucose in the last 24 to 48 hours
> - Having diabetes for over 10 years
> - Alcohol intake in the last 12 hours
> - Stress, depression, and situations where self-care becomes less of a priority
> - Excessive fear of complications and controlling glucoses too tightly

A low glucose with shaking and sweating depletes stored stress hormones. This makes it harder to recognize a second low over the next 72 hours or so while stress hormone supplies are being restored. The reduced awareness in people without diabetes in the study above makes it is even more likely that similar lows would cause hypoglycemia unawareness in someone with diabetes and a history of repeated low readings.

Symptoms for lows become weaker in people who have had Type 1 diabetes for several years and as people age. Symptoms also decrease in anyone after repeated lows lessen the body's ability to release stress hormones. Women are more prone to hypo unawareness because they have less counterregulatory hormone response and less obvious symptoms of lows than men.[112] Drinking alcohol also makes symptoms harder to recognize and slows recovery. Having more than one or two drinks can block the natural glucagon response that causes the liver to make glucose in order to raise a low glucose level.[113]

How to Reverse Hypoglycemia Unawareness

Avoidance of all lows is key to regaining warning symptoms. In one research study, researchers reduced the frequency of lows in people with hypo unawareness to see whether they could regain awareness.[114] *Preventing all lows for about three months returned them to nearly normal hypoglycemia responses.* The researchers raised the subjects' pre-meal glucose target to 140 mg/dl (7.8 mmol/L) to lessen hypoglycemia from

20.2 How to Reverse Hypoglycemia Unawareness

- Wear a CGM or check your glucose often to avoid lows.

- Keep your glucose above 70 mg/dl (4 mmol/L) for 3 to 12 weeks.

- Lower your basals and boluses so they match daily events and lifestyle changes.

- Set your correction target higher, such as 140 or 150 mg (7.8 or 8.3 mmol/L).

- Be careful to avoid subsequent lows that are more likely for up to 72 hours after a first low.

- Test in the middle of the night once or twice a week to prevent night lows.

- Do not drink alcohol, or reduce intake to one or two servings a day.

once every other day to once every 22 days. After avoiding low glucose readings for this long, people regained their low glucose symptoms and recognized when they were low.

To prevent lows and regain awareness, wear a CGM, set your target glucose higher temporarily, and lower basal and/or bolus doses to closely match your diet and exercise. Remember to be more alert for warnings of a subsequent low for up to 72 hours after a low glucose occurs. Consider any glucose below 60 mg/dl (3.3 mmol/L) as serious. Immediately reduce your boluses or basal rates so your readings do not go that low in the future, unless there is an obvious cause for the low like an error in carb counting or inappropriately overriding the bolus calculator. See Box 19.4 for suggestions for preventing night lows. Most hypo unawareness disappears once appropriate adjustments in pump settings are made, and bolus and basal doses are matched as needed for carb intake, activity, and glucose patterns.

To reduce your risk, deal with issues related to stress, depression, and other circumstances that take your focus away from self-care. Avoid alcohol or limit consumption to less than one or two drinks a day. After increased activity, reduce your basals and boluses for several hours. An occasional 2 a.m. blood test can do wonders in spotting unrecognized nighttime lows, so you can avoid them. Using a CGM can alert you and your health care team to unrecognized hypoglycemia and its timing. A CGM warns of nighttime lows and can awaken you for earlier treatment. Frequent testing or wearing a CGM enables the basal or bolus reductions that are needed and help prevent lows before they happen.

If you require help from someone else to get out of a severe low, call your doctor immediately. Hypo unawareness is very likely to occur again unless you change your pump settings. You may be told to raise your correction target, make immediate dose reductions, and check your glucose frequently, including a 2 a.m. test. A little lost sleep is a minor problem compared to an exhausting or dangerous low.

Avoid Death in Bed

The most serious complication of hypoglycemia is death. Though uncommon, this can happen to otherwise healthy people who have frequent or severe lows, sometimes in an overzealous attempt to stay "normal." The term "death in bed" is derived because death occurs at night in bed when hypoglycemia goes undetected for a long time and becomes severe. These deaths may be caused when hypoglycemia or stress hormone release triggers a cardiac arrhythmia. Death in bed causes 3% to 6% of all deaths among people with diabetes under the age of 40.[115,116]

> **20.3 How to Stop Frequent Lows**
>
> 1. Find the time of day most of your lows occur.
> 2. Identify whether it is your basal, carb boluses, or correction boluses that cause these lows.
> 3. Check your basal/bolus balance to make sure each makes up about 50% of your TDD. If one is larger, that would usually be the one to reduce.
> 4. If lows are frequent and severe, find your current average TDD and lower this by 10% or more. If lows are occasional and mild, a 5% reduction may work. See Table 10.2.

How to Avoid Death in Bed:

- Wear a CGM to prevent unrecognized night lows, or test your glucose level in the middle of the night often enough to eliminate them.
- Avoid having glucoses below 50 mg/dl (2.8 mmol/L).
- Use the Auto-Off feature available in most pumps or the basal suspend feature available in some pumps if you live alone.
- Use a temp basal reduction at night following any day with increased activity.

> **20.4 Use Auto-Off or Basal Suspend for Hypo Unawareness**
>
> The Auto-Off feature in a pump lets the user set a period of time after which the pump will automatically turn off if the wearer goes low and does not push any of the pump buttons. Normally, it is set for 8 or 9 hours to cover the nighttime hours, but it may also be set for 4 to 6 hours for daytime protection. This helps anyone who lives alone, has gone unconsciousness due to hypoglycemia, or who is prone to this. The downside is that if the alert is not heard, the pump shuts off and stays off.
>
> The basal rate suspend feature, available in the Medtronic Veo™ pump worn with their CGM, sounds an alert if the glucose goes low. If the wearer does not clear the alert, basal delivery is automatically shut for two hours. The basal then turns on for four hours, but will again turn off for two more hours if there is still no response.

People who want to share their religious views with you almost never want you to share yours with them.

Dave Barry

Reduce Skin and Site Problems

An infusion set is a foreign body placed through the skin. It can cause irritation, discomfort, infection, or other problems. Many pumpers rarely encounter a serious problem, while others have to pay close attention to avoid them.

This chapter discusses handling skin and infusion site problems

- Infections
- Site bleeding
- Pump lipohypertrophy
- Scarring and poor absorption
- Pump bumps
- Allergies

Infections

Many people with diabetes face a higher risk of infection after a history of high glucose levels or other factors have weakened the immune system, but infections also occur in relatively healthy people. Most pump-related infections can fortunately be prevented with good insertion technique, such as washing your hands with soap and water, changing the infusion site every 3 days, not breathing or blowing on the infusion set or site, not touching the infusion needle or top of the insulin bottle, cleaning the site with IV Prep, Betadine™, or Hibiclens®, and protecting the site with a bio-occlusive adhesive like IV3000.

Watch for these signs of an infection at the infusion site:

- Redness or inflammation
- Pain
- Warmth
- Swelling

Contact your physician immediately if signs of an infection are seen. Early treatment with an antibiotic keeps a small infection from developing into an abscess that may require surgery or hospitalization. You will prefer your physician calling in a prescription rather than having to lance an abscess or write hospital admission orders. Do not wait until it becomes a crisis. If you are prone to skin infections, discuss with your physician the practice of keeping a prescription on hand for a broad spectrum antibiotic to use for early treatment. The first sign of a site infection may be unexplained high glucose levels. *Always check the infusion site if two unexplained high readings occur in a row to see if the infusion set has come out or there might be an early infection.*

Staph bacteria are the most common cause for site infections. Antibiotic resistant staph, called methacillin-resistant staph aureus or MRSA are becoming increasingly common and can turn a site infection into a serious health risk. Although rare, toxic shock has been caused by an infusion site infection.[97] Assume that an infection can happen and take care that it does not. Use sterile technique described in "Prepare The Skin Site" on page 84 to prepare the site and insert the infusion set or patch pump. Sterile technique and good hygiene are your best insurance against infection.[98]

Bleeding

On the Skin

When an infusion set is inserted, the needle can nick a small blood vessel near the surface of the skin. This shows up as a bloodstain under the tape or dressing. Surface bleeding can be ignored as long as the site is not inflamed, painful, enlarged, threatening to discolor your wardrobe, or causing high readings.

Inside the Infusion Line

Blood leaking into the infusion tubing from the catheter under the skin means that bleeding is occurring around the tip of the infusion set. When insulin mixes with blood, its activity is greatly reduced. A high glucose may be the first sign of this problem. Any time you see blood inside the infusion tubing, immediately remove the entire infusion set and insert a new set at another location.

At the Infusion Tip

Bleeding may also occur beneath the skin near the end of the infusion set and cause a *hematoma* without blood appearing in the infusion line. This lump of blood under the skin may feel uncomfortable or sore like a bruise, but the skin above it usually appears normal. A lump can usually be felt under the skin after the infusion set is removed. A high glucose may be the first sign of this problem. A hematoma may allow bacteria to grow and increase your risk of an infection or abscess.

Change to a new infusion set at a new site any time you feel a lump under the skin. Wash your hands with soap and water, and then firmly squeeze the lump to extract as much matter as you can. If the discharge comes out bright red, it is likely a relatively harmless hematoma. If any other color is seen, it could be an abscess and may require an antibiotic. If you have any doubts about whether a sore spot or lump under the skin is a hematoma or an infection, call your physician or health care team immediately. Early treatment is always best.

> ### 21.1 Site Problem? Inspect It!
>
> If soreness or redness occurs at an infusion site and a lump can be felt under the skin, firmly squeeze out any fluid underneath the skin after the set is removed. If bright red blood comes out, it is likely just bleeding or a hematoma under the skin. Change to a new infusion site using a new infusion set.
>
> However, if the fluid is whitish, discolored, or appears to be pus, the infection may spread through the blood if you simply change your set and site. Call your doctor or visit a clinic right away to discuss the need for an antibiotic. Your doctor may need to see your site and do a culture to make this decision. Watch the old site to ensure the antibiotic is working. Don't use it again until the inflammation and swelling are gone.

Pump Lipohypertrophy

When infusion sets are placed into only one area of the body, excess insulin exposure causes fat cells to grow and results in a large fatty bump, called *pump lipohypertrophy*, under the skin. A simple solution for this cosmetic issue is to rotate infusion sites through other parts of the abdomen and buttocks. Change infusion sites every three days and avoid the involved area for 4 to 8 weeks to allow the enlargement to disappear.

Scarring and Poor Absorption

Visible scarring is obvious, but scarring underneath may be present if an area of skin feels firm and unyielding, has undergone surgery, or was the site of an abscess in the past. Luckily, the skin is our largest organ and there are many locations in which an infusion set can be placed.

Poor absorption of insulin at infusion sites due to scarring can occur, but scarring and poor absorption get an excessive amount of the blame for control problems caused by poor infusion set design and other issues. When other sources for high readings are carefully reviewed, your skin will rarely be the real cause.

If your glucose rises soon after inserting a new set and remains difficult to control, a kink in the Teflon line caused by the use of an autoinserter may be a likely cause. If the glucose is well controlled at first but rises 24 or more hours later, an insulin leak from the site, caused by movement or lifting of the Teflon catheter from tugs on the infusion line, may be the reason.

Pump Bumps

A pump bump sounds like a dent found in your pump after it's dropped on the floor. Instead, it is a slightly red, raised, pimple-sized, non-itching spot found at the infusion site after an infusion set is removed. The spot gradually disappears after you change to a new infusion site, but a reddish-brownish discoloration may linger for a few days or weeks. Pump bumps are usually caused when the Teflon catheter or metal needle is moved by tugs on an infusion line that is not anchored with tape.

The best way to prevent pump bumps is to always anchor the infusion line with a short length of 1" tape placed about 2 inches away from the site adhesive. This stops tugging at the insertion site. For further skin protection, you can place an IV 3000 or other adhesive on the skin before inserting the infusion set, or by placing this on top of one of the low profile metal sets. Take care to anchor your infusion line, use sterile technique, and change the infusion site every 3 days.

Allergies

Your skin may not like every infusion set, plastic infusion line, tape or dressing you use to keep insulin flowing. These are more likely than insulin to trigger an allergic reaction and are easy to diagnose because the itchy area, irritation, or redness forms a pattern with the same shape as the tape, dressing or infusion line that causes it.

When an infusion set or insulin is the culprit, redness, irritation, and usually itching will occur at the point where the Teflon or metal needle enters the skin. However, when there is only redness and residual reddish-brown spots where the catheter was inserted without itching or infection, this is likely a pump bump, discussed above.

Allergies usually start a few days or weeks after a particular tape or adhesive material is first used. Treatment involves switching to another brand of tape, dressing, or infusion set. A protective dressing like Skin Prep™ can also be used under the offending product before it is inserted or applied to the skin. If an allergy or itching occurs, discuss changing to another brand of infusion set or using Skin Prep™ with your physician.

Allergies to human insulin are extremely rare with today's highly purified insulins. An insulin allergy starts as a localized reaction with itching and redness at the spot where the insulin is infused, usually within 5 to 15 minutes after the first bolus at that site is given. If a skin reaction does not occur at the infusion site, an insulin allergy is unlikely to be the cause for any other symptoms that may be happening. Although rare, a serious systemic insulin allergy can trigger widespread itching or possibly anaphylactic shock. Insulin antibody tests are available to check for rare insulin allergies. A trial with another brand of insulin or desensitization to insulin by an allergy specialist may be necessary.

If you can't stand solitude, maybe you bore others too.

Bob Gordon

Exercise

CHAPTER

22

Exercise sharpens the mind, tones the body, and strengthens the heart. It combats depression, improves well being, increases endurance, minimizes stress and fatigue, and lowers body fat and cholesterol levels. Exercise is important for everyone's health and especially in diabetes.

With some planning, glucose monitoring, and balancing of carbs and insulin, you can exercise with renewed confidence, knowing that you are strengthening your body, improving your ability to manage your diabetes, and offsetting your risk of complications.

This chapter explains

- Benefits of exercise
- Things that affect glucose during exercise
- How to use carb equivalents called ExCarbs to increase carbs, decrease boluses or basals, or lower high readings during exercise
- Tips on avoiding exercise-related lows
- Why your glucose may rise after exercise
- When a reading is too high to exercise
- Cautions of exercise

Benefits

The more active and the more fit you are, the lower your risk for *cardiovascular disease (CVD)* and the longer you will live. This protection becomes especially important with the higher risk for heart disease in diabetes. Researchers studying Harvard alumni found that lifespan increases steadily as exercise levels rise from burning 500 calories a week (couch potato) to 3,500 calories per week (physically fit).[100] The exercise needed to burn 3,500 calories is equivalent to walking three miles an hour for seven hours (27 miles) a week, bicycling 10 miles an hour for five hours (50 miles) a week, or running nine miles an hour for 2.7 hours (24.3 miles) a week.

If burning 3,500 calories a week is too much, getting off the couch and starting to exercise protects against CVD. In the Health Professionals' Follow-Up Study, 2803 men with no physical impairments but with diabetes were followed for many years. One quarter of these men with the highest level of total physical activity had 33% less CVD and 42% fewer

239

deaths than the lowest quarter. Interestingly, walking was associated with less risk of mortality, while walking faster was associated with less cardiovascular disease and less risk of dying, regardless of how long people walked. [101] These researchers found that there was

22.1 Your Goal Determines How You Exercise			
Your Goal:	**Frequency**	**Intensity**	**Duration**
Reduce Risk of Heart Disease and Illness	2-3 times a week	40% max heart rate	15–30 min
Get Physically Fit	4 times a week	70–90% max heart rate	15–30 min
Lose Weight	5 times a week	45–60% max heart rate	45–60 min
220 – your age = your maximum heart rate			

© 2012 Diabetes Services, Inc.

a 70% reduction in cardiovascular disease among those who walked an hour 4 to 7 times/wk. Table 22.1 reviews the frequency, intensity, and duration of exercise required to reach different goals.

Even the amount of oxygen you breathe depends on your glucose level. Austrian researchers found when glucose levels are routinely elevated that airflow through the lungs is reduced as much as 15 percent, sufficient to impede performance.[103]

Managing your glucose level during and after exercise depends on how well you manage your carb intake, and basal and bolus adjustments. The section that follows provides the basic information you'll want to know, while the section after that provides the tools you'll need to appropriately lower insulin doses and add carbs.

22.2 Glucose and Insulin Levels Impact Performance		
Blood Glucose	**Effects of Glucose and Insulin on Metabolism**	**Impact on Performance**
< 70 mg/dl (3.9 mmol/L)	Too much insulin and not enough glucose available to cells	Fatigue, poor performance
70 to 180	**Efficient fuel flow**	**Maximum performance**
> 180 mg/dl (> 10 mmol/L)	If insulin level is OK, glucose comes down	Performance might be reduced – exercise OK.
> 250 mg/dl (13.9 mmol/L)	If insulin level is OK (ketone level is not moderate or large) – exercise should lower glucose	Fatigue, poor performance – moderate exercise is OK if ketones are not present.

© 2012 Diabetes Services, Inc.

Important Things to Know about Exercise

Glucose and Fat Are Your Main Fuels

Although glucose and glycogen are easily accessible and rapidly released during exercise, the supply of these fuels in the body is somewhat limited. For example, during strenuous exercise, a normal blood glucose level can be depleted in about four minutes, compared to 30 minutes at rest.[104] Additional glucose is available in the interstitial fluid around cells. Muscle cells have their own glycogen stores from which they can withdraw glucose for some time. Other cells like the nerve cells that provide coordination to these muscles depend on glucose from the blood. As these blood glucose levels are drawn down, the liver plays a critical role in supplying additional glucose by breaking down its glycogen stores and releasing glucose into the blood. Even the liver's glycogen stores can be depleted after 20 to 30 minutes of very strenuous exercise.

Fat is the body's largest fuel reserve. Fat stores are about 2,000 times as large as glucose stores and are nearly impossible to deplete even in a thin person.

> **22.3 Control During Exercise Depends on:**
> - Your current BOB, glucose, and glucose trend
> - Timing of the exercise relative to recent meals and boluses
> - The duration and intensity of exercise
> - Your training level
> - Whether the exercise is aerobic or anaerobic
> - Stress hormone release in competitive sports

Your Insulin Level during Exercise

During long periods of activity, blood insulin levels have to be lowered to access fat stores and prevent the blood glucose from dropping. When someone without diabetes starts a strenuous exercise like running a marathon, the blood insulin level drops to half of its pre-exercise level within the first 15 to 30 minutes.[105] During moderate exercise, about an hour passes before the same drop in the blood insulin level is seen.

A reduced insulin level for exercise:
- Lets the liver make and release new glucose
- Allows more fat to be released from fat cells

If your blood insulin level is too high, more glucose enters exercising muscles from the blood and less fat is available to replace the glucose. To maintain glucose levels, you have to eat or drink carbs to offset the high insulin level, or are forced to start with a high glucose level. In contrast, if your blood insulin level is too low, excess glucose and free fatty acids are released into the blood and the glucose level rises.

The right insulin level avoids these fuel delivery problems. Performance and glucose stability improve when the insulin level is lowered enough so that muscles can easily access internal stores of fat and glucose, but not so low that glucose levels rise.

22.4 How Your Insulin Level Affects Performance			
Insulin Level	**Effect on Glucose and Fat Stores**	**Effect on Glucose**	**Effect on Performance**
Low	Less glucose enters muscles, more release from fat stores and liver glycogen.	High or rising	Poor performance, possible ketosis
Ideal	Glucose enters muscles, glucose and fat are released as fuel normally.	Level	Optimal performance
High	More glucose enters muscles, less release from glucose and fat stores.	Low or falling	Poor performance, probable hypoglycemia

Table 22.4 summarizes the impact of the insulin level on glucose and fat stores, glucose levels, and performance.

A normal glucose level during and after exercise is the best indicator that your insulin doses and carb intake are in balance.

Impact of Exercise Intensity and Duration on Glucose

Walking or running a mile both consume almost the same number of calories, but where the calories come from differs. At rest, free fatty acids supply most of our fuel. During mild exercise like walking, energy is still largely obtained from fat, so the glucose is less likely to fall.

In a one-mile walk, 25 percent of the calories come from glucose with the rest coming from fat. When running the same mile at a strenuous pace, as much as 80 percent of the calories come from glucose. Strenuous exercise requires more carb intake or a larger reduction in insulin doses than mild exercise even though the same number of calories is consumed.

Just as the length of a car trip determines how many gallons of fuel will be consumed, the duration of exercise determines how many grams of carbs will be consumed. Longer activities are more likely to cause the glucose to fall. For instance, a leisurely 30-minute walk has little impact on the glucose, but a 60-minute walk may require extra carbs or a small reduction in a previous bolus. In someone with a normal pancreas, as moderate or strenuous exercise extends beyond 40 to 60 minutes, the blood insulin level gradually falls. This allows the body to preserve its limited stores of glucose and glycogen and switch to using more fat for fuel.

For example, a 150 pound person without diabetes will use 3,350 calories during six hours of moderately strenuous exercise. Near the start of exercise, glucose supplies 80 percent of the fuel they need. After 3 hours, about equal amounts of energy come from glucose and fat, and after 6 hours, almost 80 ee percent of energy will be derived from fat. Over the full 6 hours, about half the calories come from carb intake or release from internal glycogen stores, while the other half comes from internal fat stores.

Higher insulin levels require that more carbs be eaten to keep the glucose from falling. 3,350 calories is equivalent to almost two pounds of pure sugar or twenty 12-ounce cans of regular soda. A reduction in insulin doses for long periods of exercise prevents low glucoses as well as stomach aches. If you lower it too far, however, glucose will begin to climb.

Very intense or competitive exercise, on the other hand, releases counter-regulatory (stress) hormones. High intensity anaerobic exercise, like the 100-yard dash, and some competitive events release stress hormones that raise the glucose. Someone with diabetes who runs the 100-yard dash would want to start the race with a normal glucose level, and may need to take a bolus of insulin afterward to lessen the coming spike in glucose. The release of stress hormones during anaerobic exercise can be turned to your advantage during longer bouts of exercise to prevent lows. For example, when running a marathon or during a long bike ride, 10 to 20 second spurts of anaerobic exercise appear to release enough stress hormones that the glucose is less likely to go low.

In Table 22.5, the number of grams needed for each 100 lb. of weight for various lengths and intensities of exercise is shown, and this would be adjusted for your weight. Unless your insulin level is excessively high during the activity, these estimates should be the maximum number of grams you require for the exercise. As you become trained for this activity and reduce your basal and bolus doses appropriately, fewer carb equivalents than these amounts will be needed. If you find you need more than the carb amounts in the table, carefully review whether your basal rates or boluses may be too high.

Another estimate, based on body weight, says that intense activity requires about one half gram of carb per pound (or about 1 g/kg) of body weight per hour.[106] This means that someone who weighs 100 lbs would need 50 grams of carb or less per hour for strenuous exercise.

The longer and more strenuous an activity, the more you need to lower your bolus and basal doses to keep from going low.

Training Status

If you are untrained for an activity, you'll need as much as 25 percent more glucose than when you are trained. Training builds glycogen stores in the muscles being used so fuel will be readily available when these muscles are used again. One benefit to training is that large glycogen stores tend to reduce glucose fluctuations. Like shock absorbers, large glycogen stores minimize falls in glucose with less rise after meals as more glucose is shifted into these larger stores. Once basal rates and boluses are appropriately adjusted, the fit person tends to have more stable readings.

New activities like hoeing a garden in the spring or starting a new exercise typically require more carb intake, and a slightly larger reduction in basal rates and boluses doses, especially when the activity last longer than 45 to 90 minutes. Even when different muscles in the legs or arms are used, a larger reduction in insulin doses will be needed. For example, someone who runs regularly will experience a greater drop in glucose when they ride a bike, even though the total energy they use during the run and the bike ride are the same.

With new activities, a larger fall in the glucose occurs for several hours afterward as glycogen stores are enlarged in these relatively untrained muscles. During this glycogen buildup, more glucose is drawn from the blood as the body prepares to do the same activity again. The blood glucose can fall more than usual for a day or two after prolonged exercise as glycogen rebuilding and enlargement occurs.

Glycogen stores developed during routine exercise get smaller when the exercise is missed for three days or more. If a runner or biker has their normal schedule interrupted by weather or circumstances, more glycogen rebuilding occurs when they return to their exercise, and a larger than normal fall in glucose may occur.

The less trained you are, the larger the insulin reduction you will require. When you start a new exercise or activity, or return to your usual routine after a lapse, larger reductions in boluses and basal rates will be needed. More information on how to quickly restore glycogen and lessen the risk of a delayed low is covered in the next section.

The less trained you are for an activity, the more you need to lower your bolus and basal doses to keep from going low.

Convert Exercise into Grams of Carb with ExCarbs

A good way to determine how many grams of carb and how much insulin reduction you need for an exercise is to first convert its intensity and duration into grams of carb called ExCarbs. *ExCarbs quantifies how many carbs an exercise is likely to consume.* For instance, if someone weighs 150 pounds and runs 30 minutes (duration) at 7 miles per hour (effort or intensity), exercise physiologists know this run will consume 320 calories. The total calories consumed in an activity or exercise are relatively easy to calculate, similar to calculating how many gallons of gas your car will consume on a trip.

If the 320 calories came only from glucose, 320 calories divided by 4 calories per gram equals 80 grams of carb. However, the human body is similar to a hybrid car engine in that it uses two fuels. Both internal stores of glucose and fat, as well as carbs that are eaten can be used as fuel for exercise, so 80 grams of carb will not be needed.

Many decades ago, exercise physiologists measured how many calories are used in different activities per 100 lbs. of body weight, and what percentage of these calories come from glucose compared to fat. More intense exercise uses a higher percentage

This ExCarb table shows the maximum grams of carbs required for one hour of specific exercises for people who weigh 100, 150, and 200 lbs. When insulin doses are appropriate, these should be the maximum needed per hour to prevent a low glucose.

of carbs, while longer exercises begin to use more fat for fuel. This lets us closely approximate how many grams of carb will be consumed based on the intensity and the duration of various activities for each 100 lbs. of body weight. The approximate number of carbs needed for 1 hour of various intensities of activity is listed in Table 22.5. The impact of exercise duration is covered in Table 22.9.

An exercise's length is easy to determine with a watch, but its intensity is specific to the person doing the exercise. If two people run side by side, one may be running at maximum intensity while the other may be relaxed and carrying on an animated conversation. Personal intensity can to be estimated on

22.5 ExCarbs: Grams of Carb per Hour of Activity °

Activity		100 lbs.	150 lbs.	200 lbs.
baseball		25	38	50
basketball	moderate	35	48	61
	vigorous	59	88	117
bicycling	6 mph	20	27	34
	10 mph	35	48	61
	14 mph	60	83	105
	18 mph	95	130	165
	20 mph	122	168	214
dancing	moderate	17	25	33
	vigorous	28	43	57
digging		45	65	83
eating		6	8	10
golf (pull cart)		23	35	46
handball		59	88	117
jump rope 80/min		73	109	145
mopping		16	23	30
mountain climbing		60	90	120
outside painting		21	31	42
raking leaves		19	28	38
running	5 mph	45	68	90
	8 mph	96	145	190
	10 mph	126	189	152
shoveling		21	45	57
skating	moderate	25	34	43
	vigorous	67	92	117
skiing	crosscountry 5mph	76	105	133
	downhill	52	72	92
	water	42	58	74
soccer		45	67	89
swimming	slow crawl	41	56	71
	fast crawl	69	95	121
tennis	moderate	23	34	45
	vigorous	59	88	117
volleyball	moderate	23	34	45
	vigrorous	59	88	117
walking	3 mph	15	22	29
	4.5 mph	30	45	59

a 1 to 7 scale. The number 1 represents a slight increase in activity, such as a casual walk, while a 7 would be all-out exercise, such as running so hard that you are barely able to talk between breaths.

Lower numbers are given to activities that are relatively easy to do, such as casual walking. Middle numbers are given to things that make you breathe hard but you are able to do for some time, such as brisk walking or jogging. The highest numbers would apply to exercise that causes deep breathing but you can still carry on a conversation. Examples might be race walking or cross-country skiing.

> ## 22.6 Quick and Slow Carbs for Exercise
>
> Not all carbs are the same. Knowing how quickly different foods will raise the blood sugar can be useful.
>
> Fast carbs are ideal for raising low blood sugars before or during exercise, and for exercise that consumes carbs rapidly. Fast carbs include glucose tablets, Sweet Tarts, honey, corn flakes, raisin bran, athletic drinks (Gatorade™, Power Ade™), dried or ripe fruits, and regular soft drinks.
>
> Slow carbs help prevent a blood sugar drop during longer periods of activity. They can be eaten at the start of exercise and every 45 minutes thereafter. Slow carbs also help replenish glycogen stores after exercise. Slow carbs include PowerBars™, oatmeal, Swiss muesli, fruit, ginger snaps, pasta *al dente*, brown rice, and many candy bars.

You can use ExCarbs equivalents to:

1. **Eat more carbs**
2. **Take less insulin**
3. **Lower a high glucose**
4. **Or a combination of these**

Eat More Carbs

The simplest way to balance exercise is to eat extra carbs. No carb bolus is needed to cover these carbs. To use ExCarbs, look up your planned exercise in Table 22.5 and find out how many carbs you need each hour to balance it. This number of carbs would usually be the maximum number you need to eat before, during and after the exercise to maintain control. Often less than these maximum amounts are needed if you are already trained for the activity and have reduced your insulin doses appropriately.

For instance, if you weigh 150 pounds and take a one hour walk at 3 miles an hour, you will use 22 grams of carbs in your walk as shown in Table 22.5. This is equal to an average-size apple or a cup of milk plus a graham cracker. If you walk at the same pace for two hours rather than one, you will need 44 grams of carbohydrate, while if you walk only 30 minutes, 11 grams are required.

If you run the same 3 miles at 8 m.p.h. rather than walk, you will need 53 grams of carbohydrate (145 grams times 22 min. ÷ 60 min.), even though it takes only 22 minutes

22.7 ExCarbs Needed for Exercise per 100 lbs. (45 kg) of Weight

For intensity, the number 1 represents a slight increase in activity, such as a casual walk. A 7 would be all-out exercise, such as running so hard that you are barely able to talk between breaths.

Duration (minutes)	Exercise Intensity						
	1	2	3	4	5	6	7
15	4 g	9 g	13 g	17 g	21 g	26 g	30 g
30	9 g	17 g	26 g	34 g	43 g	51 g	60 g
45	13 g	26 g	39 g	51 g	64 g	77 g	90 g
60	17 g	34 g	51 g	69 g	86 g	103 g	120 g
75	21 g	43 g	64 g	86 g	107 g	129 g	150 g
90	26 g	51 g	77 g	103 g	129 g	154 g	180 g
105	30 g	60 g	90 g	120 g	150 g	180 g	210 g
120	34 g	69 g	103 g	137 g	171 g	206 g	240 g
150	43 g	86 g	129 g	171 g	214 g	257 g	300 g
180	51 g	103 g	154 g	206 g	257 g	309 g	340 g
210	60 g	120 g	180 g	240 g	300 g	360 g	420 g
240	69 g	137 g	206 g	274 g	343 g	411 g	480 g

A = carb intake   B = carb intake + bolus reduction
C = carb Intake + bolus reduction + basal reduction

to complete the run. This is more than twice the amount needed for the leisurely one-hour walk over the same ground! Though walking or running 3 miles requires nearly the same calories, a higher percentage of these calories come from carbohydrates while running because it is more intense than walking.

In the first 30 minutes of moderate or strenuous exercise, local muscle glycogen contributes five times as much glucose as the blood. For example, during the first 30 minutes of running at 6 m.p.h., only about 10 percent of the glucose needed is removed directly from the blood. This glucose is replaced by eating carbs during the run or by production of glucose from the liver. Even when insulin levels are high during a 30 minute run, only about 16 percent of the calories come directly from glucose in the blood. Most of the glucose used during exercise comes directly from muscle glycogen stores. In the hours following the exercise, glycogen stores are gradually rebuilt from glucose removed from the blood.

As running continues beyond 30 minutes, more and more glucose is drawn from the blood. The percentage of glucose withdrawn from the blood gradually climbs to a maximum of about 40 percent over the first couple of hours. This makes it more and more necessary to eat or drink carbs to avoid a fall in glucose. An appropriate fall in the blood insulin level lets the liver release more glucose so that fewer carbs need to be consumed right away.

Because most of the carbs that muscles use come from their local glycogen stores, immediate replacement of all the carbs used in exercise is unnecessary. For example, someone who weighs 150 lbs. and rides a bicycle at 10 m.p.h. for one hour will require about 48 grams of carbs for the ride. This person might eat or drink 24 grams of carbs before and during the ride, and consume an equal number over a few hours after the ride.

One exception to this approach comes when insulin levels are so high that the liver cannot make enough glucose to keep the blood glucose from falling. Here, eating becomes the only way to avoid a low glucose, and to deliver the fuel needed by exercising muscles and the nerves that control them.

Lower Your Bolus and Basal Doses

Eating extra carbs is the easiest way to handle short, less intense exercise, but for longer and more intense activity, a reduction in insulin doses is required. How many units to reduce your insulin can be determined by dividing the ExCarbs an exercise requires by your carb factor. This converts grams of carb into equivalent units of insulin that can then be used to reduce basal rates or boluses.

Translate ExCarbs into an insulin reduction:

ExCarbs ÷ CarbF = units of insulin that might be reduced.

If someone weighing 150 lbs. plans to dance at a moderate intensity for one hour, Table 22.5 shows that this will require about 25 grams of carb. If this person's carb factor is one unit for every 12 grams of carb, 25 grams divided by 12 grams per unit gives a maximum of 2 units that may need to be subtracted from bolus or basal doses. This person could also combine eating carbs and lowering insulin by choosing to eat 12 grams of free carbs and lower a bolus or basal rate by 1 unit.

A reduction in bolus or basal delivery during exercise lets more fuel be produced by the liver and more fat be released from fat stores. An insulin reduction means that fewer carbs have to be eaten. This helps weight loss when someone does not want to consume the large portions of carbohydrate that long periods of increased activity would otherwise require.

Keep in mind that these ExCarb equivalents should be the *maximum* amount needed. Someone who is trained for an exercise and has appropriately reduced their insulin doses may need fewer ExCarbs than those in Table 22.5. Keep in mind that it takes some time for a basal or bolus reduction to be seen in the blood. Table 22.9

22.8 Rapid Glycogen Rebuilding Reduces the Risk of a Delayed Low Glucose

After long or strenuous exercise, rebuilding muscle glycogen quickly after stopping is important. There is a 20 to 30 minute window following exercise when muscles are primed to restore their depleted glycogen. Consuming carbs and protein (for muscle repair), like those found in chocolate milk, right after exercise lets muscle glycogen stores quickly rebuild.

A small carb bolus insulin may be needed to cover these carbs, but less glucose will be withdrawn from the blood in the hours that follow. Rapid rebuilding of muscle glycogen reduces the risk for having a delayed low glucose many hours after an exercise, which often occurs at night. Drinking chocolate milk or eating other carbs just after exercise reloads your glycogen and gets you ready to exercise the next day.

Carb intake increases the amount of glucose stored in muscle glycogen. The body uses these stores for exercise endurance and performance. On a high carb diet, a trained marathon runner can run for about four hours before exhaustion sets in. Contrast this with a runner on a low carb diet where exhaustion begins in less than an hour and a half, well before the finish line.

To improve performance, many athletes "fuel up" muscle glycogen stores by eating a high carb meal covered with a carb bolus on the evening before major exercise events.

shows some suggested changes in carb intake, carb boluses, and basal rates for different intensities and durations of exercise.

Whether you reduce basal rates, bolus doses, or both will depend on the duration of the activity, its timing in relation to meals, and whether the exercise was planned. When exercise follows a meal, a carb bolus can be lowered to help reduce the insulin level. The carbs eaten in a meal work quickly to raise the glucose, so timing of the carb bolus is not critical. Ideally, the exercise would begin within an hour of the bolus so that the glucose does not rise too high before the exercise begins. A breakfast bolus can be reduced for exercise that starts after breakfast, but if you walk, run, or go to the gym before breakfast, you may need to eat carbs or try a temporary basal reduction to help handle this.

For strenuous exercise that lasts 60 minutes or longer, or moderate exercise lasting 90 minutes or longer, a reduction in the basal rate will likely be needed. Basal rates are ideally lowered one to two hours *before* an activity begins to allow enough time for the insulin level in the blood to start to drop. After long, intense periods of exercise, both basal rates and boluses may need to be reduced for 24 to 48 hours afterward.

The blood insulin level falls fast if the basal rate is completely stopped, but a basal reduction is better. A pump should never be stopped longer than 60 to 90 minutes to avoid ketosis and having the glucose spike afterward. For long periods of exercise, a basal reduction that is 20% lower than normal (80% of the usual rate) for moderate, and as 50% lower than normal for long periods of strenuous exercise can be tried.

Basal reductions are most effective when started well before the exercise begins. If an exercise is spontaneous or unanticipated, a short and sharp reduction in the basal rate can be considered. The basal rate is generally not lowered more than 40 to 50% for

22.9 Carb and Insulin Adjustments to Balance Exercise per 100 lbs. Weight

Exercise Duration	Exercise Intensity								
	Mild			Moderate			Intense		
	Carbs*	Bolus	Basal	Carbs*	Bolus	Basal	Carbs*	Bolus	Basal
15 min	+ 0g	normal	normal	+ 0 g	normal	normal	+ 20g	- 10%	normal
30 min	+ 10g	normal	normal	+ 20g	- 10%	normal	+ 40g	- 20%	normal
45 min	+ 18g	- 10%	normal	+ 30g	- 20%	normal	+ 50g	- 30%	normal
60 min	+ 25g	- 15%	normal	+ 40g	- 30%	normal	+ 60g	- 40%	- 10%
90 min	+ 38g	- 20%	normal	+ 55g	- 45%	- 20%	+ 90g	- 50%	- 20%
120 min	+ 50g	- 30%	normal	+ 70g	- 60%	- 20%	+ 110g	- 70%	- 30%
240 min	+ 80g	- 50%	- 10%	+ 120g	- 60%	- 20%	+ 200g	- 70%	- 40%

These are estimates. They have to be adjusted by each individual through testing.

* Important: These carb values above are for someone who weighs 100 lbs. If you weigh 200 lbs, you will need twice these amounts. If you are not trained, you may need slightly more than these amounts. Once trained, you may need less.

long periods of exercise, but a larger reduction, such as 75% for 60 to 90 minutes can be used to partially cover an hour of moderate or strenuous exercise before breakfast.

Example

Once you know how many ExCarbs are needed for an exercise, you can use your carb factor to translate some or all of these carbs into an appropriate insulin reduction.

Let's say someone weighing 150 pounds wants to run for 30 minutes at 8 m.p.h. Table 22.5 shows they will need about 72 grams of ExCarbs (145 grams per hour times a half hour) for this run. We can divide these carbs by their carb factor to find out how much insulin this exercise is equal to. Dividing 72 grams by this person's carb factor, which is 16 grams per unit of insulin, tells us that the run is equal to about 4.5 units of insulin (72 grams ÷ 16 carbs per unit = 4.5 units). Knowing the carbs and the equivalent insulin reduction required for the run, our runner can choose to eat extra carbohydrates, lower a meal bolus, or both. (A basal reduction would ordinarily not be used for a run that lasts only a half hour.)

Using only carbs, our runner could consume 24 grams of carb before the run, 24 after the run, and the remaining 24 as needed later in the day. These carbs are not covered with insulin unless your experience tells you that your glucose will rise without a carb bolus. If our runner chooses to only reduce carb boluses, one or two meal boluses close in timing

22.10 How Far Can Insulin Be Reduced for Exercise?

Can basals and boluses be totally eliminated if you exercise long enough? This may be possible for someone with Type 2 diabetes who retains adequate internal insulin production. With Type 1 diabetes, however, basal and bolus doses can be lowered only so far.

Consider what happens to insulin during maximum training in a marathon runner who does not have diabetes. Their blood insulin level drops no further than to about half of its original level. So with Type 1 diabetes, basal and bolus doses would normally be lowered no more than 40 to 50 percent for longer periods of intense exercise if the current basals and boluses are appropriate.

Insulin can be lowered only so far because some is always needed:

1. As basal delivery to enable glucose to enter cells and to keep internal stores of glucose and fat from being released in massive amounts, and ultimately prevent ketoacidosis, which results from this uncontrolled release.

2. To cover some of the carbohydrates eaten in meals.

to the exercise can be lowered by 4.5 units. For a run an hour after breakfast, coverage for the carbs at breakfast could be reduced by 3 units with the remaining 1.5 units taken out of boluses for carbs eaten at lunch or in a midmorning snack.

Our runner could also reduce the breakfast bolus by 2 units (32 grams) and the lunch bolus by 1 unit (16 grams) for a total insulin reduction of 48 grams an have the other 24 grams as free carbs during or after the run.

Lower a High Glucose

Exercise can also be used to lower a high glucose. For example, Jeremy weighs 175 pounds, uses 50 units of insulin a day, and is generally in good control. He uses one unit for each 10 grams of carbohydrate and one unit for every 40 mg/dl above his target glucose of 100 mg/dl.

If Jeremy finds his glucose is 180 mg/dl (10 mmol/L) before dinner with no BOB, he can exercise to lower his glucose. If he plans to eat 60 grams of carb for dinner, he would usually take 6 units for dinner plus 2 units for the high glucose (80/40 = 2.0). He plans to ride his bike at 10 m.p.h. for an hour after dinner. From Table 22.5, the ExCarbs for a 175 lb. person riding one hour at 10 m.p.h. is about 54 grams of carb.

These 54 grams of ExCarbs used by the exercise can be replaced by:

- Eating 54 grams of carb not covered with a bolus during or after the exercise,
- Giving 5.4 fewer units of insulin (54 grams of carb ÷ 10 grams per unit) in basal or bolus doses,
- Or a combination of these.

251

Jeremy wants to lower his glucose by 80 mg/dl (4.4 mmol/L) with exercise. This would use 2.0 of the 5.4 units of glucose lowering capacity (80 mg/dl drop ÷ 40 mg/dl per unit = 2.0 units). The remaining 3.4 units could be converted into 20 free grams of carb eaten sometime after the bike ride (20 grams ÷ 10 grams per unit = 2.0 units), plus a reduction of 1.4 units from the normal carb bolus. He is already lowering his high glucose, so instead of 6.0 units for 60 grams at dinner, Jeremy could give only 4.6 units.

Ways to Avoid Exercise Lows

Exercise and increased activity can cause lows during and for several hours after it ends. The longer and more intense an activity, the more likely that your glucose will go low in the hours that follow. See Box 22.8 for how to rebuild glycogen quickly and lower your risk for delayed and nighttime lows after exercise. Use *Smart Charts* or notes to record exercise and match it to your food or pre-meal boluses to improve glucose outcomes.

A low glucose during or shortly after exercise can be difficult to recognize because sweating and tiredness are similar to hypoglycemia and exercise. Warning signs that occur may go unnoticed when someone is focused on the activity or sport at hand. Water sports can be especially difficult because they mask sweating and shaking. Frequent glucose testing or wearing a CGM are the best ways to keep your readings in your target range when you exercise.

Have quick-acting, high carb snacks on hand to prevent or treat a low glucose. Be especially careful during and after exercise that is intense and for which you are not trained. Canoe trips, backpacking, skiing, horseback riding, spring cleaning, snow shoveling, home remodeling, heavy work in the garden, or even washing the car can create an unusually fast drop in the glucose if the exercise or activity is not done regularly. Infrequent activities that use the arm and shoulder muscles are especially likely to cause lows. A larger carb intake or greater insulin reduction is needed for any strenuous activity that is done infrequently.

Test often or use a CGM after any long period of strenuous activity to avoid delayed lows. Strenuous exercise can cause a low up to 36 to 48 hours later and will be most likely to happen during the first night. Delayed lows are caused when the muscles and liver gradually remove glucose from the blood to replenish their glycogen stores depleted during the activity. Delayed lows can be prevented by testing often, using a temporary basal rate reduction that night, and adding extra carbs at dinner and bedtime not covered by bolus insulin.

A low can also creep in when exercise conditions change. If you usually walk two miles on flat ground but decide to walk the same distance in hilly country, you will use more fuel climbing the grades. A strong headwind can increase fuel consumption by about one percent for each extra mile per hour of headwind (i.e., for a 10 m.p.h. headwind, increase carbs by 10 percent). Walking in dry sand or soft snow can double the amount of carbs you need compared to the same walk on firm ground.

> ### 22.12 Trust Your Experience
> Never take a dose of insulin that seems inappropriate. If you usually take five units for your meal prior to the start of your exercise and when you do this your control has been good, don't take more or less than this if a different dose is suggested by the ExCarbs system or other rule. Your own experience is always your best guide.

Activities that have an uneven pace like spring cleaning or playing football can also cause problems in estimating carb need. With cleaning, it's hard to predict whether you will spend the next hour sorting through the closet for throwaways or moving furniture. In football, you could sit on the bench during the entire game or give your all on the field. Luckily, most activities are not this unpredictable.

The impact that extra activity has on your glucose depends on:

1. How strenuous it is,

2. How long it lasts, and

3. What your BOB is when you start.

Mild to moderate activity that lasts less than 30 to 45 minutes will not require as much extra carb intake or as much reduction in insulin doses as longer and more intense forms of exercise. Table 22.9 provides guidance for carb and insulin adjustments for the amount of activity.

Strenuous and anaerobic activities can at times release glucose into the blood from the liver faster than it can be moved into muscle cells by the current insulin level.

How High Is Too High to Exercise?

High glucoses impair performance during exercise in people with Type 1 diabetes. A high glucose likely means that some dehydration has already begun. A high glucose during exercise has been associated with a lower secretion of beta–endorphins and an increased RPE (a measure of difficulty) for leg and whole body effort. Exercise under these conditions likely leads to discomfort and stress.

If the glucose is 250 mg/dl (13.9 mmol/L) or above, exercise often is not recommended. If the insulin level is dangerously low at this time, exercise will cause the glucose to rise much higher. Although the insulin level cannot be directly measured, you can accurately guess it is low in many situations.

If a glucose were normal at bedtime but rises to 280 mg/dl (15.6 mmol/L) on waking because an infusion set became dislodged, the insulin level is likely to be very low and the person may even be in early ketosis. Exercising at this time will cause the glucose to rise and *put you at risk of ketosis* unless an injection is taken and enough time passes for the insulin to begin to lower the glucose.

> ### 22.13 Simple Exercise Tips
> **For Casual or Light Exercise**
> (i.e. casual walking, biking, softball)
>
> - No adjustment to insulin
> - Keep fast carbs and your meter and test strips with you.
>
> **For Heavy or Aerobic Exercise**
> (i.e. tennis, baseball, football, jogging, swimming vigorously)
>
> - Test your blood sugar before the exercise and every 30 minutes after you start
> - If less than 120 mg/dl (6.7 mmol/L), eat 30 grams of carb before exercise.
> - If between 120 and 200 mg/dl (6.7 to 11.1 mmol/L) eat 15 grams of carb.
> - If over 200 mg/dl (11.1 mmol/L), don't eat anything, but retest in 30 minutes.
> - Test every 30 minutes and follow these tips each time you test.

Contrast this situation to one where the glucose is raised to 250 mg/dl (13.9 mmol/L) in preparation for a four-hour athletic event. ExCarbs covered by a reduced carb bolus before the event creates this high glucose, but the person can start the event confidently because the glucose will begin to drop shortly after the exercise starts. Even though the glucose is high, enough insulin is available to move glucose from the blood into exercising muscles.

Rather than raising the glucose high, basal and bolus doses can be reduced so fewer carbs have to be eaten to exercise safely. With the insulin level lower at the start of the event, the starting glucose can remain at or near the normal range more safely. Additional carbs will be needed, but fewer than if the insulin level had not been lowered.

Exercise Cautions

Any current medical problem you have with nerve damage, eye changes, kidney disease, or a history of heart or blood vessel problems must be evaluated by your physician before you start to exercise. Blood flow in involved muscles may increase 15 to 20 times above resting levels during strenuous exercise, and cardiac output may increase fivefold. Increased blood flow and blood pressure move oxygen and fuel to muscles but also place extra strain on the heart. This could harm organs and blood vessels weakened by previous high glucoses, high blood pressure, or high cholesterol.

22.14 Glucose Trending during Intense Exercise

Rather than occasional monitoring, many professional athletes with diabetes want to know their glucose trend before, during, and after an athletic event. They need to know where their glucose is, what direction it's headed, and how quickly it's changing.

Athletes like Jay Leeuwenburg, former offensive lineman for the Cincinnati Bengals, would test every 20 to 30 minutes for about two hours before a football game, during the game as often as possible, and again for the same period after the game. Frequent testing allowed him to see his glucose trend and correct as needed with carbs or insulin to keep his readings as normal and level as possible. Post game readings helped him avoid unexpected highs and lows after his very strenuous exercise.

Trending, of course, becomes easier with a CGM. Team Type 1 has competed in the Ride Across America bike ride for several years and won the team competition in 2009 in record time, even though they were the only team with diabetes. They wore CGMs and insulin pumps on their ride to avoid highs and lows.

If feeling in the feet is reduced, the type and level of exercise has to be chosen carefully to prevent foot injuries. Swimming or biking, which are non-weight-bearing activities, may be better choices than jogging. Proper footwear is essential for avoiding blisters or calluses that exacerbate a high risk for foot problems.

Autonomic neuropathy involves damage to the nerves that control processes like digestion, heart rate, and blood vessel tone. It can create an artificially low heart rate and reduce blood flow to exercising muscle. With autonomic neuropathy, a heart rate monitor may not accurately measure exercise intensity, but the person exercising can still feel how intense their activity is. A gradual training program under supervision is strongly advised when autonomic neuropathy is present.

Autonomic neuropathy can be detected by changes that appear in an EKG or by measuring the change in blood pressure from a reclining to a standing position. If you suspect you have this disorder because you have had diabetes for a long time or have a history of poor control, discuss how to diagnose it with your physician.

Consider any heart or blood vessel risk you may have before beginning an exercise program, especially if it includes an exercise like heavy weight lifting or scuba diving that can significantly raise blood pressure. A gradual increase in training level or modified goals may be required if blood vessel damage is a concern. Discuss your exercise plans with your physician before you start.

22.15 Things that Make the Glucose Rise during and after Exercise

Exercise usually lowers the glucose. Here are four things that can make glucose rise:

Lack of insulin	This is the most common cause for a glucose rise during exercise. For example, if a person goes for a run before breakfast and their fasting glucose is above 160 mg/dl (8.9 mmol/L), their glucose may rise somewhat as the relatively low insulin level causes their liver to start making glucose. If the same run is done on another morning with a fasting glucose below 140 mg/dl (7.8 mmol/L), the glucose is likely to fall.
Anaerobic exercise	With short, intense anaerobic exercises, like running the 100-yard dash or power weight-lifting, glucose is almost the only fuel used. Glucose is rapidly released into the blood by rising adrenaline levels. Adrenaline causes glucose production to rise seven or eight times higher than normal, while uptake of glucose into cells rises only three to four fold.[107] A normal pancreas releases insulin rapidly into the blood in this situation, but a pump cannot do this.
Competition	Large amounts of stress hormones are released in competitive events, like a swim meet, a 10K run, or a century bike ride. Stress hormones cause release of large amounts of glucose in these "fight or flight" situations. The person without diabetes quickly releases insulin to balance this, but the person with diabetes may have their glucose rise rapidly even if their starting glucose was normal and they don't eat. Nervousness at the starting line suggests that stress hormones are at work.
Dehydration	Dehydration from hot weather or strenuous exercise can mimic a high glucose. If your urine looks like lemonade, dehydration is unlikely, but if it looks like apple juice, dehydration can cause the glucose to appear higher than it actually is. Drink ample non-caloric fluids and retest your glucose 30 minutes later before you decide whether you need a correction bolus.

Summary

The need for insulin and carb adjustments before, during, and after exercise vary greatly from individual to individual. Although this chapter covers many aspects of control during exercise, these variations are complex and not completely understood. Some people may need to lower their boluses and basals only slightly for exercise, while others find that a large insulin reduction is the only way to control their glucoses for the same exercise. For some, a breakfast bolus may not need to be lowered for morning exercise, but when they do the same exercise later in the day, they have to reduce their lunch or dinner bolus.

Be sure your insulin doses and carbohydrate intake are matched to your normal daily lifestyle before attempting to make adjustments for exercise. ExCarbs won't work if glucose control is not good when you are not exercising. Discuss your exercise program with your physician or health care team. Keep in mind your personal experience with similar exercise in the past.

The only way to determine your own response is to experiment, record your results, and discuss these with your physician. Remember, the ExCarb tables and the carb and basal and bolus adjustments that you make based on these tables are only designed as a starting point to help you safely exercise and be active – your own experience is your ultimate guide! Experience will help you only if you look back over your records before deciding how to manage a particular situation.

22.16 Easy Way to Measure Heart Rate/Pulse

Feel your pulse at the wrist and count it for 10 seconds, then use this table to find beats per minute.

10 Second Pulse Count	Beats per Minute
10	60
11	66
12	72
13	78
14	84
15	90
16	96
17	102
18	108
19	114
20	120
21	126
22	132
23	138
24	144
25	150
26	156
27	162
28	168
29	174
30	180

The biggest problem with communication is the illusion it has taken place.

Anon

Exercise Tips

- Test your glucose often before, during, and for 24 to 36 hours after exercise or use a CGM for accurate and timely insulin and carb adjustments.
- Performance is improved with the glucose between 70 and 150 mg/dl (3.9 to 8.3 mmol/L) with proper insulin and carb adjustments.
- Vigorous exercise or heavy work may require major reductions in meal boluses of 50 percent or more before and after the exercise or activity. For example, if you normally take one unit for each 10 grams of carbohydrate, try taking one unit for every 20 grams while working or exercising hard.
- Correction boluses may also need to be lowered by 50 percent or more.
- For longer, intense activities like a weekend backpacking trip, try a temporary basal rate that is 20 percent to 40 percent lower. Keep it somewhat lower for 24 to 36 hours after the activity ends.
- A basal reduction is often needed when you start a new exercise.
- Before adjusting insulin for exercise, discuss these changes with your physician.
- Test your glucose often both during and after exercise,
- Always carry fast carbs, like glucose tablets, SweetTarts™, or a sport fluid like Gatorade™ to rapidly correct low glucoses.
- Stay hydrated. Always have water or a glucose-containing or sport fluid available.
- For strenuous activities like triathlons, marathons, or century bike rides, try to get tips from other athletes with diabetes who have already done them.
- For weight loss with exercise, lower your basal rates and boluses so you need fewer carbs to meet your fuel needs, but keep your glucose well controlled. Remember there is a limit to how far your insulin doses can be lowered.

Laughter is inner jogging.

Norman Cousins

Children and Teens

With Co-Author Jen Block, R.N., C.D.E
Stanford Univ. Dept. of Pediatrics

23

Kids, teens, and their parents all benefit from pump therapy. Small children are highly sensitive to insulin and often require small doses, while teens often face a strong Dawn Phenomenon that must be met with specific, well-timed basal adjustments and increasing overall insulin requirements. Children require flexible, individualized approaches to maintain control in the very dynamic environment of growth.

When basal and bolus doses are carefully matched to carb intake, exercise, hormones, and changes in weight, the improved control enhances growth and school performance. The early years are also a time when healthy lifelong patterns need to be set. An insulin pump can make these challenges easier.

This chapter explains
- Why choose pump therapy
- Roles and responsibilities in care
- Setting the TDD, basals and boluses for kids and teens
- Special child and teen issues

Why Choose Pump Therapy

Glucose regulation is challenging in small children who are often sensitive to insulin and unpredictable and impulsive about their eating and activity. Recognizing this difficulty in matching insulin to need in children, and their greater risk for hypoglycemia, the ADA recommends that glucose targets and A1c goals be set higher for kids than adults as shown in Table 23.1.

Parents and health care providers will want to consider pump therapy for any toddler or child who experiences frequent episodes of severe hypoglycemia, has wide fluctuations in their readings, is in poor control with a high A1c, or requires flexible insulin doses to match their lifestyle, such as in college. Fear of needles and participation in competitive sports are additional reasons to consider a pump.

23.1 ADA Glucose Goals for Children and Teens			
	Toddler Preschoolers (0-6 yrs)	**School Age (6-12 yrs)**	**Adolescents/ Young Adults (13-19 yrs)**
A1c (%)	≤ 8.5% but ≥ 7.5%	< 8%	< 7.5%*
Before meal glucose	100 - 180 mg/dl (5.5-10 mmol/L)	90-180 mg/dl (5-10 mmol/L)	90-130 mg/dl (5-7.2 mmol/L)
Bedtime/overnight glucose	110-200 mg/dl (6.1-11.1 mmol/L)	100-180 mg/dl (5.5-10 mmol/L)	90-150 mg/dl (5-8.3 mmol/L)

*A lower goal (<7%) is reasonable if it can be achieved without excessive hypoglycemia.

Diabetes Care. 2005; 28 (suppl 1): S4-S36.

The International Society for Pediatric and Adolescent Diabetes (ISPAD) recommends an HbA1c of less than 7.5% for all age groups. In Sweden, the recommendation is to get as close to 7.0% as possible without problematic hypoglycemia.

Additional considerations for the parents, child, or teen in choosing pump therapy include quality of life issues that are important to consider. These can include:

- If the need for basal insulin varies throughout the day.
- If you have days when more carbs are desired but will require additional injections.
- If changes in glucose as a result of exercise, sleep or eating are challenging to adjust for on injection therapy.
- If you need small doses of insulin that may be hard to deliver with a pen or syringe.
- If you are willing and able to use and wear an insulin pump. Parents and children generally prefer to change an infusion set every 2-3 days over multiple injections a day.
- Injections can be difficult to manage when a toddler refuses to eat, is napping at shot time, or is ill. A pump makes these situations easier to handle.
- Insulin pumps can track bolus on board (BOB) and lessen insulin stacking in growing children and teens who eat and bolus frequently, a great advantage over injections.
- Bolus calculators can assist in calculating insulin doses and the ability to download insulin pumps allow both parents and health care providers to see when and how bolus doses are given, such as those for snacks after school.

The flexibility and precision of pump therapy can improve quality of life, but parents and the child or teen have to be realistic about what a pump can do. Some common myths and realities about what a pump can do are listed in Table 2.1.

Roles And Responsibilities

Parents want to do their part to provide better control of their child's diabetes now and to promote better health in the future. Although insulin pumps can improve lifestyle flexibility, a child or teen may think that the extra planning, thought, attention, training, and finger sticks associated with pump therapy are too much bother or are too limiting to their spontaneity. It is important that the child or teen is willing and able to use pump therapy and that the decision to do so involve their input. Regardless of a child or teen's mental state or motivation, diabetes management is challenging at any age, so parents must remain involved in the care of diabetes to ensure their child does what is needed to maintain their health.

A thorough discussion of the roles of the parent and the child or teen with the health care team is helpful for clarifying responsibilities. Any child or teen going on a pump needs at least one adult who is trained in its use. The diabetes health care team provides training, and sets the pump up with basal rates, CarbF, CorrF, DIA time, and a correction target. The parent or primary caregiver must acquire the skills to test basal rates and other settings, calculate and give carb boluses, record data, analyze patterns, and troubleshoot when problems arise. In other words, the child or teen does not have to shoulder full responsibility at first, and the parent turns over control as their maturity allows.

It is important to be aware that a child or teen's motivation to carry out self-care behaviors essential to safe pump therapy may change over time. Checking in regularly to be sure that safeguards like regular blood glucose testing and appropriate pump use are continued can support the continuation of healthy behaviors and provide early identification of problems.

After switching to a pump, the health care team is typically available for frequent consultation while the starting basal and bolus doses are being tested and adjusted. Problems with insulin doses for children and teens are not terribly different from those encountered by adults. The real difference is in the pumper's problem solving skills. Very young children are incapable of self-care and older children may not be ready to analyze problems. Children and teens can be taught the basics, but they require good supervision from a knowledgeable adult.

A parent needs to know how to verify whether carbs are being counted and that insulin doses are accurate and are being given. Verification of regular blood glucose testing is also important, as are ongoing discussions of how best to handle glucose values outside of the target range. It can be helpful for the parent to periodically review how and when to test for ketones, the signs of DKA, steps to take to prevent DKA, and how to manage sick days. Like driving or any other critical skill, parents need to provide appropriate control, supervision, and discipline to insure safe pumping and successful outcomes.

The child's glucose readings need to be regularly evaluated and issues must be discussed with an older child or teen in ways that produce positive outcomes. Recording and analyzing carbs, glucoses, and basal and bolus doses create opportunities to adjust the amount and timing of insulin doses and carbs for the best results. Through all stages, a parent's compassion and readiness to forgive mistakes can be critical in steady improvement in a child or teen's skills. Getting support from family and friends, as well as family or personal counseling is essential if a child's diabetes begins to take a toll on family life or relationships. Counseling and guidance help minimize the toll of a chronic issue like diabetes that requires daily involvement.

23.2 When Is a Child Ready for Self-Care?

Children differ greatly in the age at which they can manage the self-care required on a pump. After acquiring a skill, relapses may occur, but the desire to manage the pump on their own is often reintroduced by the desire to stay overnight at a friends or go camping.

When is a child ready to:

count carbs:	about 9 years
test blood sugar:	about 10 years
give a bolus:	about 10 years
insert an infusion set :	about 12 years
determine a carb bolus:	about 12 years

For insulin dose adjustments, parents need phone access to their health care providers. Some clinics and diabetes centers prefer to have pump, CGM, and other data downloaded over the internet, or have reports emailed or faxed. Some meters will automatically text a glucose reading to the parent each time their child or a baby-sitter checks it. Use any system that gets your child's data to the person who monitors dosing decisions.

Caregivers, teachers, baby sitters, school nurses, camp nurses, and coaches need to be trained on the insulin pump, know usual bolus doses and how to give them, appropriate foods, the symptoms and treatment for hypoglycemia and hyperglycemia, and who to call for help. Diabetes supplies are provided in a bag for school nurses and coaches and stored in the nurse's office or carried in a fanny pack or backpack by the child or teen. It is critical to make caregivers aware that an insulin pump should not be stopped and that a dislodged infusion set or a patch pump must be replaced quickly.

Once essential skills are taught and demonstrated back to the trainer, the child or teen is ready to go on a pump. Children often have the motor skills to handle giving doses on their own by age 10. Judgment and problem solving come at a later age. The encouragement of self-care that is appropriate to the pumper's age and maturity is an important part of engaging them in their own diabetes management. For example, allow a young child to clean the skin with IV Prep and push the buttons on the pump while you supervise. After the child shows full proficiency in these and other skills, the parent may decide to check occasionally to make sure the technique is accurate. Table 23.2 shows suggested ages to recommend different self-management skills.

Selecting Starting Doses For Kids And Teens

Setting basal and bolus doses is covered in Chapters 11, 12, and 13, but there are some differences when selecting basal rates and initial pump settings for children and teens. One difference is they require snacks in addition to meals to provide enough calories for growth and development. Depending on their growth cycle, a child may need to snack a little or a lot. How to best cover snacks with boluses and avoid insulin stacking needs to be individualized when setting doses.

Teens are notorious for inconsistent routines and random eating, with or without diabetes. While a pump is the ideal tool for a varied or even erratic lifestyle, a teen will need to keep a consistent schedule for at least four weeks after the pump start to set insulin doses correctly. When schedules change, as at the start of school or vacation, basal rates and boluses often need to be retested and adjusted.

> ### 23.3 Testing and Kids
>
> When giving an injection or drawing blood from young children for monitoring, remember that their imagination can be vivid, and reassurance about their fears may be needed. Let them know that an infusion needle will not affect their heart or puncture a large blood vessel and cause bleeding, and that their bodies easily replenish the small amounts of blood removed for blood tests. Encourage them to ask questions so their fears are allayed.

Hormonal changes at puberty can make one month's insulin program obsolete by the next month. During puberty, growth spurts occur, and hormones like growth hormone and cortisol levels rise. This often requires that basal and bolus doses also rise. Managing hormonal changes of puberty, growth spurts, attitudes, and peer pressure bring humility to the best diabetes clinicians. The most effective advice is to be prepared to adjust basal and bolus doses frequently to keep up with growth, and to discuss issues openly.

Although a reduction in the TDD is generally recommended when starting on a pump, this may not be appropriate for a teen who has had inadequate glucose control before switching to a pump, or a child who has recently experienced a growth phase and now requires more insulin.

Some pediatricians believe the DIA for children is shorter than that of adults, but research has shown similar DIA times in young children and adults at about 5.5 hours. Although activity can speed up insulin uptake through increased blood flow and lower glucose independently of insulin, this happens only occasionally in both adults and children. A pediatrician may choose to shorten the DIA time to increase the size of carb and correction boluses because kids and teens often don't bolus as often as they should, but the child may encounter excess hypoglycemia if they begin to cover all meals with boluses. Kids eat and bolus more often, making the handling of BOB more difficult and its tracking more important.

Basal/Bolus Balance

Basal/bolus balance can differ between small kids and adults. Adults and teens typically do better with basal insulin making up about half of the TDD. Breast-fed and bottle-fed infants on a pump that feed every few hours often have only small rises and falls in their blood glucose levels. During the day, they may benefit from a slightly higher basal dose to cover their carbs. Young children can be more sensitive to insulin at night and require lower basal rates than adults.

In the PedPump study conducted in Europe with 1,086 kids and teens between the ages of 1 and 18 on pumps, the participants had better glucose control and lower A1cs when boluses made up more than 50% of the TDD.[108] In this study, an average of 6.7 boluses were given a day to cover meals and snacks. Carb and correction boluses averaged 58% of the TDD, compared to 52% for adults. The frequent daytime bolus doses in this study may allow some bolus insulin to replace part of the basal delivery.

A lower starting basal percentages, such as 40% of the TDD, can be tried for an active child or teen who has even a small portion of their own insulin production remaining, usually seen in those who have had diabetes less than five years. Prior to puberty, a high intake of carbohydrate and calories relative to weight necessitates a greater use of bolus insulin compared to basal. Teens, especially boys, often eat six high carb meals a day. Matching these snacks and meals with boluses creates good control. Alternatively, some teens do best when 60% or more of their TDD is basal to offset to their higher levels of circulating pubertal hormones. Basal testing is essential for sorting out a child or teen's basal needs.

> ### 23.4 Prevent Afternoon Highs
>
> A common problem among school age children and teens is a high blood sugar in the late afternoon or before dinner, usually caused when the child neglects to take boluses for after school snacks. A parent can often follow the paper trail of wrappers and containers in the trash, then compare these with the history of boluses actually delivered.
>
> If afternoon highs are a problem for your child, review bolus history regularly and provide guidelines for how much bolus to take for each snack. It helps to label each food container with how many grams it contains and the bolus dose it requires.
>
> One way to cover lunches or afternoon snacks when a child or teen is forgetful about taking carb boluses is to raise the afternoon basal rate. A pump can also be set up with a reminder to take a bolus at a certain time, and some will warn if a bolus was not taken within a certain time period.

Setting And Testing Basal Doses

Children may have a slight Dawn Phenomenon, but teens often have a pronounced one due to early morning surges in growth hormone and cortisol. Frequent nighttime monitoring or using a CGM is necessary to determine whether the Dawn Phenomenon is present and what its impact is. After this initial testing phase, a glucose taken periodically between 1:00 and 3:00 a.m. helps determine when basal doses need to be adjusted. This can be done once a week or more often if nighttime hypoglycemia or breakfast hyperglycemia begins. Wearing a CGM continually provides quick guidance on setting accurate basal rates and boluses.

If the basal rate is not working well, raise or lower the basal in increments of 0.05 or even 0.025 units per hour unless a larger increase or decrease is obviously needed.

Test the glucose every one to two hours during basal testing, if possible. See Chapter 11 for a full discussion of setting and testing basal doses.

Setting And Testing Carb Boluses

See Chapter 12 for a full discussion of how to select and test carb boluses. All meals and most snacks (any carbs not used to treat or prevent a low) are typically covered with a full bolus. A small carb snack of 8 to 15 grams may not need a bolus if it does not affect the glucose. Whether a particular bedtime snack needs to be completely covered will only be known after adequate testing. Look at how much BOB is present when the bedtime glucose is checked for your best guidance on whether free carbs or a correction bolus is needed. Any carbs above those covered by the BOB can be covered with a carb bolus. For instance, the first 10 to 20 grams in bedtime snacks may not need to be covered and more carbs might not be covered after an active day. This decision becomes easier after some experience with how the day's activity affects the overnight glucose.

Smart pumps allow different CarbFs and CorrF to be set for different times of the day. These are especially convenient to reduce bedtime boluses and to reduce boluses when sports or other increased activities typically occur during the day.

Have the child or teen practice carb counting and bolus dosing. Be sure the child or teen calculates correctly several examples of counting and covering various carb amounts in meals and snacks. This ensures they understand how to determine bolus doses for a variety of foods and snacks.

The timing of meal boluses is very important. Typically, boluses are given prior to eating carbs that are not used to treat or prevent a low. While rapid acting insulins are just that, most carbs raise glucose levels faster, especially with meals that have simple carbs. The most effective timing is delivery of meal boluses 10 to 20 minutes before eating begins when the glucose is not low and a meal's carb count and timing are known. This helps lower the peak glucose after a meal.

Meal boluses may need to be tailored for specific situations:

Split boluses: Sometimes it is safer to bolus part of a meal now and the rest later. This is useful when you do not know how much food a fussy eater will consume or the time a meal will be served, such as during parties, restaurant dining, or all-you-can-eat buffets. It may also happen during holiday feasts, snacking on chips and salsa, or expecting to eat more than you really can, the "my eyes are bigger than my stomach" phenomenon. A child or teen should always keep in mind that using an extra bolus when food intake turns out to be more than expected is far better than having a high glucose later.

Combo or dual-wave boluses: Here, part of the entire bolus is given right away and the rest is delivered gradually over a period of time. If the carb amount turns out to be less than expected or not all of the food is eaten, the remaining part of the bolus can be cancelled. This helps picky eaters, low GI carbs, or foods like pizza that digest slowly because of their fat and protein content.

After-meal boluses: Though generally not recommended because it may cause post-meal highs, a meal bolus may be given immediately after a meal when a child is a picky eater or when an illness is underway and the child may not be able to keep food down.

Setting And Testing Correction Boluses

See Chapter 13 for steps to set and test correction boluses in adults. The procedure is similar in children and teens, but keep in mind that an active child or teen will lower high glucose readings faster through exercise than most adults. This glucose lowering with exercise usually requires a smaller correction bolus.

Setting The Duration Of Insulin Action

How long a bolus lowers the glucose after it is given is called the DIA. Setting an accurate DIA time is critical for calculating carb and correction boluses so they will account for BOB. Several studies have shown that the DIA for children is no different than it is for adults. Box 8.6 gives additional information.

Evaluating Outcomes

The overall goals for pump therapy for children and teens are similar to those for adults – less exposure to high glucose (a lower A1c) without encountering lows and less glucose variability (a lower SD). Meeting individual goals is also important. How well pump therapy is working depends on matching the original reasons a pump was chosen to a program that will accomplish this. For example, if the goal was for fewer hospital admissions, then one measure of success will be fewer or no hospitalizations.

Other measures of success can be identified by questions regarding satisfaction and quality of life. Are the child or teen and the parents happy with the program? How often do they report complaints or problems with the pump, infusion set, and glucose tests? Does the child or teen proudly show their pump to friends and relatives? Has the child or teen benefitted medically, emotionally or socially? Has the child or teen's general confidence and competence grown in proportion to success with the pump?

If any of these goals are not being met, it is important to discuss the challenges and issues with your healthcare team.

Special Control Issues

Growth And Growth Spurts

Growth spurts in children and teens almost always present a challenge for glycemic control. Growth spurts where insulin doses need to be increased over a short period of time are followed by periods of more gradual growth through childhood. The onset of puberty also signals a time of rapid growth and glucose upheaval. Hormones produced during puberty cause glucose to be released and impair insulin action, necessitating increases in basal and bolus doses. An insulin pump allows teens and parents to make the basal and bolus adjustments that are needed to keep up with changes in control during this transition time.

During the growth years and puberty, anticipate increasing basal and bolus doses every few weeks or months as the need becomes apparent. Children require a quarter to a half unit of insulin per pound of body weight each day, while teenagers can require up to one unit per pound. This need for extra insulin does not indicate that the teen's diabetes has become "worse." It is simply a physiological change caused by normal growth, something the teenager needs to be told frequently.

An endocrinologist may recommend that a teen who requires large insulin doses try a prescription medication called metformin. This medication, approved for adults with Type 2 diabetes, reduces the excess glucose release from the liver when growth hormone levels are high. Metformin lowers glucose production to more normal levels, reduces the amount of insulin needed for control, and often makes the teen feel better. Discuss this with your child's doctor if your teen is having a difficult time with control.

Teens will be glad to know that these high insulin doses will taper off as they reach the late teen years and puberty subsides. Their TDD may fall to half that used during puberty. The FDA does not approve metformin for use in teens, so discuss this with your healthcare professional. Metformin may not be recommended for a teen with a history of repeated DKA because of the possibility that DKA in the presence of metformin might trigger a very serious medical condition called lactic acidosis.

23.5 Grams of Carbs for Lows in Children and Teens			
Age	**1-6 yrs**	**6-10 yrs**	**10 yrs-Adult**
Grams of Carbs	**5-10 grs**	**10-15 grs**	**15-20 grs**
Glucose Tabs 5 grams each	1 - 2 tabs	2 - 3 tabs	3 - 4 tabs
Glucose Tabs 4 grams each	1 - 2 tabs	3 - 4 tabs	4 - 5 tabs
Orage Juice 1/3 cup = 10 grams	1/4 - 1/2 cup	1/2 - 3/4 cup	3/4 - 1 cup
Apple Juice 1/3 cup = 10 grams	1/4 - 1/2 cup	1/2 - 3/4 cup	3/4 - 1 cup
Table Sugar 4 grams per tsp.	2 tsps.	3 tsps.	4-5 tsps
Regular Soda 3 grams per oz	2 - 3 ozs	4 - 5 ozs	5 - 6 ozs
Lifesavers 3 grams each	2 - 3	4 - 5	5 - 7
Milk 8 oz = 12 grams	4 - 5 ozs	6 - 7 ozs	8 - 10 ozs

Adapted from Understanding Diabetes, 10 ed., by H. Peter Chase, M.D., 2002

Relatively normal glucose levels are necessary to realize full growth, especially height. This can be a motivator to the child or teen, particularly teenage boys, to manage their diabetes well if they are made aware that short height often results from poor glucose control during these growth years.

Menses

Some young women find their glucose levels are not affected by their cycle, or that their periods are so irregular that it is difficult to tell what affects them. Others experience drastic changes in glucose levels that typically occur a few days prior to the beginning and during the first day or two of their menstrual periods. High glucose levels may require increased insulin doses at this time. The need for more insulin may drop dramatically after the first day of a menstrual period and care must be used to avoid lows. A good practice is to test glucose levels more often and record results prior to and during the period. Keep a record of menses and glucose levels to find patterns and discover how the cycle may affect glucose control.

Many teens do not have regular, predictable cycles for several months after the onset of puberty. After the first period, it is wise to start recording dates of the periods even though they may be irregular so that any pattern in their effect on the glucose may be seen. With accurate records, the impact of regular cycles on the glucose can be anticipated and adjustments can be made. See page 204 for more information.

Considerations For Parents Of Infants And Toddlers

Cooperation between diligent, well educated parents and their diabetes team is critical for success with a toddler on pump therapy. Education and evaluation is similar for people of all ages on pump therapy and should include carbohydrate counting, insulin needs, sick day management, and troubleshooting skills.

Basal and bolus doses in toddlers are much smaller, often in fractions of units compared to those for older children. A diabetes care team that is experienced in working with small children must carefully monitor these doses. Basal delivery can be as low as 0.025 units per hour, and boluses as low as 0.05 unit, making precise dosing easier than ever before.

On a pump, ketoacidosis can result from a clogged infusion line, detachment of the infusion set, or leakage of insulin at the hub or elsewhere. There may be little outward sign of this, so frequent glucose monitoring and checking for ketones to detect an infusion failure is essential for toddlers and children on a pump. For young children, a blood ketone meter is the best way to measure ketones. Talk with your healthcare team about this option. To reduce the risk for accidentally pulling out an infusion set, always anchor a child's infusion line with 1-inch tape. Despite all precautions, constant monitoring for problems is essential, especially during any presumed "illness." The symptoms of ketoacidosis (DKA) may be confused with illness, and DKA is more likely to occur during illness.

Toddlers and children often need to be monitored while they are asleep. To test a child's glucose at night, uncover your child's toe from the blankets, prick the side of the toe or the heel, and get a reading without waking them. A headlamp can also be used to illuminate the meter to reduce the chances of a child being awakened.

Parents and the diabetes care team should have realistic expectations for age appropriate goals regarding glucose control. Infants and toddlers are unable to perceive and treat hypoglycemia or hyperglycemia. An adult around them will have little success in sensing their glucose status. Therefore, setting a goal of 'tight control' or trying to achieve an A1c less than 7% may be dangerous. Instead, rely on safer measures of success: Is your child having fewer episodes of hypoglycemia? Are the fluctuations in blood glucose levels more controlled? Has your child's quality of life improved? Are you less fearful and anxious? Is your child growing and developing normally? If the answers to these questions are "Yes," pump therapy has proven to be a success. See Table 23.1 for ADA age-appropriate goals for control.

Babysitters and Day-care

Babysitters and day-care providers can be trained to deliver appropriate boluses and to recognize when a glucose reading indicates there is a problem and how to respond. The parent or health care personnel should always directly supervise pump use and training. Simple worksheets with instructions can be created for the childcare provider regarding how to test the glucose, give boluses, and what to do if an infusion set becomes detached. Carb boluses can be given after meals for toddlers who may be finicky or unpredictable eaters.

Both written and verbal instructions should be given for when to immediately contact a parent, such as when the blood glucose is abnormally high or low, if the child is vomiting, or there is another critical issue. A parent must be accessible at all times. Any delay in response time can cause significant harm to a child as a result of ketoacidosis or severe hypoglycemia. A simple piece of advice for caretakers is to always give fast-acting carbs if something is wrong and they cannot test. Stopping a low is more important than treatment of a high when waiting for help.

School Concerns for Children and Teens

Key school personnel need to know about diabetes, the pump, the procedures typically followed, and what to do in case of emergencies. Many schools (in the US) have zero tolerance for medications and syringes. However, to receive federal funding schools must follow a 504 Plan that is an agreement between the parents of children and teens who have diabetes or other medical issues and the school they attend.

Sample 504 Plans for different grades and ages are available at www.childrenwith-diabetes.com/504/. To minimize problems, the child or teen and parent should provide the school nurse, coach, teachers, and principal with printed materials about the insulin pump, and treatment of high and low glucoses, including a 504 Plan. A diabetes educator or physician can also write a letter to the school concerning the child's diabetes.

Check with school officials about where a child's glucose can be tested and by whom. It greatly encourages good care if a child or teen is able to test their glucose wherever they are instead of having to go to a nurse's office. Although the school policy may require that all diabetes care be done in the nurse's office, this is open to the 504 Plan that is developed. Work out a health program with school officials that enables the child with diabetes to stay healthy while at school and to have the freedom other children and teens have with respect to outings and sports.

If an insulin pen is used at school as well as a pump, let the school administration know. Have your physician write a letter to the school explaining why it may be needed if an infusion set gets pulled out or a pump problem occurs.

Keep your school kit filled and handy with these necessities:
- Insulin
- Insulin syringes and/or an insulin pen with needles as backup
- Spare infusion sets, reservoirs and any tape or related supplies
- Blood testing supplies
- Urine ketone test strips or a Precision XtraTM Blood Ketone meter and test strips
- Fast-acting carbs for lows
- Glucagon and glucose gel for lows
- Crackers and cheese or other snack to cover exercise and activity
- Extra batteries for both the insulin pump and blood glucose meter
- Emergency contact phone numbers and information

Physical Exercise and Athletics

Activity levels during P.E. classes at school are never consistent. One day may be spent playing a vigorous game of soccer and the next day watching a movie. It is important to monitor glucose levels before exercise. When vigorous exercise is planned, an additional snack of free carbs (carbs not covered with insulin) may need to be eaten at the beginning of class. A request to test the glucose and have a snack as needed before exercise should be covered in the child's 504 plan. A snack can be available in a pocket or backpack. If no snack is available, the workout may need to be skipped. If the child's glucose is high, blood or urine ketones should be tested. If ketones are present, exercise should be avoided and the plan to manage ketones should be activated.

If a sport has a practice session or game every day after school, reduce basal or bolus doses so that insulin levels are lower at that time. Eating carbs not covered by a carb bolus also works for practices. Practice sessions should be prepared for because lows and highs harm performance and may jeopardize the child's place on the team. Pumps are ideal for most athletes because adjustments in carbs, basal rates, and carb boluses are easily made on a pump. It helps to have good guidance on fine-tuning the pump for success. Chapter 22 provides guidelines about adjusting basal rates, boluses, and carb intake for various durations and intensities of exercise.

Dining Out at Fast Food and Chain Restaurants

Children and teens often eat at fast food restaurants. To cover these carbs with confidence, consult the nutritional information provided by these restaurants in their pamphlets. Excellent lists of the carb content in fast food and chain restaurant meals are in a book called The Calorie King Calorie, Fat, and Carbohydrate Counter. See Box 3.6 for more reference books and how to order. Chapter 3 in this book provides helpful information on carb counting and eating out. Apps for phones and other mobile technology allow carb counts to be easily looked up.

Certain pizzas and high fat or high protein meals may require a combo bolus with an initial carb bolus to match part of the carbohydrate intake followed by a delayed bolus to match the digestion of carbs slowed by the fat. Never be afraid to experiment with combination and extended boluses, but when you do, be sure to base decisions on past glucose patterns and test blood sugar frequently during and after completion of the full bolus. Write down what works or what you tried that did not work to help plan for the next time you eat the same food.

Sleep-Overs

Have a sleep-over plan to help relieve some of the anxiety when your child spends a night or weekend away from home. It is difficult to predict which direction the glucose may go during a sleep-over. With the excitement and extra snacks, glucose levels may be higher than usual. On the other hand, being awake during usual sleep time with extra activity may cause lower glucose levels. The only way to know for certain is to test frequently and be prepared to eat carbs to raise a low or to take an extra bolus if a high occurs. Always take your supplies if you stay overnight with a friend so that you are ready for anything. Discuss whether or not you want to set different glycemic targets that may be less aggressive than usual as you gain experience with this.

Sleeping In

After starting on a pump, it is better to follow a specific routine of waking, eating, and sleeping until the basal rates have been tested. The overnight basal rate needs to be tested and adjusted to maintain a safe glucose through the night and into the morning before attempting to sleep late. Only when these rates have been tested can a child safely hit the snooze button and go back to sleep, although doing a test before going back to sleep is best!

Diabetes Camp

Diabetes camp is a great way to meet other children and teens with diabetes. The American Diabetes Association maintains a listing of camps throughout the U.S., as does Children With Diabetes at www.childrenwithdiabetes.com. Camp is a great way to contact others with diabetes. Lifelong friendships can be developed, especially if you start young as a camper and attend for several years or become a junior counselor.

Special Issues for Teens

Acceptance

The physical, emotional, and social demands of the teen years often lead to neglect of glucose testing, carb counting and giving boluses. Depression, denial, and rebellion may contribute to neglect. Work with your diabetes team by telling them what gives you the most trouble with and how they can help you. They want to make your life easier if they can, but they have to understand your needs to be able to help.

Work with your team to identify any specific causes of poor control and develop a plan to deal with them. Negotiate reasonable and specific goals, and track how well you are meeting your goals. Let your parents, friends, and diabetes team know how you are really doing. Try to involve your parents to help you stay on track. Confiding your struggles to your best friend may lead to some new approaches as well. Remember diabetes management is challenging for everyone. Working together as a team with your friends, your family and your health care team can help.

Driving

Always check your blood glucose before driving. Discuss with your healthcare team what your target blood sugar should be before driving and how best to avoid a low. Before short trips, eat a snack of at least 15 grams of carbohydrate, such as 3 glucose tablets, before you put the keys in the ignition to ensure that a low reading does not occur. Keep snack foods available in the car at all times. On long trips, stop every hour if you are driving and check your blood glucose. Always check your BOB along with your glucose to make sure you won't go low from residual insulin action. A CGM can help you identify trends and give you a rate and direction of change, but be sure to do a finger stick test to confirm your glucose level.

Dating

When to tell someone that you have diabetes is a personal decision. Friends and dates are often inquisitive about diabetes if they see an insulin pump, see you testing your glucose, or counting carbs. This can serve as an "ice breaker" to start talking about and explaining diabetes. On the other hand, you may not feel ready to share or talk about diabetes for a while. Even if you do not feel ready to talk about your diabetes at first, continue to wear identification, like a medic alert and do not skip testing and taking your boluses. Excuse yourself and go to the restroom for these procedures, if necessary.

Eating Disorders

With all the focus on food in diabetes care, it is not surprising that some teens with diabetes have eating disorders. This often occurs with young women who may have a distorted image of themselves and who want to lose inappropriate amounts of weight. They may discover a quick weight-loss technique by eating what they want while decreasing their insulin doses. This soon causes glucose, calories and ketones to spill into the urine. This results in weight loss but carries with it an extreme risk for ketoacidosis in the short run, as well as a shorter, medically challenged life in the long run.

Parents and diabetes professionals must stay aware of teens who are overly concerned about food and weight. These teens typically have poor glucose control because they do not calculate basal rates and boluses appropriately. For teens with these behaviors, psychological assessment and intervention are imperative.

If you are using any of these harmful weight-loss techniques or think that you have problems with food and weight, seek professional help. Untreated eating disorders are very dangerous and can be life threatening, especially with diabetes.

Pregnancy

Young women with diabetes need education about their options for contraception. This is especially important because of the risk of becoming pregnant while diabetes control is poor, especially if the pregnancy is unplanned. If oral contraceptives are used, often a low dose is used to offer protection with less effect on glucose levels. A series of unexplained low glucoses in a young woman may be the earliest sign of pregnancy. Excellent glucose control in the weeks or months prior to conception and throughout pregnancy is critical for a healthy pregnancy. Refer to Chapter 25 for details.

Teens with Type 2

Teens with Type 2 diabetes who use insulin can equally benefit from insulin pump therapy. Therapy for Type 2 starts with adequate exercise and appropriate eating with carb counting. An overnight basal rate from a pump can be matched to the Dawn Phenomenon and meals and snacks can be covered with boluses. Type 2 teens on pumps are better able to reduce eating and match this with a smaller bolus, thus avoiding overeating. A pump also makes it easier to adjust insulin doses for planned and unplanned exercise or activity.

Summary

Success and safety with insulin pump therapy occurs when therapy is matched to the needs of the young pumper, and the child or teen and their family are well trained and properly supported. The well being of the child or teen makes all the training and care worthwhile. A child or teen wearing a pump has the opportunity for excellent glucose control during the most challenging years of diabetes. Success during this critical time occurs when the family, the child or teen and their healthcare team work together. This is a time of life when the child and then the teen learns about diabetes and gains independence in diabetes tasks as they demonstrate ability to care for themselves. At all ages it is important for parents to remain appropriately involved in diabetes care. It is vital for parents to remember to complement children and teens on their diabetes successes, identify challenges, and work together to overcome them.

Happiness is health and a short memory.
Audrey Hepburn

Pumping with Type 1.5 and Type 2 Diabetes

Benefits of an insulin pump are obvious with Type 1 diabetes, but most adults with Types 1.5 and 2 make equally good candidates for a pump once they need insulin to maintain control. Like Type 1s, they benefit from easy, precise, and convenient insulin delivery, helpful dose recommendations, reminders, and data tracking.

This chapter explains

- Why Type 1.5 diabetes is often mistaken for Type 2
- What is unique about Type 2 diabetes
- Insulin need and the advantages of pumps in Type 1.5 and 2

What is Type 1.5 Diabetes and Why is it Often Misdiagnosed as Type 2?

Type 1 diabetes used to be called "juvenile onset" diabetes but this term is no longer used because so many people develop it when they are adults. Even so, adults who are considered "too old" for the onset of Type 1 and do not immediately require insulin for treatment are often mistakenly told they have Type 2 diabetes. Many actually have a slower form of Type 1 diabetes, referred to as *Type 1.5 or LADA* (latent autoimmune diabetes in adults) because fewer antibodies are destroying the beta cells. They can often be treated with oral medications at first, while their insulin production continues over a few years.

One in every seven to ten people said to have Type 2 diabetes actually has antibodies that indicate they have Type 1.5. Those with Type 1.5 number over 2 million people in the U.S. or double the million or so people with Type 1 diabetes.

Type 1.5 starts in adults when antibodies slowly destroy beta cells. The only difference from Type 1 is that only one or occasionally two antibodies are involved, rather than three or more. The primary antibody involved in Type 1.5 is the GAD65 or glutamic acid decarboxylase antibody as shown in Table 24.1.

Type 1.5 differs from Type 2 in that insulin resistance is often not involved. Type 1.5 starts about 15 years earlier at an average age 46 instead of 61, usually without excess

275

24.1 Differences in the Three Major Types of Diabetes			
	Type 1	**Type 1.5 / LADA**	**Type 2**
Avg. age at start	12	46	61
Typical age at start	3 - 40*	20-70*	35-80*
% of all diabetes	10% (25%**)	15%	75%
Insulin problem	absence	deficiency	resistance
Antibodies	ICA, IA2, GAD65, IAA	mostly GAD65	none
Early Treatment	insulin is vital, diet & exercise changes helpful	pills or insulin vital, diet & exercise changes helpful	pills helpful, diet & increased activity essential
Late Treatment	insulin, diet, exercise (occasionally pills)	insulin, pills, diet, exercise	insulin, pills, diet, exercise

* may occur at any age
** if all antibody positive cases are included, ie Type 1 and Type 1.5

weight, but often with a personal or family history of an autoimmune disease.[110] It should be suspected when an adult does not have other classic signs of Type 2 diabetes, such as high triglyceride or low HDL levels, abdominal obesity, or a family history of high blood pressure. Many people with Type 1.5 are not overweight, while others are, making a "visual" diagnosis difficult. As the population increases in weight, people with Type 1 and 1.5 can have traits of Type 2, such as excess weight, insulin resistance and cholesterol problems.

Correct diagnosis of Type 1.5 is important because insulin treatment will be required much sooner in Type 1.5 than Type 2 diabetes. If Type 1.5 is suspected, a GAD65 antibody test should be done. When GAD65 or islet cell antibodies are present, the decline in insulin production is faster and the person requires insulin earlier than in Type 2. In the UKPDS study, 94% of those with Type 1.5 diabetes required insulin six years after being diagnosed compared to only 16% of those with Type 2 diabetes and no antibodies.[111]

Those with Type 1.5 diabetes obtain the same benefits from a pump as those with Type 1. Because relatively low insulin doses are needed in early Type 1.5 while internal insulin production remains, a pump is better able to provide these precise doses and may also help preserve beta cell production. As beta cell production declines and Type 1.5 turns into Type 1, small increases in basal and bolus delivery are more conveniently delivered with a pump.

What Is Unique about Type 2 Diabetes?

In contrast to Type 1 diabetes where the immune system destroys beta cells and the need for insulin becomes obvious very quickly, true Type 2 diabetes results from a slower mismatch between the beta cells ability to produce insulin and an increasing need for insulin caused by insulin resistance. The blood glucose usually rises slowly over several years as the beta cells become more and more damaged by higher glucose levels and the excessive demand on insulin production.

Type 2 is often part of a metabolic syndrome that includes insulin resistance, plus a variety of other problems: high blood pressure, high triglycerides, low levels of HDL (protective cholesterol), and abdominal obesity.

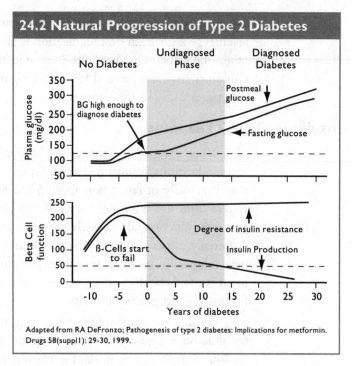

24.2 Natural Progression of Type 2 Diabetes

Adapted from RA DeFronzo; Pathogenesis of type 2 diabetes: Implications for metformin. Drugs 58(suppl1): 29-30, 1999.

Type 2 is a progressive disease in which insulin production ramps up in an attempt to keep up with insulin resistance for the first few years but then gradually falls off as beta cells become exhausted.

Can Type 2 be prevented? Absolutely, if you remain diligent about staying physically active and avoid gaining weight. In the Diabetes Prevention Program conducted by the NIH, the diagnosis of diabetes was reduced by 58% in the group that did these two things.[112] Also, two classes of diabetes medications, GLP-1 agonists and glitizones, have been shown to slow the loss of beta cells in Type 2 diabetes. When started early, these medications prevent loss of glucose control and delay the need for insulin for at least several years. It is truly unfortunate that these medications do not work in antibody positive or Type 1 diabetes.

An epidemic new cases of Type 2 diabetes throughout the world has led groups like the WHO, ADA, and AACE to lower glucose levels for diagnosis and treatment goals in an attempt to increase awareness and help people avoid heart attacks, blindness, amputations, and other health complications. Suggested treatment goals in Type 2 diabetes include:

- A fasting plasma glucose of 110 mg/dl (6.1 mmol/L) or less

- Glucoses of 140 mg/dl (7.7 mmol/L) or less 2 hours after eating

- An A1c of 6.5% or less

During the first years after diagnosis, the glucose may be brought down to goal through lifestyle changes. However, many people fail in this effort because beta cell failure is progressive and they have difficulty improving their diet, exercising regularly, and losing weight for their lifetime. When a person cannot control glucose levels well enough to reach Type 2 goals, an oral medication is prescribed and increased or supplemented with other oral diabetes medications. New injectable medications, such as Symlin® and GLP-1 inhibitors, may also be used for both weight loss and to lower glucose levels after meals. (See pages 213-215 for information.)

Insulin for Type 2 Diabetes

When glucose control can no longer be maintained with lifestyle modification and medications, insulin is started. Type 2 diabetes is typically diagnosed about 10 years after it actually began, when about 50 to 80% of insulin production is already lost.[111] *Excess insulin* is often produced by the body in early stages of Type 2, but the stress of overproduction, along with the toxic effects of excess glucose and free fatty acids, eventually causes damage to beta cells and causes insulin output to fall. After diagnosis, beta cell insulin production typically declines about 4% to 5% per year. Insulin replacement is most effective when started early where its use can slow damage to beta cells from stress and glucose toxicity.

Though not routinely done, giving insulin for Type 2 at the first clinic visit if the glucose is high can overcome glucose toxicity and rapidly bring down the high reading. Sometimes an initial injection may be enough to regain glucose control and medications and lifestyle changes can then be prescribed. An injection of insulin also helps alleviate the anxiety many people have about injections, and ease the transition to insulin later when needed.

Over half of those with Type 2 diabetes eventually require insulin using injections or a pump. Starting on insulin does not mean you have failed to control your diabetes. Rather, needing insulin results from a natural progression in Type 2 that we do not yet have the tools to stop (See Figure 24.2). Starting on insulin as soon as it is needed simply improves quality of life and health, and often prolongs beta cell productivity.

Over 20 million people in this country have Type 2 diabetes, but only about 34% use insulin. Resistance to prescribing and taking insulin means that many start on insulin only after their beta cells have already been severely damaged. Early use of insulin appears to preserve some beta cell activity and make control easier. Beta cell preservation is also seen with use of GLP-1 agonists like Byetta®, Victoza®, and Bydureon®, as well as insulin-sensitizing agents like Actos®.

Advantages of a Pump in Type 2

Insulin pump use benefits glucose control in Type 2 diabetes as well as many other health issues that arise in the metabolic syndrome, including cholesterol problems, high blood pressure, and excess inflammation and oxidation. Use of insulin helps glucose control and some of these associated problems.

Many people with Type 2 diabetes resist using insulin. When they finally agree to start using it, they want a simple approach with as few injections as possible. For convenience and ease of use, they are often started on one or two injections of premixed 70/30 insulin. This mixture of 70% slower background insulin and 30% rapid insulin is used to reduce the number of injections and simplify the calculation required for dosing. It attempts to cover background and meal needs, but doses are never exact and the user is tied to eating enough to offset the activity of the rapid insulin every time they take the combined insulin to cover their background need.

A pump offers the convenience of 70/30 insulin with a much more precise and flexible method of meeting insulin need. A pump uses only one type of insulin adjusted to provide a basal profile that matches background insulin need and easy bolusing for every snack and meal. It provides precise dosing without increasing the number of injections and improves the user's control. When insulin is needed, an insulin pump offers the most convenient and natural way to deliver the insulin that is lacking.

The small number of studies that have been done with people with Type 2 using pumps suggest that these people prefer pumps to multiple injections. One small study in 1993 found that people preferred pumps because they experienced less pain, fewer social limitations, less life interference, and less burden. They also experienced more general satisfaction, flexibility, and convenience.[113] These positive aspects help Type 2s overcome their reluctance to using insulin.

Another interesting way to help Type 2 diabetes is with short-term use of an insulin pump to prolong good control in early stages of the disease. In one French study, 82 people with Type 2, who were unable to control their glucoses with a low calorie diet and maximum doses of Glucophage (metformin), were temporarily placed on insulin pumps for periods of 8 to 32 days.[114]

Glucoses were brought down to target in the few days they were on pumps, but what was more interesting was that the glucose stayed under control for several months after the pump treatment stopped! Brief use of an insulin pump appears to give an overworked pancreas a "vacation" and helps it again produce adequate amounts of insulin.

A Turkish study tried the same approach in people with newly diagnosed Type 2 diabetes who did not respond to diet control. After two weeks on a pump, six of 13 patients were able to stay well controlled on diet alone for between 16 and 59 months, although four people required a second two-week treatment, and one required a third treatment.[115]

Helps Overcome the Metabolic Syndrome

Elements of the metabolic syndrome that affect many people with Type 2 can be dealt with more effectively by a pump than with injections. The better control of a pump reduces insulin resistance, as well as how much insulin is required. A pump helps lower high triglyceride levels as rapid insulin is matched to the carbs in meals.[116,117] This lessens elevated cholesterol levels and reduces blood clotting which can be dangerously high in Type 2 diabetes and lead to heart problems.

Lowers High Morning Glucose Levels

In Type 2 diabetes, a high waking glucose is common, even when the person has gone to bed with a normal reading. The rise in glucose during the night occurs when the liver makes and releases glucose into the bloodstream because it cannot "sense" that the insulin level is low. High glucose levels increase the resistance to insulin and make it even harder for the beta cells to keep up.

Oral medications may work for a while at controlling the high morning glucose of a person with Type 2, but eventually the addition of insulin to oral medications is required. The insulin may be delivered with one or more injections, but a pump does the job better. Basal insulin from a pump can be precisely adjusted so that it is delivered in the exact amount and at the exact time it is needed during the night to prevent the liver's production and release of glucose.

Studies done in the early 1980's found that increasing insulin levels in Type 2 diabetes by over 40% in the early morning was needed to prevent high glucose readings on rising.[118] This increase is about double that required to control the Dawn Phenomenon in Type 1 diabetes. This need for extra basal insulin in early morning hours is caused by insulin resistance and the release of free fatty acids that block insulin's effect. An injection of "flat" long-acting insulin may not control these as well. High morning glucose readings are easier to prevent by the precise dosing and exact timing of basal delivery on a pump.[116,117]

Decreases Weight Gain

Excess weight is common with Type 2 diabetes and insulin use can lead to more weight gain. Someone with Type 2 often goes for years with high readings that flush excess calories into the urine. They may have adapted by eating an extra 500 to 1000 calories a day with no weight gain. When treatment with medications or insulin begins to lower the glucose level, these calories previously lost in the urine start to move into cells. Unless calorie intake is reduced as soon as glucose control improves, a rapid increase in weight will be seen.

Weight gain does not have to happen with improved control. The road to real glucose control lies in eating only what you need and adjusting your insulin to handle it. Less insulin is required on a pump to achieve control, resulting in less exposure to glucose and insulin. The data in a pump provides easy access to a history of carb intake and can even act as a coach for weight loss. Smart use of a pump encourages the user to account for all meals and snacks, making mindless eating less likely.

Pumps help avoid weight gain because the user does not need to eat to avoid lows. A lower calorie intake is easier with a pump that calculates and reduces carb boluses based on the number of carbs to be eaten. Choosing carbs from a carb database in a pump, a linked PDA or a smart phone also helps reduce calories and carbs.

Improves Control and Lowers A1c

Precise basal and bolus delivery helps glucose control in Type 2 diabetes. Fasting glucoses are stabilized with precise overnight basals matched to need. Post-meal readings are lowered by using a variety of boluses, from extended to combination, that match insulin-to-carbs better. A carb database and a carb factor in the pump BC provides a recommendation for a carb bolus and tracks the history of how well control is maintained. With this, successful insulin delivery is reproducible.

Use of U-500 Insulin in Pumps

Many Type 2s are very resistant to insulin and may require 150 units or more of insulin a day. To handle the need for large insulin doses, such as 30, 50, or more units for a meal, U-500 Regular insulin is often used in a pump, although this has not been approved by the FDA. U-500 is concentrated and 5 times as strong as the U-100 insulin that most people use. Although U-500 Regular insulin has a slower onset and longer action than U-100 Novolog®, Humalog®, or Apidra®, the ability to give less volume at a time makes it more comfortable and in some ways more effective. When large doses of U-100 insulin are needed, the volume required slows down its action and makes it act like less voluminous U-500 Regular insulin.

One study looked at all the published research on U-500 insulin given by injection or with a pump. With injections, the U-500 lowered A1c levels by 1.59% but the injectors gained 9.6 lbs (4.38 kg) and required 52 more units of insulin a day. Those using pumps, however, had the same A1c reduction but had no significant change in weight or TDD.[119]

If you require 150 or more units a day, U-500 insulin in your pump may be ideal for you. Work closely with a physician who is familiar with U-500 to set basal rates, CarbF, and CorrF appropriately. With U-500 insulin, each one unit delivered by your pump actually delivers 5 units of this concentrated insulin. This requires that settings be carefully programmed to avoid getting too much insulin.

Medicare Pump Coverage

People with Type 2 or Type 1.5 who are eligible for Medicare are candidates for coverage for an insulin pump if they meet certain criteria. They can qualify for an insulin pump if they meet Medicare's definition of diabetes as shown by the C-peptide test or the beta cell autoantibody test. Medicare's addition of the autoantibody test allows people with Type 1.5 or LADA to start on a pump when antibodies to GAD65 or islet cells are present. They can qualify before they lose all beta cell insulin production, which is indicated by a very low C-peptide level. Pump candidates must meet a second criterion that establishes the need for a pump based on the failure in some respect of MDI to provide good control, as shown in Box 24.3.

24.3 Medicare Requirements for Pump Coverage (2002)

In order for a person with Type 1.5 or Type 2 diabetes to be eligible for coverage of an insulin pump, they must have either:

1. A low C-peptide
   For kidney insufficiency of creatinine clearance < 50 ml/min, a C-peptide < 200% of labs lower limit
   For other people, C-peptide < 110% of lab's lower limit of normal and fasting glucose is < 225 mg/dl

2. Or a positive beta cell autoantibody (GAD65, IA2a, etc.)
   Test result out of normal range documented by lab report, including lab's normal range

Criterion A: New pump for a person currently on MDI (2005)

- Completed diabetes education

- At least 3 injections of insulin a day

- Documented self-adjustment of insulin doses for 6 months

- Documented self testing of glucose at least 4 times a day for 2 months

PLUS one of these while on MDI:
  - A1c > 7%
  - Recurring hypoglycemia
  - Unstable blood sugars before meals
  - Dawn Phenomenon with fasting blood sugar > 200 mg/dl
  - Severely unstable blood sugars

Criterion B: On pump prior to Medicare enrollment

- Documented self-testing of glucose at least 4 times a day during the month prior to Medicare enrollment

Any fool can have bad luck; the art consists in knowing how to exploit it.

Frank Wedekind

Pregnancy

CHAPTER

25

Three types of diabetes can complicate pregnancy: Type 1, Type 2, and gestational diabetes. Diabetes affects 10,000 pregnancies each year in women who have Type 1 diabetes prior to conception. The number of women with preexisting Type 2 diabetes who become pregnant nearly equals this number as women now develop Type 2 at younger ages and become pregnant in their 30's and 40's.

Gestational diabetes (GDM), the third type, begins during pregnancy as an abnormal glucose elevation. This affects 7% of all pregnancies, with over 200,000 women affected each year in the U.S. GDM is a form of Type 2 diabetes that begins during pregnancy, often near the end of the second trimester or during the third trimester, and often disappears for a number of years once the pregnancy is over. Insulin pumps are helpful in pregnancies involving all three types of diabetes.

This chapter covers
- Why glucose control is important in pregnancy
- What makes control more difficult during pregnancy
- Testing for prediabetes and diabetes before pregnancy
- Pregnancy management in Type 1, Type 2, and GDM
- How to distribute carbs through the day with the Rule of 18ths
- Insulin adjustments during pregnancy
- Labor, delivery, and follow-up after delivery

Why Glucose Control Is So Important in Pregnancy

All pregnant women have a compelling reason for controlling their diabetes – only strictly controlled glucose levels create the environment needed to produce a healthy baby. High glucose levels before conception and during the first eight weeks of pregnancy are associated with serious birth defects. High levels in the second and third trimesters may result in fetal complications and problems during delivery or in the first few days after.

First trimester complications include
- Birth defects
- Spontaneous miscarriage

A special thanks to Lois Jovanovic, M.D. for her many contributions to better pregnancy outcomes.

25.1 Glucose Targets before and during Pregnancy		
Time	**Before pregnancy & 1st trimester**	**2nd trimester & 3rd trimester**
Before meals and at bedtime	60–119 mg/dl 3.3-6.6 mmol/L	60–99 mg/dl 3.3-5.5 mmol/L
1 hour after meals	100–149 mg/dl 5.6-8.3 mmol/L	100–129 mg/dl 5.6-7.2 mmol/L
2 to 6 am	65-119 mg/dl 3.6-6.6 mmol/L	65-99 mg/dl 3.6-5.5 mmol/L

A1c should be less than 6% during both stages.

Adapted from **Managing Preexisting Diabetes and Pregnancy**, ADA, 2008

Risks for these complications increase in women who have Type 1 or Type 2 diabetes when glucoses have been poorly controlled near the time of conception.

Second and third trimester complications include

- Premature delivery
- Delayed growth and development
- Large birth weight or macrosomia (over 9 pounds), often requiring a C-section

Problems for the child at birth if mother's glucose is poorly controlled include

- Injury during delivery
- Severe low glucose after delivery
- Seizures
- Respiratory distress syndrome
- Enlarged heart
- Low calcium level and tetany (jitters or spasms)
- Jaundice
- High red blood cell count (polycythemia)

These complications can arise with poor control in Type 1, Type 2, or gestational diabetes. High glucose levels during pregnancy may cause the baby to have under-developed lungs at birth even though it is full term and normal weight. Underdeveloped lungs, in turn, cause the baby to have respiratory distress or difficulty in breathing after delivery.

High glucoses in the mother near the time of delivery can also cause severe hypoglycemia in the newborn baby after delivery. While in the womb during the third trimester, the fetus produces large amounts of insulin whenever the mother has a high glucose. If the mother's glucose is high near delivery, the baby will continue to produce excessive amounts of insulin after delivery, which trigger severely low glucoses in the baby.

Tight Glucose Management for a Healthy Pregnancy

Glucose control has been directly linked to the survival of the infant since 1949, when Priscilla White, M.D. of the Joslin Clinic in Boston reported that 18 percent of the babies of mothers with diabetes were stillborn or died shortly after birth. She noted that "good treatment of diabetes" clearly improved the outcome.[121] In 1965, Jorgen Pedersen, M.D., studying pregnant women in Copenhagen, reported that 130 women who had one of the Bad Signs in Box 25.2 had a 31 percent rate of fetal and neonatal death.[122] In contrast, women who had none of these signs, the death rate was only 6.9 percent.[123,124]

During the late 1960's and early 1970's, it became clear that the higher the average glucose level of the mother, the more likely a child would die near birth. By the 1980's, the mother's glucose and the child's metabolic environment could be normalized through glucose testing at home, helping reduce complications once the mother knew she was pregnant, but the problems caused by high glucoses at conception still existed.

25.2 Dr. Pedersen's Bad Signs

Things to avoid in pregnancy:
1. Ketoacidosis
2. Preeclampsia or toxemia of pregnancy: a combination of high blood pressure, headaches, protein in the urine, and swelling of the legs, usually occurs late in the pregnancy
3. Kidney infection
4. Neglect of prenatal care

Around this time, birth defects emerged as a major cause of infant deaths in babies born to women with Type 1 diabetes.[125,126] In several studies, birth defects were found to occur in 4% to 11% of infants born to women with Type 1 diabetes, compared to a rate of 1.2% to 2.1% in the general population.[127,128] Researchers and physicians realized that for best results glucose levels need to be normalized prior to conception. The child's organs form rapidly during the first eight weeks after conception, often before a woman realizes she is pregnant.

Researchers also noticed that higher A1c values in the first trimester were associated with more spontaneous miscarriages than in nondiabetic women.[129,130] An A1c that is in the normal range or no higher than one percent above the upper limit of a normal range minimizes the risk of both birth defects and miscarriages. Interestingly, one researcher found that women with diabetes who have excellent control throughout pregnancy actually have a lower rate of miscarriage than nondiabetic women.[130]

The conclusion from these early studies was that maintaining normal glucoses before and throughout pregnancy reduces the risk of complications. Women with Type 1 or Type 2 diabetes who plan to conceive should keep their glucose at the lower levels recommended for pregnancy even before conception and maintained through delivery. The guidelines that follow provide a good way to maintain tight control during pregnancy.

Diabetes Control Is More Important During Pregnancy – All Diabetes Types

During pregnancy, day-to-day glucose levels in a woman without diabetes are naturally lower than prior to pregnancy, apparently to protect the fetus. Research shows that a normal waking glucose for a woman who is pregnant but does not have diabetes is 55 to 65 mg/dl (3 to 3.6 mmol/L) after an overnight fast. The glucose level is always less than 120 mg/dl (6.6 mmol/L) even one hour after eating a high carb meal. For good control and a healthy baby, A1c levels need to stay within a normal range throughout pregnancy. Although A1c levels for pregnancy are 20 percent lower than the normal range for healthy adults, an A1c between 5.5% and 6.5% appears good for a healthy outcome with diabetes.

These normal glucoses during pregnancy come very close to a hypoglycemic range, as shown in Table 25.1. Control may become complicated when morning sickness causes nausea and vomiting, and makes eating and insulin coverage difficult. Other factors that must be balanced are a rising placental hormone release that raises the glucose, and a gradual weight gain that requires additional insulin during the course of the pregnancy.

A pump is better able to deliver the precise insulin doses required for tight glucose management and makes it more convenient to give frequent boluses for frequent small meals that can greatly improve post-meal control while keeping track of BOB. A CGM is a great asset for keeping glucose levels within the tight range required for pregnancy.

Preparing for Pregnancy – Type 1, Type 2

If you have Type 1 or Type 2 diabetes, you should have your glucose under good control before you try to conceive. If you have Type 2 diabetes, metformin appears safe through the first trimester, and glyburide may be used through the entire pregnancy as long as glucose levels are well controlled. A program for Type 2's using diet, exercise, and insulin, if needed, can be worked out with your physician to achieve optimal control before conception.

Until your glucose is controlled, use adequate birth control. Low dose birth control pills appear to be both safe and effective. Once your A1c is below 7.0% and preferably below 6.5%, you are ready for pregnancy. At this time, birth control can be discontinued.

Achieving optimal control before conception is necessary because the fetus begins to develop specialized organs and tissues from the time the egg is fertilized through the first three months of pregnancy. High glucoses at this time interfere with cell division and can lead to DNA damage and birth defects. There is a 20 percent chance that the infant will develop complications or die if control was poor prior to conception and optimal control is achieved only in the second trimester.[131]

If you plan to become pregnant, follow a healthy food plan, exercise regularly, and supplement your diet with a prenatal vitamin. If you have any complication caused by diabetes prior to pregnancy, such as damage to the eyes, kidneys, or vascular system, there is a greater risk of complications in pregnancy for yourself and the baby.[132] This does not rule out a healthy pregnancy, but should be carefully considered before pregnancy begins.

Testing for Prediabetes or Diabetes prior to Pregnancy

If you might have diabetes or you have any of the high-risk factors for GDM listed in Box 25.4 and are attempting to conceive, you should be tested to determine if you have prediabetes or diabetes before you conceive. If the glucose tests in Table 25.5 show a positive result, follow Preparing for Pregnancy in the previous section. If these tests are negative, they should be repeated as soon as your pregnancy is confirmed and, if again negative, repeated at 24 to 28 weeks of gestation. A diagnosis of prediabetes or diabetes warns that your glucose levels are higher than normal and are above the optimal levels desired for a healthy pregnancy.

Gestational Diabetes

The most common form of diabetes during pregnancy is *gestational diabetes mellitus (GDM)*, which is defined as glucose intolerance that is first recognized during pregnancy. It typically develops late in the second trimester or early in the third trimester of an otherwise normal pregnancy due to the increasing demand for insulin production at this time. Gestational diabetes puts both the mother and baby at risk for serious complications during the pregnancy if not managed carefully.

Gestational diabetes is often early Type 2 diabetes uncovered by the increased insulin requirements found in pregnancy. A mother with GDM faces a high risk of developing Type 2 diabetes later in life. Glucose elevation during pregnancy can also result from early Type 1.5 diabetes (pages 275-276). If a woman with GDM tests positive for GAD65 antibodies, she has Type 1.5 diabetes and will be seven times as likely to need insulin compared to Type 2 diabetes.[133] Often, glucose levels return to normal after delivery, but the underlying problem remains and needs to be addressed through lifestyle changes and/or adding metformin. Follow-up screening is done at 6-12 weeks after delivery and then every 3 years for life.

Screening for GDM

An accurate diagnosis of gestational diabetes is important to reduce health risks to the mother and baby, especially to prevent having a large baby, called *macrosomia*.

Macrosomia often necessitates a C-section and causes problems for the newborn. Pregnant women who are at high risk of GDM should be tested at the first prenatal visit. A pregnant woman with any of the higher risk factors in Box 25.4 should be screened for GDM at the first prenatal visit using the thresholds in Table 25.5.

> ## 25.4 High Risk Factors for GDM
>
> - Over 35 years of age
> - Overweight with a body mass index over 25
> - An inactive lifestyle
> - Family history of Type 2 diabetes
> - Prior history of gestational diabetes
> - History of polycystic ovary syndrome (PCOS)
> - A previous baby weighed over 9 lbs (4.1 kg)
> - High blood pressure
> - Abnormal cholesterol levels with an HDL less than 35 or triglycerides greater than 250 mg/dl (2.83 mmol/L)
> - African-American, Hispanic, American Indian, Asian-American, or a Pacific Islander

A pregnant woman who does not have high-risk characteristics can be screened for GDM with a 1-hour glucose tolerance test done between the 24th and 28th weeks (the sixth month) of pregnancy. All pregnant women should be screened for GDM because traditional risk factors have a low probability of predicting who will develop GDM, especially during the first pregnancy.[134] Both fasting and glucose tolerance tests are used to detect GDM because an elevation of either one may be the only clue that GDM is present.

Fasting hyperglycemia may be particularly important. One research study involving over 145,000 births in Dallas, Texas, found that a fasting plasma glucose of 105 mg/dl (5.8 mmol/L) or higher was over three times as likely to be associated with fetal malformations compared to women without diabetes and surprisingly to women who did have GDM but whose fasting value was below 105 mg/dl. Women who had diabetes prior to pregnancy were at the highest risk of fetal malformations at 6.1%, followed by those with GDM and an elevated fasting plasma value at 4.8%, then women without diabetes at 1.5%, and finally those with GDM and a low fasting plasma glucose value at 1.2%.[135]

Table 25.5 shows appropriate glucose values during pregnancy. Screening to detect GDM is done in two steps with a fasting glucose first, followed by glucose tests at one and two hours after drinking 75 grams of glucose. Gestational diabetes is diagnosed if the fasting plasma glucose is 92 mg/dl (7 mmol/L) or higher, the one-hour test is 180 or higher, or the two-hour test is 153 or higher. Any one of these gives the diagnosis.[136]

Pregnancy Management Program – All Diabetes Types

Regardless of whether you have Type 1, Type 2, GDM, or marginal glucose values during testing, you want to make every effort to keep your glucose within the targets in Table 25.1 throughout your pregnancy. You need to manage your diabetes in these ways:

- Frequent glucose and A1c tests to determine your exact level of control
- An eye exam for retinopathy
- A 24-hour urine collection for creatinine clearance, total protein, and microalbumin to assess the health of your kidneys, done each trimester
- An evaluation of your cardiovascular system
- A detailed diet program, using the Rule of 18ths in Table 25.8 or a similar plan
- A regular exercise program

25.5 ADA Screening and Diagnosis of Gestational Diabetes (GDM)				
Any combination of two values for a fasting plasma glucose level ≥126 mg/dl (7.0 mmol/l) or a random plasma glucose ≥200 mg/dl (11.1 mmol/l) is a diagnosis of diabetes. No further testing is needed.				
If a diagnosis of diabetes (above) has not been done, two lab plasma glucose values greater than the following values gives a diagnosis of GDM: *				
	Fasting	**1 hr**	**2 hr**	**3 hr ** **
75 or 100 gram OGTT	95 mg/dl (5.3 mmol/L)	180 mg/dl (10 mmol/L)	155 mg/dl (8.6 mmol/L)	140 mg/dl (7.8 mmol/L)
* Home glucose meters are not accurate enough to diagnose diabetes.				
** A 3 hour test is not done with the 75 gram OGTT test				
OGTT = oral glucose tolerance test				

Glucose Monitoring

As weight is gained and the child grows during pregnancy, more and more insulin is needed. In order to adjust insulin to need in Type 1 diabetes, use a CGM or check at least eight times a day: before each meal, an hour after each meal, at bedtime, and at 2 a.m. These tests alert yourself and your health care team quickly to any increased need for insulin. Table 25.6 shows the typical rise in insulin requirements throughout pregnancy for women with Type 1 diabetes.

The glucose at one hour after eating should be the highest reading of the day. Your desired target at one hour is to be less than 130 mg/dl (7.2 mmol/L). A glucose in the lower end of the target range indicates more carbs may be needed to avoid a low glucose.

For women with Type 2 and GDM, using a CGM or testing the glucose four to seven tests a day is required to reduce exposure of the fetus to elevated glucose readings. Readings done while fasting and one hour after each meal are the most important times to test to ensure adequate glucose control during pregnancy. Some tests before meals and at bedtime are also very helpful. Adjustments in insulin, diet, and activity are made based on how well the glucose targets are being met.

The last three months of the pregnancy when the baby can produce its own insulin is an especially critical time to test. The baby will overproduce insulin if the mother's glucose is higher than normal for pregnancy. The mother's excess glucose easily crosses the placenta, but the excess insulin that the baby makes cannot cross the placenta to lower the mother's high glucose. This insulin causes unwanted weight gain in the baby, often makes a C-section necessary for delivery, and creates other problems for the child after delivery.

Other Pregnancy Tests

Certain tests are essential for all women with diabetes and pregnancy:

- In the first trimester, an eye exam is done to check for retinopathy, and urine and blood tests are done to detect any kidney disease that might worsen during pregnancy.
- Screening tests for Down's syndrome and spina bifida may be done in the 1st or early 2nd trimester.
- Measure blood pressure at home and at each clinic visit to detect a severe disorder called preeclampsia or toxemia of pregnancy. This is a combination of very high blood pressure, swelling, and protein in the urine that starts late in the second trimester or third trimester in about 5% of pregnancies.
- An ultrasound is a safe procedure that may be done before 13 weeks to determine the delivery date, at 18 to 20 weeks to screen for birth defects, or at other times to check for polyhydramnios (excess amniotic fluid). It is repeated early in the third trimester to assess fetal size, screen for heart defects, and warn if macrosomia (large baby) is present.
- In the last month of pregnancy, the mother may wear a small ultrasound device for 30 to 40 minutes to check that normal changes in the baby's heart rate are present.

Insulin Adjustment

If you have well-controlled Type 1 diabetes when you become pregnant, you can begin adjusting your normal basal doses and boluses through the pregnancy. If you are not in good control, you'll need expert guidance to select better doses and adjust them to maintain a healthy pregnancy.

Insulin requirements rise steadily throughout pregnancy and will usually double by the last month.[138] The rising need for insulin is caused by several factors, including weight gain, increased caloric intake, creation of new tissue, and an increase in hormones made by the enlarging placenta. The action of placental hormones, especially estrogen, cortisol, and human placental lactogen, conflict with the action of insulin. Each woman's experience varies, so an insulin program must be tailored to each individual's need.

There are two periods prior to delivery when insulin doses may be reduced. The first period occurs in Type 1 diabetes during a five-week interval between weeks 7 and 12 of gestation. In one clinic's experience, after an initial rise in insulin doses of 18% between weeks 3 and 7, a significant drop in insulin requirement averaging 9% was seen in weeks 7 through 12.[139] The fall in insulin requirements in early pregnancy was first noted in the 1950's when physicians noted that unexpected, sudden hypoglycemia in women with Type 1 diabetes was often the first sign of pregnancy. It may be caused by a decline in progesterone secretion at this time.

The second exception occurs in the last four weeks of pregnancy when the fetus starts to draw more glucose from the mother's blood for its own use, and the mother starts to eat smaller portions as her abdomen enlarges.

At these times, basal rates and boluses may need to be reduced. A reduced overnight basal and a larger bedtime

25.6 Typical Rise in Total Daily Insulin Doses by Trimester for Type 1 Diabetes				
If your weight is:	At this trimester:			
	Pre	1st*	2nd	3rd**
100	27 u	32 u	36 u	41 u
120	33 u	38 u	44 u	49 u
130	35 u	41 u	47 u	53 u
140	38 u	45 u	51 u	57 u
160	44 u	51 u	58 u	65 u
180	49 u	57 u	65 u	74 u
200	55 u	64 u	73 u	82 u

In contrast to Type 1 diabetes, the TDD for women with Type 2 diabetes and recently diagnosed gestational diabetes varies greatly.

* From week 7 to 12, the need for insulin may decrease about 9%.
**In the last 4 weeks, the need for insulin may decrease slightly.

Adapted from Jovanovic L, et al. Am J Med. 71: 925-927, 1981

snack may be required to keep the glucose from dropping during the night at this time. Carb boluses are reduced as needed as the meal size shrinks with an enlarging uterus.

The flexibility of an insulin pump works well for maintaining control when insulin need constantly rises, especially in the last four months of pregnancy. With Type 1 diabetes, basal insulin delivery usually makes up 50 to 60% of the TDD through the pregnancy. The basal percentage may be lower or higher in women who have GDM or Type 2 diabetes, where significant insulin production remains.

Correction boluses are used whenever they are needed to bring down high readings. This should be done quickly so that the fetus is not harmed. Any time your glucose remains above your targets, your basal and bolus doses should immediately be raised. An increase in the TDD is usually required every 5 to 15 days through most of the pregnancy. A graphic charting system like *Smart Charts* or a comprehensive logbook should be used during pregnancy to track everything that affects your control. Include your weight in your charts.

Insulin Choices

No insulin has ever been formally approved for use during pregnancy, although human Regular insulin and NPH are considered safe and effective. Studies suggest that Novolog® (aspart) and Humalog® (lispro) are reasonably safe for pregnant women. Less is known about Apidra® (glulisine), and the long-acting insulins Lantus® (glargine) and Levemir® (detemir) in pregnancy, but no problems have been noted up to this point.

Caution: If you have an unexpected drop in your insulin need not caused by an obvious reason, contact your obstetrician for consideration of immediate delivery.

Nutrition Therapy and Carb Adjustments

Good nutrition is critical for every pregnant woman with diabetes. This should include nutritional counseling by a registered dietitian. Foods eaten during pregnancy have to be selected carefully to keep glucose readings after a meal with safe limits for the child. Many of the foods eaten in the past need to change.

Eating a balanced diet every day with adequate calories and nutrients for the pregnant woman based on her weight, height, and activity is important. The fetus continually removes glucose from the mother's blood for its growth, so it is important that the mother eat many meals and snacks throughout the day. More frequent eating also reduces the amount of carbs at each meal and makes glucose control easier as glucose spiking is avoided. During pregnancy, a diet made up of 40 percent carbohydrate, 40 percent fat, and 20 percent protein is generally recommended.

One way to spread carbohydrates is to use the Rule of 18ths. To do this, estimate your total daily caloric need

25.7 Carb Distribution with the Rule of 18ths		
Meal or Snack	**Portion of the Day's Total Carbohydrate:**	**Percent of Total Daily Carbs**
Breakfast	2/18	11.0%
Midmorning Snack	1/18	5.5%
Lunch	5/18	27.5%
Midafternoon	2/18	11.0%
Dinner	5/18	27.5%
After-Dinner Snack	2/18	11.0%
Bedtime Snack	1/18	5.5%

with the help of your dietitian. Then distribute the carbohydrate portion of these calories through the day in seven meals and snacks based on the number of 18ths of total carbs needed at each time, as shown in Table 25.8.

For example, if you require 1800 calories a day, you would need 180 grams of carbohydrate for the entire day. Your breakfast in Table 25.8 has two 18ths that equals 20 grams of carb.

Breakfast carbs are kept low compared to other meals of the day because most women with Type 1 diabetes have at least a mild Dawn Phenomenon and are more resistant to insulin at the beginning of the day. Women with Type 2 and gestational diabetes

25.8 Rule of 18ths: Grams of Carb per Meal Based on Total Calorie Need

Meal	Carbs as 18ths	Total Calories per Day							
		1600	1800	2000	2200	2400	2600	2800	3000
Breakfast	2/18 =	19 g	20 g	22 g	24 g	26 g	29 g	30 g	34 g
Morning Snack	1/18 =	9 g	10 g	12 g	14 g	14 g	14 g	16 g	17 g
Lunch	5/18 =	44 g	50 g	55 g	60 g	66 g	72 g	78 g	82 g
Afternoon Snack	2/18 =	18 g	20 g	22 g	24 g	27 g	30 g	31 g	82 g
Dinner	5/18 =	44 g	50 g	55 g	60 g	66 g	72 g	78 g	34 g
Evening Snack	2/18 =	18 g	20 g	22 g	24 g	27 g	29 g	31 g	82 g
Bedtime Snack	1/18 =	9 g	10g	12 g	14 g	14 g	14 g	16 g	34 g
Total Carbs/Day =		160 g	180 g	200 g	220 g	240 g	260 g	280 g	300 g
40% of Total Cal/Day =		640 cal	720 cal	800 cal	880 cal	960 cal	1040 cal	1120 cal	1200 cal

often have insulin resistance that can also cause high morning readings. Keeping carb intake low until noon helps prevent the post-meal glucose spiking that is common at this time of day. Avoid high glycemic foods that spike the glucose at all times. Select foods with a glycemic index of 60 or less. A CGM helps find the foods least likely to spike your glucose and quickly lets you know it's time to increase your basal and/or bolus doses during the course of the pregnancy.

An extra 500 to 1,000 calories per day are needed by the end of the nine months. These calories supply fuel for your higher metabolic rate and your required weight gain. The distribution of carbohydrates changes along with the calorie change. Table 25.8 provides guidance for distributing the carb portion of these calories.[137]

Exercise

Exercise is a critical part of glucose control during pregnancy. An ideal way to do this is to walk for 15 to 20 minutes after each meal. When this can be done, post-meal readings are greatly improved. A total of 45 to 60 minutes of walking a day is ideal during pregnancy. Starting or continuing an exercise program is highly recommended to improve control of glucose, blood pressure, weight and circulation during pregnancy, and ease delivery.

Oral Diabetes Medications in Type 2 or GDM

The FDA has not approved oral diabetes medications for use in pregnancy. Some oral agents may have a negative effect on the fetus, while others may be safe. One study of glyburide showed it could achieve tight control in a head to head study with insulin in women with GDM. The study involved over 400 women with gestational diabetes who were not able to achieve glucose control with diet alone, and the glyburide was started after conception. No differences were found in control or outcomes between the two groups.[142] Older sulfonylureas are known to cause fetal damage and are avoided. Glyburide is usually stopped before delivery to avoid hypoglycemia.

Many women of child-bearing age with polycystic ovary syndrome (PCOS) have been treated with metformin to improve fertility, and pregnancy has often occurred while the metformin was still being used. Although metformin is used in pregnancy, it can lower levels of folic acid and vitamin B12 in the blood. A lack of folic acid during pregnancy can cause spina bifida and other neural tube defects in the child. Poor absorption of vitamin B12 caused by metformin may be corrected by taking a calcium supplement.[141] Women of childbearing age on metformin should take a calcium supplement along with their prenatal vitamin that contains B12 and 400 mg. of folic acid.

When to Start Insulin in Type 2 or GDM

Ten to fifteen percent of women with gestational diabetes require insulin to control high glucoses. If you have Type 2 diabetes or GDM, diabetes medications are usually replaced immediately with insulin, and insulin should be started anytime that the glucose rises above the target levels required for a healthy pregnancy as shown in Table 25.9

Some pregnancy specialists recommend that insulin be started as soon as home blood glucose tests (or plasma values) are greater than 100 mg/dl (5.6 mmol/L) fasting, or above 130 mg/dl (7.2 mmol/L) one hour after a meal.[142] Home glucose values are more indicative of actual control and are easier to obtain during pregnancy than lab tests.

Another indication that it is time to begin insulin therapy is when a fetal ultrasound at 29 to 33 weeks shows the fetal weight to be greater than the 70th percentile. Insulin is started at this time regardless of the mother's glucose levels.[141] When macrosomia is controlled, the need for a C-section becomes less likely. Gestation should last 38 weeks

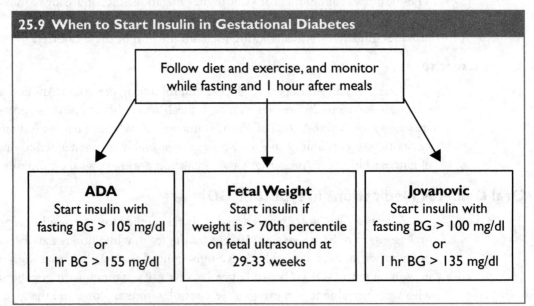

25.9 When to Start Insulin in Gestational Diabetes

Follow diet and exercise, and monitor while fasting and 1 hour after meals

ADA
Start insulin with fasting BG > 105 mg/dl
or
1 hr BG > 155 mg/dl

Fetal Weight
Start insulin if weight is > 70th percentile on fetal ultrasound at 29-33 weeks

Jovanovic
Start insulin with fasting BG > 100 mg/dl
or
1 hr BG > 135 mg/dl

when possible, but not go beyond 38 weeks because longer pregnancies increase the risk of macrosomia and do not decrease the risk of a C-section.

Glucagon Can Be Used to Offset Insulin with Nausea

Nausea and vomiting often occur in the first trimester and become a concern when a pregnant woman with diabetes on insulin cannot eat. If you become nauseated, your basal delivery is still required to keep the glucose from rising. If nothing is eaten, a bolus is needed only to lower a high glucose that may occur. Always check for ketones if your glucose is unexpectedly high to avoid ketoacidosis caused by an infusion set problem.

If nausea occurs often, as it will in some pregnancies, part of the carb bolus can be taken and eating attempted. If food or liquids with carbs can be kept down, the rest of the bolus can be taken as soon as the meal is finished. If the food or liquid won't stay down after a meal bolus is given, a temp basal reduction equal to your BOB can be tried, or a partial dose of glucagon can be injected to quickly raise the glucose.

See Box 25.10 to see how much glucagon is needed to prevent a low glucose. Keep glucagon available at all times to treat severe lows, as well as to raise the glucose when a carb bolus has been taken but nausea prevents eating. Glucagon raises the blood glucose by releasing stored glucose from the liver.

> **25.10 Glucagon: How Much Do You Need?**
>
> Each 0.15 mg of glucagon or 1/6 of a standard dose raises the glucose about 30 mg/dl. Avoid taking too much glucagon – this raises the glucose too high and can also cause nausea.

Prevent Ketoacidosis during Pregnancy

With Type 1 diabetes, the greatest threat to the fetus and the mother are high glucoses that lead to ketoacidosis. Ketoacidosis occurs in 1-3% of pregnancies in women with diabetes,[140] and 9% of these fetuses are lost. Use these precautions to avoid ketoacidosis:

- Test the glucose frequently to ensure that control is constant
- Take a correction bolus to lower any glucose over 160 mg/dl (8.9 mmol/L)
- Check for ketones each morning and when the glucose is above the target level
- Give an injection of long-acting insulin at bedtime. NPH insulin can be given by injection at bedtime equal to 30% of the entire day's normal basal delivery. For instance, if basal rates equal 30 units per day, give 9 units (30 u X 0.3 = 9 u) of NPH at bedtime. Lower the night basal rate at the same time, giving 40% of the current basal starting at bedtime for the next 10 hours. Then adjust these doses as needed.
- Lantus® or Levemir® insulins are used by some clinicians to replace about half the basal delivery because they offer a more consistent insulin activity than NPH.

Labor and Delivery

Labor got its name because muscle contractions during active labor are equivalent to strenuous exercise. This reduces insulin need dramatically. The goal is to maintain blood glucose levels between 60 and 100 mg/dl (3.3 and 5.6 mmol/L). If you have Type 1 diabetes, you might attain this level of control by reducing your basal doses quickly and discontinuing all boluses during labor. Hospital personnel find it far easier, however, to disconnect the pump and start an intravenous line to give insulin as needed to lower the glucose or to give glucose to raise it. Glucose levels need to be monitored very closely during this time.

Women who have pre-existing Type 2 diabetes or GDM generally discontinue both basal delivery and carb boluses when active labor begins. If insulin or glucose is needed, they can be given through the IV line.

Care after Delivery

After delivery, the hormones from the placenta that antagonized insulin are no longer present. Insulin requirements drop rapidly right after delivery. A reduced demand for insulin after delivery, together with the prolonged "exercise" of labor, may dramatically reduce insulin need, even in Type 1 diabetes, for a day or two. If a woman has had a C-section, her eating will be limited for the next two to three days, which also limits insulin need. In a few days, the woman with Type 1 will be back to her pre-pregnancy insulin requirements if weight gain during pregnancy has been minimal.

Most women with GDM who required insulin during their pregnancy no longer need it. Some will continue to have diabetes and require treatment, but most return to impaired glucose tolerance, impaired fasting glucose, or to normal glucoses. Over the next 20 years, half of women with gestational diabetes develop Type 2 diabetes.

In GDM, tests are performed six weeks after birth to determine whether the mother's glucose has returned to normal. The criteria for a diagnosis of diabetes at this time are the same as for diagnosing the general population. See Screening for GDM on page 288. Women with a diagnosis of prediabetes or diabetes should be counseled on diet, exercise and medications to treat the condition.

Babies born to women with GDM should be followed closely to prevent the development of obesity or abnormal glucose tolerance.

Breast Feeding

Breast feeding benefits the baby's immune system and also lowers the mother's insulin requirements, as her glucose is diverted into breast milk. Adjust your calorie intake to match the child's breast-feeding habits. If the baby consumes most of its calories at bedtime or in the middle of the night, you must do the same. Many Type 1 women with this breast-feeding pattern need only a low basal rate to cover eating in the evening hours.

While breast feeding, the mother needs to keep her glucose well-controlled. Any excess glucose also goes into breast milk. With poor control, these excess calories can put the baby at risk for weight gain and the possibility of contracting Type 2 diabetes at an earlier age.[141]

If you have something of importance to say, for God's sake start at the end.

Sarah Jeannette Duncan

Wrap Up

Now that you've worked through **Pumping Insulin**, you have the information and skills to begin to control your glucose on a pump. You know good control makes you feel better and reduces your risk of complications over time. You've got the knowledge and motivation needed to take control of your diabetes, but what else do you need?

The information you've worked hard to get is never enough by itself. It has to be supplemented with hands on experience, perseverance, doing the same or similar thing over and over again until you have better results. Setting basal and bolus doses, counting carbs and matching them with carb boluses, testing blood sugars, correcting highs, avoiding lows and recording these details in a useful way are all part of the mix.

Life has a way of changing, and your glucose control will change with it. Once you attain reasonable control, this may last weeks, months, years or only a short time before you have highs and lows all over again. You may have no idea why your good control is gone. When this happens, just go back, troubleshoot, problem solve, make some changes and test until you see improvements again. Once you succeed through science or luck, you will have the confidence to try again.

If you draw a blank, seek help from an endocrinologist or trained health professional who can spot important details and patterns in your charts that you might miss. You are responsible for collecting and recording the information related to your glucoses, but you don't have to solve all your problems alone. Develop a good relationship with a knowledgeable and supportive health care team to speed your success.

We hope you're encouraged by the new advances in CGMs and pumps and get involved in learning how to use them to their fullest capacity. They make pumping easier and safer. Future developments in pumps, meters, continuous monitors and glucose lowering drugs are happening quickly, so pay attention to these new developments.

We hope the information in this book helps you move toward your goal. We learned a great deal in writing it. Thanks for being such an engaging and hardworking audience to address. We keep you in mind as we write so that the concepts we present fit your needs and are clear and understandable. We offer our wholehearted support for your success in using your pump to improve your glucoses and health. You've already come far, simply by engaging in this process. Our best to you on your adventure.

Counting Carbs with a Gram Scale & Carb Percentages

Few foods, other than table sugar and lollipops, are totally carbohydrate. The carb percentages on the following pages give the amount of carbohydrate in 1 gram of that food. To find out how much carbohydrate you are eating in a particular food, do a simple calculation:

1. Weigh the food you want to eat on a gram scale to get its total weight, or check the label to find its weight in grams.
2. Find your food and its carb percentage in the tables that follow.
3. On a calculator, multiply the food's weight in grams by its carb percentage.
4. Your answer gives the number of grams of carb you are eating.

Example: Let's say you place a small apple on a gram scale and find that it weighs 100 grams. You look up its carb percentage and find that it is 0.13. You then multiply 100 grams by 0.13 to get the carbohydrate you will be eating:

100 grams of apple X .13 = 13 grams of carbohydrate

Additional Information

Carb percentages give the actual concentration of carbohydrate in foods. For instance, apples are 13% carbohydrate (most of their weight is water); raisins are 77% carbohydrate by weight, and bagels contain 56% carbohydrate by weight. Both apple juice and regular sodas are 12% carbohydrate, although the carbohydrate in apple juice is higher in fructose, while a regular soda has more of its carbohydrate as sucrose or sugar.

Cranberry juice is even richer in carbohydrate at 16%, while grapefruit juice contains only 9% by weight. A 6-oz. glass of cranberry juice will therefore contain almost twice as much carbohydrate as an identical glass of grapefruit juice. Because it contains more carbohydrate, the glass of cranberry juice can raise the blood sugar nearly twice as far as the same amount of grapefruit juice. It will also require almost twice as much insulin to cover it.

Carb Percentages for Various Foods

Juices

apple cider	.14	frozen	.09	orange-apricot	.13
apple juice	.12	grapefruit-orange: canned	.10	papaya	.12
apricot	.12	frozen	.11	pineapple: canned	.14
apricot nectar	.15	lemon	.08	frozen	.13
cranberry	.16	lemonade, frozen	.11	prune	.19
grape: bottled	.16	orange: fresh	.11	tomato	.04
grape: frozen	.13	canned, unsweet	.10	V-8	.04
grapefruit: fresh	.09	canned, sweet	.12		
canned	.07	frozen	.11		

Dressings, Sauces, Condiments

bacon bits	.19	olives	.04	soy sauce	.10
BBQ sauce	.13	pickles, sweet	.36	spaghettie sauce	.09
catsup	.25	salad dressings: blue cheese	.07	steak sauce	.09
cheese sauce	.06	ceasar	.04	sweet & sour sauce	.45
chili sauce	.24	diet	.22	tartar sauce	.04
hollandaise sauce	.08	French	.17	tomato paste	.19
horseradish	.10	Italian	.07	Worcestershire sauce	.18
mayonnaise	.02	Russian	.07		
mustard	.04	pickle relish, sweet	.34		

Fruit

apple	.13	dried	.62	pears: fresh	.15
apple sauce	.10	fruit cocktail, in water	.10	canned in water	.09
apricots: fresh	.13	grapes: concord	.14	persimmons: Japanese	.20
canned in water	.10	european	.17	native	.34
canned in juice	.14	green, seedless	.14	pineapple: fresh	.14
dried	.60	grapefruit	.10	canned in water	.10
banana	.20	kiwi	.15	canned in juice	.15
blackberries	.12	lemons	.09	plums: fresh	.13
blueberries	.14	limes	.10	canned in water	.12
cantalope	.08	mangoes	.17	prunes: dehydrated	.91
cherries: fresh, sweet red	.16	nectarines	.17	dried, cooked	.67
fresh, sour red	.14	oranges	.12	raisins	.77
canned in water	.11	papayas	.10	rasberries, fresh	.14
maraschino	.29	peaches: fresh	.10	strawberries, fresh	.08
cranberry sauce, sugar	.36	canned in water	.08	tangerines	.12
dates, dried and pitted	.74	canned in juice	.12	watermelon	.06

Vegetables

artichoke	.10	cooked	.07	potatoes: baked	.21
asparagus	.04	cauliflower: raw	.05	boiled	.15
avacado	.05	cooked	.04	hash browns	.29
bamboo shoots	.05	celery	.04	French Fries	.34
beans: raw green	.07	chard, raw	.05	chips	.50
cooked green	.05	coleslaw	.12	sweet	.24
beans: kidney, lima, pinto,		corn: canned	.06	pumpkin	.08
red, white, baked	.21	steamed, off cob	.19	radishes	.04
beans sprouts	.06	sweet, creamed	.20	sauerkraut	.04
beets, boiled	.07	cucumber	.03	spinach: raw	.04
beet greens, cooked	.03	eggplant, cooked	.04	cooked	.08
broccoli	.06	lettuce	.03	soybeans	.11
brussel sprouts, cooked	.11	mushrooms	.04	squash: summer, cooked	.03
cabbage: raw	.05	okra	.05	winter, baked	.15
cooked	.04	onions	.07	winter, boiled	.09
Chinese, raw	.03	parsnips	.18	tomatoes	.05
Chinse, cooked	.01	peas	.12	turnips	.05
carrots: raw	.10	peppers	.05		

Cold Cereals, Dry

All Bran™	.78				
Cheerios™	.70				
Corn Chex™	.89				
Corn Flakes™	.84				
Frosted Flakes™	.90				
Fruit and Fiber™	.78				
granola	.68				
Grapenuts™	.83				
NutriGrain™	.86				
Product 19™	.77				
Puffed Wheat™	.77				
Raisin Bran™	.75				
Shredded Wheat™	.81				
Special K™	.76				
Rice Chex™	.86				
Rice Krispies™	.88				
Total™	.79				
Wheaties™	.80				

Combination Dishes

beef stew	.06
burrito	.24
chicken pie	.17
chili: with beans	.11
no beans	.06
con carne	.09
coleslaw	.14
enchilada	.18
fish and chips	.18
fish sticks	.37
hot dog	.18
lasagna	.16
macaroni and cheese	.20
pizza	.28
potato salad	.13
spaghetti with meat sauce	.15
tossed salad	.05
tuna casserole	.13

Sandwiches

BLT	.19
chicken salad	.24
club	.13
egg salad	.22
hot dog with bun	.26
peanut butter and jelly	.50
tuna salad	.24

Soups

clam chowder	.07
cream of mushroom	.04
tomato	.09
vegetable beef	.04
bean w/ pork	.09
chicken noodle	.07
chicken w/ rice	.07

Carb Percentages for Various Foods Cont.

Desserts and Sweets

apple butter	.46	lollipops	.99	ice cream: plain	.21
banana bread	.47	peanut brittle	.73	cone	.30
brownie	.71	gum drops	.99	bar	.25
brownie with nuts	.50	chocolate syrup	.65	ice milk	.23
cakes: angel food	.60	cookies: animal	.80	jams	.70
chocolate	.55	chocolate chip	.73	jellies	.70
coffee	.52	fig bar	.71	pies: apple	.37
fruit	.57	gingersnap	.80	blueberry	.34
pound	.61	oatmeal & raisin	.72	cherry	.38
sponge	.55	vanilla wafers	.74	lemon meringue	.47
white	.63	danish pastries	.46	pecan	.57
candies: caramel	.76	doughnuts: cake	.52	pumpkin	.23
fudge with nuts	.69	jelly filled	.46	preserves	.70
hard	.96	fruit turnovers	.26	pudding, chocolate	.23
jelly beans	.93	honey	.76	sherbert	.32

Breads and Grains

bagel	.56	couscous	.33	brown	.23
barley, cooked	.28	English muffin	.51	white	.25
biscuits	.45	French toast	.26	rolls	.60
bread: italian	.50	lentils	.19	spaghetti: plain	.26
rye	.47	macaroni: plain	.23	with sauce	.15
wheat	.47	cheese	.20	toast	.70
white	.49	muffins	.45	tortillas: corn	.42
bread crumbs	.74	noodles	.25	flour	.58
bread sticks	.75	pancakes & waffles: dry mix	.70	wheat flour	.76
buns	.50	prepared	.44		
corn starch	.83	rice, cooked	.24		

Alcoholic Beverages

beer: regular	.04
light	.02
champagne	.01
liqueurs	.30
wine: dry	.04
sweet	.12

Beverages

carbonated soda	.12
chocolate milk	.11
eggnog	.08
flavored instant coffee	.06
milk	.04
punch	.11

Hot Cereals, Cooked

corn grits	.11
Cream of Wheat™	.14
Farina™	.11
oatmeal	.10
Roman Meal™	.14
Wheatena™	.12

Carb Percentages for Various Foods Cont.

Snack Foods

almonds	.19	saltines	.70	popcorn, popped, no butter	.78
cashews	.26	marshmallows	.78	with butter	.57
cola	.10	mixed nuts	.18	potato chips	.50
corn chips	.57	onion dip	.10	pretzels	.75
cheese	.58	peanut butter	.17	sunflower seeds, no shell	.19
crackers: graham	.73	peanuts	.20	walnuts	.15
round	.67	pecans	.20		
rye	.50	pistachios	.27		

Dairy

cheese: cottage	.03	ice cream: choc	.28
ricotta	.05	vanilla	.22
cheddar	.01	milk	.05
		yogurt	.08

Diabetes Resources

Insulin Pump Companies:

Accu-Chek (Roche Diagnostics)	(800) 280-7801	www.accu-chekinsulinpumps.com
Animas Corporation	(877) 937-7867	www.animas.com
Asante Solutions Inc	(408) 716-5600	www.asantesolutions.com
Cell Novo	440 (203) 058-1250	www.cellnovo.com
Insulet Corporation	(800) 591-3455	www.myomnipod.com
Medtronic Inc.	(800) 646-4633	www.medtronicdiabetes.net
Sooil Development Co LTD	(866) 747-6645	www.sooilusa.com
Tandem Diabetes Care	(858) 366-6900	www.tandemdiabetes.com

Continuous Glucose Monitoring Companies:

Dexcom Inc	(888) 738-3646	www.dexcom.com
Medtronic Inc.	(800) 646-4633	www.medtronicdiabetes.net

The latest pump information at our web site:

Current insulin pumps
www.diabetesnet.com/diabetes-technology/insulin-pumps/current-pumps

Pump models & features
www.diabetesnet.com/diabetes-technology/insulin-pumps/current-pumps/pump-comparison

Infusions sets
www.diabetesnet.com/diabetes-technology/infusion-sets

Continuous monitors
www.diabetesnet.com/diabetes-technology/meters-monitors/continuous-monitors

The Insulin Tools
www.diabetesnet.com/diabetes-tools/

Diabetes Blogs & Communities:

D-Mom Blog	www.d-mom.com
Diabetesaliciousness	www.diabetesaliciousness.blogspot.com
Diabetes Daily	www.diabetesdaily.com
Diabetes Mine	www.diabetesmine.com

Diabetes Stories	*www.diabetesstories.com*
Diabetic Connect	*www.diabeticconnect.com*
Diabetic's Corner Booth	*www.thediabeticscornerbooth.com*
Exploring Diabetes Type 2	*www.bobsdiabetes.blogspot.com*
Life After DX	*www.lifeafterdx.blogspot.com*
Life of a Diabetic	*www.thelifeofadiabetic.com*
Living In Progress	*www.living-in-progress.com/*
Scott's Diabetes	*www.scottsdiabetes.com*
Six Until Me	*www.sixuntilme.com*
Stop Diabetes	*www.diabetesstopshere.org*
TuDiabetes	*www.tudiabetes.org*
Your Diabetes May Vary	*www.ydmv.net*

Other web sites of interest in pumping or diabetes

American Diabetes Association	*www.diabetes.org*
A Sweet Life	*www.asweetlife.org*
Children With Diabetes	*www.childrenwithdiabetes.com*
Clinical Trials in Diabetes	*www.centerwatch.com/patient/studies/area4.html*
Close Concerns	*www.closeconcerns.com*
Diabetes Health	*www.diabeteshealth.com*
Diabetes In Control	*www.diabetesincontrol.com*
Diabetes Sisters	*www.diabetessisters.org*
dLife	*www.dlife.com*
Health Central	*www.healthcentral.com/diabetes/*
Insulin Pumpers Group	*www.insulin-pumpers.org*
Juvenile Diab. Research Foundation	*www.jdrf.org*
Medline	*www.ncbi.nlm.nih.gov/PubMed/*
Nutrition and Carb Data	*www.medexplorer.com/nutrition/nutrition.dbm*
Topix.net	*www.topix.net/health/diabetes*

Visit www.diabetesnet.com/diabetes-resources/diabetes-links for more great diabetes links

References

[1] Pickup JC, White MC, Keen H, Parsons JA, and Alberti KG: Long-term continuous subcutaneous insulin infusion in diabetics at home. *Lancet* 2, 8148:870-873, 1979.

[2] Weissberg-Benchell J, Antisdel-Lomaglio J, and Seshadri RW: Insulin pump therapy: a meta-analysis. *Diabetes Care* 26(4):1079-87, 2003.

[3] Willi SM, Planton J, Egede L, Schwarz S: Benefits of continuous subcutaneous insulin infusion in children with type 1 diabetes. *J Pediatr* 143:796-801, 2003.

[4] Linkeschova R, Raoul M, Bott U, Berger M, Spraul M: Less severe hypoglycaemia, better metabolic control, and improved quality of life in Type 1 diabetes mellitus with continuous subcutaneous insulin infusion (CSII) therapy; an observational study of 100 consecutive patients followed for a mean of 2 years. *Diabet Med* 19:746-751, 2002.

[5] Hanaire-Broutin H, Melki V, Bessieres-Lacombe S, Tauber JP: Comparison of continuous subcutaneous insulin infusion and multiple daily injection regimens using insulin lispro in type 1 diabetic patients on intensified treatment: a randomized study. The Study Group for the Development of Pump Therapy in Diabetes. *Diabetes Care* 23:1232-1235, 2000.

[6] Sulli N, Shashaj B: Continuous subcutaneous insulin infusion in children and adolescents with diabetes mellitus: decreased HbA1c with low risk of hypoglycemia. *B. J Ped Endocrinol Metab* 16:393-399, 2003.

[7] Weintrob N, Schechter A, et. al.: Glycemic patterns detected by continuous subcutaneous glucose sensing in children and adolescents with type 1 diabetes mellitus treated by multiple daily injections vs continuous subcutaneous insulin infusion. *Arch Pediatr Adolesc Med.* 158:677-684, 2004.

[8] Bode BW, Steed RD, and Davidson PC: Reduction in severe hypoglycemia with long-term continuous subcutaneous insulin infusion in type 1 diabetes. *Diabetes Care* 19:324-327, 1996.

[9] Hirsch IB, Bode BW, Garg S et.al: Continuous subcutaneous insulin infusion (CSII) of insulin aspart versus multiple daily injection of insulin aspart/insulin glargine in type 1 diabetic patients previously treated with CSII. *Diabetes Care* 28(3):533-538, 2005.

[10] Binder C et al.: Insulin pharmacokinetics. *Diabetes Care* 7:188-199, 1984.

[11] Hirsch IB, Farkas-Hirsch R and Cryer PD: Continuous subcutaneous insulin infusion for the treatment of diabetic patients with hypoglycemic unawareness. *Diabetes Nutr Metab* 4:1-3, 1991.

[12] Fanelli CG, Epifano L, Rambotti AM, et. al.: Meticulous prevention of hypoglycemia normalizes the glycemic thresholds and magnitude of most of neuroendocrine responses to, symptoms of, and cognitive function during hypoglycemia in intensively treated patients with short-term IDDM. *Diabetes* 42:1683-1689, 1993.

[13] Beyer J et. al.: Assessment of insulin needs in insulin-dependent diabetics and healthy volunteers under fasting conditions. *Horm Metab Res Suppl* 24:71-77, 1990.

[14] Pickup J, Mattock M, and Kerry S: Glycaemic control with continuous subcutaneous insulin infusion compared with intensive insulin injections in patients with type 1 diabetes: meta-analysis of randomized controlled trials. *BMJ* 324(7339):705, 2002.

[15] Colquitt JL, Green C, Sidhu MK, Hartwell D, and Waugh N: Clinical and cost-effectiveness of continuous subcutaneous insulin infusion for diabetes. *Health Technol Assess.* 8(43):1-186, 2004.

[16] Pickup J, Mattock M, and Kerry S: Glycaemic control with continuous subcutaneous insulin infusion compared with intensive insulin injections in patients with type 1 diabetes: meta-analysis of randomised controlled trials. *BMJ* 324(7339):705, 2002.

[17] American Diabetes Association: Standards of Medical Care In Diabetes. *Diabetes Care* 31 (Suppl 1):S12-S54, 2008.

[18] ACE Consensus Development Conf. on Guidelines for Glycemic Control. *Endocr Pract. Suppl.*, Nov/Dec 2001.

[19] Downie E, Craig ME, Hing S, et al: Continued Reduction in the Prevalence of Retinopathy in Adolescents With Type 1 Diabetes. Role of insulin therapy and glycemic control. *Diabetes Care* 34(11):2368-2373, 2011.

[20] Hermanides J, Vriesendorp TM, Bosman RJ, AZandstra DF, Hoekstra JB, Devries JH: Glucose variability is associated with intensive care unit mortality. *Crit Care Med* 38:838-842, 2010.

[21] Monnier L, Mas E, Ginet C, Michel F, Villon L, Cristol JP, Colette C: Activation of oxidative stress by acute glucose fluctuations compared with sustained chronic hyperglycemia in patients with type 2 diabetes. *J Am Med Assoc* 295:1681-1687, 2006.

[22] Fedele D et. al.: Influence of continuous insulin infusion (CSII) treatment on diabetic somatic and autonomic neuropathy. *J Endocrinol Invest* 7:623-628, 1984.

[23] Boulton AJ, Drury J, Clarke B, and Ward JD: Continuous subcutaneous insulin infusion in the management of painful diabetic neuropathy. *Diabetes Care* 5:386-390, 1982.

[24] G.Viberti: Correction of exercise-induced microalbuminuria in insulin-dependent diabetics after 3 weeks of subcutaneous insulin infusion. *Diabetes* 30:818-823, 1981.

[25] Dahl-Jorgensen K et al.: Effect of near normoglycemia for two years on progression of early diabetic retinopathy, nephropathy, and neuropathy: the Oslo study. *BMJ* 293:1195-1201, 1986.

[26] Olsen T et. al.: Diabetic retinopathy after 3 years' treatment with continuous subcutaneous insulin infusion. *Acta Ophthalmol* (Copenh) 65:185-189, 1987.

[27] Eichner HL et. al.: Reduction of severe hypoglycemic events in Type I (insulin dependent) diabetic patients using continuous subcutaneous insulin infusion. *Diabetes Research* 8:189-193, 1988.

[28] Chantelau E, Spraul M, Muhlhauser I, et. al.: Long-term safety, efficacy and side-effects of continuous subcutaneous insulin infusion treatment for Type I (insulin-dependent) diabetes mellitus: a one center experience. *Diabetologia* 32:421-426, 1989.

[29] Beck-Nielsen H, Richelsen B, Hasling C, et. al.: Improved in vivo insulin effect during continuous subcutaneous insulin infusion in patients with IDDM. *Diabetes* 33:832-837, 1984.

[30] Fioretto P, Steffes MW, Sutherland DER, Goetz FC, and Mauer M: Reversal of Lesions of Diabetic Nephropathy after Pancreas Transplantation *NEJM* 339(2):69-75, 1998

[31] R. Kowluru, S. Abbas, S. Odenbach: Reversal of hyperglycemia and diabetic nephropathy. Effect of reinstitution of good metabolic control on oxidative stress in the kidney of diabetic rats. *Journal of Diabetes and its Complications* 18(5):282-288, 2004.

[32] Edge JA, Matthews DR, Dunger DB. The dawn phenomenon is related to overnight growth hormone release in adolescent diabetics. *Clin Endocrinol (Oxf)*. 33(6):729-37, 1990.

[33] Carroll MF, Hardy KJ, Burge MR, Schade DS. Frequency of the dawn phenomenon in type 2 diabetes: implications for diabetes therapy. *Diabetes Technol Ther.* 4(5):595-605, 2002.

[34] Brinchmann-Hansen O, Dahl-Jørgensen K; Hanssen KF, Sandvik L. The Response of Diabetic Retinopathy to 41 Months of Multiple Insulin Injections, Insulin Pumps, and Conventional Insulin Therapy. *Arch Ophthalmol.* 106(9):1242-1246, 1988.

[35] Van Ballegooie E, Hooymans JM, Timmerman Z, et. al.: Rapid deterioration of diabetic retinopathy during treatment with continuous subcutaneous insulin infusion. *Diabetes Care* 7:236-242, 1984.

[36] Dahl-Jorgensen D, Brinchmann-Hansen O, Hansen KF, et. al.: Transient deterioration of retinopathy when multiple insulin injection therapy and CSII is started in IDDM patients. *Diabetes* 33(1):4A, 1984.

[37] Jeganathan VS: Anti-angiogenesis drugs in diabetic retinopathy. *Curr Pharm Biotechnol.* 12(3):369-72, 2011.

[38] Castillo MJ, Scheen AJ, and Lefebvre PJ: The degree/rapidity of the metabolic deterioration following interruption of a continuous subcutaneous insulin infusion is influenced by the prevailing blood glucose level. *J Clin Endocrinol Metab.* 81(5):1975-1978, 1996.

[39] Mecklenburg RS et al.: Acute complications associated with insulin infusion pump therapy. *JAMA* 252:3265-3269, 1984.

[40] Bending JJ, et al.: Complications of insulin infusion pump therapy. *JAMA* 253:2644, 1985.

[41] Renner R: Therapy of Type 1 diabetes with insulin pumps. *Diamet* June, 1991.

[42] Roze S, Valentine WJ, Zakrzewska KE, Palmer AJ: Health-economic comparison of continuous subcutaneous insulin infusion with multiple daily injection for the treatment of Type 1 diabetes in the UK. *Diabetic Medicine* 22(9):1239-1245, 2005.

[43] Cohen N, Minshall ME, Sharon-Nash L, et. al.: Continuous subcutaneous insulin infusion versus multiple daily injections of insulin: economic comparison in adult and adolescent type 1 diabetes mellitus in Australia. *PharmacoEconomics* 25(17):881-897, 2007.

[44] Feinle C, O'Donovan D, Doran S, Andrews JM, Wishart J, Chapman I, and Horowitz M: Effects of fat digestion on appetite, APD motility, and gut hormones in response to duodenal fat infusion in humans. *Am J Physiol Gastrointest Liver Physiol* 284: G798–G807, 2003.

[45] Boden G and Jadali F: Effects of lipid on basal carbohydrate metabolism in normal men. *Diabetes* 40:686-692, 1991.

[46] Nuttall FQ, Mooradian AD, Gannon MCet al.: Effect of protein ingestion on the glucose and insulin response to a standardized oral glucose load. *Diabetes Care* 7:465-470, 1984.

[47] Jenkins DJA, Wolever TMS and Jenkins AL: Starchy foods and glycemic index. *Diabetes Care* 11:149-59, 1988.

[48] Jenkins DJA, Wolever TMS, et al.: Glycemic index of foods: a physiologic basis for carbohydrate exchange. *Amer J Clin Nutr* 34:362-66, 1981.

[49] Van de Wiel A: Diabetes mellitus and alcohol. *Diabetes/Metabolism Research and Reviews* 20(4):263–267, 2004

[50] Juvenile Diabetes Research Foundation Continuous Glucose Monitoring Study Group: The Effect of Continuous Glucose Monitoring in Well-Controlled Type 1 Diabetes. *Diabetes Care* 32(8):1378-1383, 2009

[51] Radermecker RP, Saint Remy A, Scheen AJ, Bringer J, Renard E: Continuous glucose monitoring reduces both hypoglycaemia and HbA1c in hypoglycaemia-prone type 1 diabetic patients treated with a portable pump. *Diabetes Metab.* 36(5):409-13, 2010.

[52] Battelino JT, Phillip M, Bratina N, Nimri R, Oskarsson P, and Bolinder J: Effect of Continuous Glucose Monitoring on Hypoglycemia in Type 1 Diabetes. *Diabetes Care* 34(4):795-800, 2011.

[53] Kamath A, Mahalingam A, Brauker J: Analysis of Time Lags and Other Sources of Error of the DexCom SEVEN Continuous Glucose Monitor. *Diabetes Technology & Therapeutics* 11(11):689-695, 2009.

[54] Stout PJ, Peled N, Erickson BJ, Hilgers ME, Racchini JR, Hoegh TB: Comparison of Glucose Levels in Dermal Interstitial Fluid and Finger Capillary Blood. *Diabetes Technology & Therapeutics* 3(1):81-90, 2001.

[55] Mazze RS, Strock E, Borgman S, Wesley D, Stout P, and Racchini J. Evaluating the Accuracy, Reliability, and Clinical Applicability of Continuous Glucose Monitoring (CGM): Is CGM Ready for Real Time? *Diabetes Technology & Therapeutics* 11(1):11-18, 2009.

[56] Garg SK, Voelmle M, Gottlieb PA: Time lag characterization of two continuous glucose monitoring systems. *Diabetes Research and Clinical Practice* 87(3):348-353, 2010.

[57] Bailey T, Zisser H, and Chang A: New Features and Performance of a Next-Generation SEVEN-Day Continuous Glucose Monitoring System with Short Lag Time. *Diabetes Technology & Therapeutics* 11(12):749-755, 2009.

[58] Weil C, Lunn DJ, Acerini CL, Allen JM, Larsen AM, Wilinska ME, Dunger DB, Hovorka R: Measurement delay associated with the Guardian® RT continuous glucose monitoring system. *Diabetic Medicine* 27(1):117–122, 2010.

[59] Zisser HC, Bailey TS, Schwartz S, Ratner R, Wise J: Accuracy of the SEVEN continuous glucose monitoring system: comparison with frequently sampled venous glucose measurements *J Diabetes Sci Technol* 3:1146-54, 2009.

[60] Keenan DB: Accuracy of the Enlite 6-day glucose sensor with guardian and Veo calibration algorithms *Diabetes Technol Ther* 14:225-31, 2012.

[61] Walsh J, Roberts R, Vigersky RA, and Frank Schwartz F: New Criteria for Assessing the Accuracy of Blood Glucose Monitors Meeting. *J Diabetes Sci Technol* 6(2), 460-468, 2012.

[62] Kamath A, Mahalingam A, and Brauker J: Analysis of Time Lags and Other Sources of Error of the DexCom SEVEN Continuous Glucose Monitor. *Diabetes Technology & Therapeutics* 11(11):689-695, 2009.

[63] Walsh J, Roberts R, Bailey T: Guidelines for Insulin Dosing in Continuous Subcutaneous Insulin Infusion Using New Formulas from a Retrospective Study of Individuals with Optimal Glucose Levels. *J Diabetes Sci Technol* 4:1174-1181, 2010.

[64] International Diabetes Federation: Global Guidelines For Type 2 Diabetes, Chapter 6: Glucose control levels, pages 25-28. © International Diabetes Federation, 2005.

[65] Rewers M, Pihoker C, Donaghue K, Hanas R, Swift P, and Klingensmith GJ: Assessment and monitoring of glycemic control in children and adolescents with diabetes. *Pediatric Diabetes(Suppl 12)* 10:71-81, 2009.

[66] Brownlee M, Hirsch IB: Glycemic variability: a hemoglobin A1c-independent risk factor for diabetic complications. *JAMA* 295:1707–1708, 2006.

[67] Kilpatrick ES, Rigby AS, and Atkin SL: The effect of glucose variability on the risk of microvascular complications in type 1 diabetes. *Diabetes Care* 29:1486–1490, 2006.

[68] Kilpatrick ES, Rigby AS, and Atkin SL: A1C Variability and the Risk of Microvascular Complications in Type 1 Diabetes. Data from the Diabetes Control and Complications Trial. *Diabetes Care* 31:2198–2202, 2008.

[69] Walsh J, Roberts R, Bailey T: Guidelines for Optimal Bolus Calculator Settings in Adults. *J Diabetes Sci Technol* 5(1):1711-1717, 2011.

[70] Heinemann L: **Time-Action Profiles of Insulin Preparations**, Kirchchem & C. GmbH, Mainz, Germany, 2004.

[71] Heinemann L, Weyer C, Rauhaus M, Heinrichs S, and Heise T: Variability of the metabolic effect of soluble insulin and the rapidacting insulin analog insulin aspart. *Diabetes Care* 21(11):1910-4, 1998.

[72] Vaughn DE, Yocum RC, Muchmore DB, Sugarman BJ, Vick AM, Bilinsky IP, and Frost GI: Accelerated pharmacokinetics and glucodynamics of prandial insulins injected with recombinant human hyaluronidase. *Diabetes Technol Ther.* 11(6):345-52, 2009.

[73] Steiner S, Hompesch M, Pohl R, Simms P, Flacke F, Mohr T, Pfützner A, Heinemann L: A novel insulin formulation with a more rapid onset of action. *Diabetologia* 51(9):1602-1606, 2008.

[74] Rave KM, Nosek L, de la Peña A, Seger M, Ernest CS 2nd, Heinemann L, Batycky RP, Muchmore DB. Dose response of inhaled dry-powder insulin and dose equivalence to subcutaneous insulin lispro. *Diabetes Care* 28(10):2400-2405, 2005.

[75] Rave K, Bott S, Heinemann L, Sha S, Becker RH, Willavize SA, Heise T. Time-action profile of inhaled insulin in comparison with subcutaneously injected insulin lispro and regular human insulin. *Diabetes Care* 28(5):1077-1082, 2005.

[76] Heinemann L: The future of pumps and sensors, Chap. 9, pg.103, in **Insulin Pump Therapy And Continuous Glucose Monitoring**, edited by John Pickup. Oxford Diabetes Library, Oxford, 2009.

[77] NovoLog® Physician Insert – Approved October 21, 2005

[78] Mortensen HB, Lindholm A, Olsen BS, Hylleberg B: Rapid appearance and onset of action of insulin aspart in paediatric subjects with type 1 diabetes. *European Journal of Pediatrics* 159(7);483-488, 2000.

[79] Buckingham BA, Block J, Wilson D, Rebrin K, Steil G: Novolog Pharmacodynamics in Toddlers. *Diabetes* 54(Suppl 1): Abstract 1889-P, 2005.

[80] Apidra Product Monograph; Version 9.0, April 4, 2011. Internet: products.sanofi.ca/en/apidra.pdf

[81] Becker R, Frick A, Heinemnn L, Nosek L, Rave K: Dose response relation of insulin glulisine (GLU) in subjects with type 1 diabetes (T1DM). *Diabetes* 54 (Suppl. 1): A332 (Abstract 1367-P), 2005.

[82] Walsh J: Internet: www.diabetesnet.com/diabetes_presentations/proposedinsulinpumpstandards.html.ppt Slides 59-61.

[83] Walsh J, Wroblewski, D, Bailey, TS. Disparate Bolus Recommendations In Insulin Pump Therapy. Poster at American Association of Clinical Endocrinology Meeting, 2007. Internet: www.diabetesnet.com/pdfs/AACE2007Poster.pdf.

[84] Hanaire-Broutin H, Melki V, Bessières-Lacombe S and Tauber JP: Comparison of continuous subcutaneous insulin infusion and multiple daily injection regimens using insulin lispro in type 1 diabetic patients on intensified treatment: a randomized study. The Study Group for the Development of Pump Therapy in Diabetes. *Diabetes Care* 23:1232-1235, 2000.

[85] Heinemann L, Schweitzer M, Nozek L, Krinelke L, and Kapitza C: Changes in basal insulin infusion rates with subcutaneous insulin infusion. *Diabetes Care* 32:1437-1439, 2009.

[86] Self reported data from pumpers at InsulinPumpers.org. Internet: http://www.insulin-pumpers.org/about.shtml

[87] Bruns W et. al.: Nocturnal continuous subcutaneous insulin infusion: a therapeutic possibility in labile Type I diabetes under exceptional conditions. *Z. Gesamte Inn Med* 45:154-158, 1990.

[88] Haakens K et. al.: Early morning glycaemia and the metabolic consequences of delaying breakfast/morning insulin. A comparison of continuous subcutaneous insulin infusion and multiple injection therapy with human isophane or human Ultralente at bedtime. *Scand J Clin Lab Invest* 49:653-659, 1989.

[89] Perriello G, De Feo P, Torlone E, et. al.: The Dawn Phenomenon in Type I (insulin-dependent) diabetes mellitus; magnitude, frequency, variability, and dependency on glucose counterregulation and insulin sensitivity. *Diabetologia* 42:21-28, 1991.

[90] Vella S, Buetow L, Royle P, Livingstone S, Colhoun HM and Petrie JR: The use of metformin in type 1 diabetes: a systematic review of efficacy. *Diabetologia* 53:809–820, 2010.

[91] American Diabetes Association: Postprandial blood glucose (Consensus Statement). *Diabetes Care* 24(4):775-778, 2001.

[92] Bonora E: Postprandial peaks as a risk factor for cardiovascular disease: epidemiological perspectives. *Int J Clin Pract* Suppl 129:5-11, 2002.

[93] Internet: www.idf.org/webdata/docs/Guideline_PMG_final.pdf.

[94] Dencker Johansen M, Gjerløv I, Sandahl Christiansen J, and Hejlesen OK: Interindividual and Intraindividual Variations in Postprandial Glycemia Peak Time Complicate Precise Recommendations for Self-Monitoring of Glucose in Persons with Type 1 Diabetes Mellitus. *J Diabetes Sci Technol* 6(2):356-361, 2012.

[95] Walsh J. Changes In Diabetes Care: A History Of Insulin And Pumps, Past, Present, and Future. Internet: www.childrenwithdiabetes.com/presentations/DMCare-Past-Future-0904_files/outline.htm

[96] Bondia J, Dassau E, Zisser H, Calm R, Vehí J, Jovanovic L, Doyle III FJ: Coordinated basal-bolus for tighter postprandial glucose control in insulin pump therapy. *J Diabetes Sci Technol* 3(1):89-97, 2008.

[97] Ahern JA, Gatcomb PM, Held NA, Petit WA Jr, Tamborlane WV. Exaggerated hyperglycemia after a pizza meal in well-controlled diabetes. *Diabetes Care* 16(4):578-80, 1993.

[98] Brodows RG, Williams C, Amatruda JM. Treatment of insulin reactions in diabetics. *JAMA* 28;252(24):3378-81, 1984.

[99] Bergenstal R, Callahan T, Johnson M, et. al.: Management principles that most influence glucose control: a follow-up study of former DCCT participants. *Diabetes* 45 (Suppl. 2):124a, 1996.

[100] Kerr D, Morton J, Whately-Smith C, Everett J, and Begley JP: Laboratory-Based Non-Clinical Comparison of Occlusion Rates Using Three Rapid-Acting Insulin Analogs in Continuous Subcutaneous Insulin Infusion Catheters Using Low Flow Rates. *J Diabetes Sci Technol* 2(3):2008.

[101] Fredrickson DD, Guthrie DW, Nehrling JK, Guthrie R: Effects of DKA and severe hypoglycemia in cognitive functioning: a prospective study. *Diabetes* 44 (suppl 1):Abstract 97, 1995.

[102] Snorgaard O, Eskildsen PC, MacCuish AC. Diabetic ketoacidosis in Denmark: epidemiology, incidence rates, precipitating factors and mortality rates. *J Intern Med* 226:223–228, 1989.

[103] Tamás G, Tabák AG, Vargha P, Kerényi Z. Effect of menstrual cycle on insulin demand in IDDM women. *Diabetologia* 39 (Suppl 1): A52 (abstract 188), 1996.

[104] Brink S, Laffel L, Likitmaskul S, Liu L, Maguire AM, Olsen B, Silink M, Hanas R: Sick day management in children and adolescents with diabetes. *Pediatric Diabetes* 10 (Suppl. 12):146–153, 2009.

[105] Cox D, Gonder-Frederick L, Polonsky W, Schlundt D, Kovatchev B and Clark W: Recent hypoglycemia influences the probability of subsequent hypoglycemia in Type I patients. *Diabetes* Abstract 399, ADA Conference 1993.

[106] ter Braak EW, et. al.: Clinical characteristics of type 1 patients with and without severe hypoglycemia. *Diabetes Care* 23(10):1467-1471, 2000.

[107] US DOT: Medical Conditions and Driving: A Review of the Literature (1960 - 2000) at http://www.nhtsa.dot.gov/people/injury/research/Medical_Condition_Driving/pages/Sec9-HypogUA.htm.

[108] Anderson J, Symanowski S, and Brunelle R: Safety of [Lys(B28), Pro(B29)] human insulin analog in long-term clinical trials. *Diabetes* 43(1):Abstract 192, 1994.

[109] The Diabetes Control and Complications Trial Research Group: Hypoglycemia in the Diabetes Control and Complications Trial. *Diabetes* 45:271–286, 1997.

[110] Bhatia V and Wolfsdorf JI: Severe hypoglycemia in youth with insulin-dependent diabetes mellitus: frequency and causative factors. *Pediatrics* 88(6):1187-1193, 1991.

[111] Veneman T, Mitrakou A, Mokan M, Cryer P and Gerich J: Induction of hypoglycemia unawareness by asymptomatic nocturnal hypoglycemia. *Diabetes* 42:1233-1237, 1993.

[112] Davis SN, Fowler S, and Costa F: Hypoglycemic Counterregulatory responses differ between men and women with Type 1 diabetes. *Diabetes* 49:65-72, 2000.

[113] Avogaro A, Beltramello P, Gnudi L, Maran A, Valerio A, Miola M, Marin N, Crepaldi C, Confortin L, Costa F, MacDonald I and Tiengo A: Alcohol intake impairs glucose counterregulation during acute insulin-induced hypoglycemia in IDDM patients. *Diabetes* 42:1626-1634, 1993.

[114] Fanelli CG, Epifano L, et al: Meticulous prevention of hypoglycemia normalizes the glycemic thresholds and magnitude of most of neuroendocrine responses to, symptoms of, and cognitive function during hypoglycemia in intensively treated patients with short-term IDDM. *Diabetes* 42:1683-1688, 1993.

[115] Ramsli HM, Therkelsen SP, Sovik O, and Thordarson H: Unexpected and unexplained deaths among young patients with diabetes mellitus. *Tidsskr Nor Laegeforen* 124 (23):3064-3065, 2004.

[116] Sovik O and Thordarson H: Death-in-bed syndrome in young diabetic patients. *Diabetes Care* 22 (Suppl 2): B40-42, 1999.

[117] Tanner MH et. al.: Toxic shock syndrome from staphylococcus areus infection at insulin pump infusion sites. *JAMA* 259:394-395, 1988.

[118] Pietri A and Raskin P: Cutaneous complications of chronic continuous subcutaneous insulin infusion therapy. *Diabetes Care* 4:624-627, 1981.

[119] Powell KE et al.: Physical activity and chronic disease. *Am J Clin Nutr* 49:999-1006, 1989.

[120] Tanasescu M, Leitzmann MF, Rimm EB, et al.: Physical activity in relation to cardiovascular disease and total mortality among men with type 2 diabetes. *Circulation* 107:2435–2439, 2003.

[121] A. Festa, C.H. Schnack, A.D. Assie, P. Haber and G. Schernthaner: Abnormal pulmonary function in Type I diabetes is related to metabolic long-term control, but not to urinary albumin excretion rate. *Diabetes* 43 (1): abstract 610, 1994.

[122] Wahren J: Glucose turnover during exercise in healthy man and in patients with Diabetes Mellitus. *Diabetes* 28(1):82-88, 1979.

[123] Felig P and Wahren J: Role of insulin and glucagon in the regulation of hepatic glucose production during exercise. *Diabetes* 28(1):71-75, 1979.

[124] Perkins BA and Riddell MC: Diabetes and exercise: Using the insulin pump to maximum advantage. *Canadian J of Diabetes* 30(1):72-79, 2006.

[125] Marliss EB and Vranic M: Intense exercise has unique effects on both insulin release and its role in gluco-regulation: implications for diabetes. *Diabetes* 51 (Suppl 1): S271-283, 2002.

[126] The PedPump Study: A Low Percentage of Basal Insulin and More Than Five Daily Boluses are Associated With Better Centralized A1c in 1041 Children on CSII in 17 Countries, *Diabetes* Abstract #1887-P, 2005.

[127] Fourlanos S, Perry C, et. al.: A clinical screening tool identifies autoimmune diabetes in adults. *Diabetes Care* 29:970-975, 2006.

[128] U.K Prospective Diabetes Study 16: Overview of 6 years of therapy of Type II diabetes – a progressive disease. *Diabetes* 44:1249-1258, 1995.

[129] DPP Research Group: 10-year follow-up of diabetes incidence and weight loss in the Diabetes Prevention Program Outcomes Study. *Lancet* 374:1677–1686, 2009.

[130] Raskin P, Bode BW, Marck JB, et al: Cont. subcutaneous insulin infusion and multiple daily injection therapy are equally effective in type 2 diabetes: a randomized, parallel-group, 24-week study. *Diabetes Care* 26:2598 -2603, 2003.

[131] Valensi P, Moura I, Le Magoarou M, Paries J, Perret G, Attali JR: Short-term effects of continuous subcutaneous insulin infusion treatment on insulin secretion in non-insulin-dependent overweight patients with poor glycaemic control despite maximal oral anti-diabetic treatment. *Diabetes Metab* 23:51-57, 1997.

[132] Ilkova H, Glaser B, Tunckale A, Bagriacik N, and Cerasi E: Induction of long-term glycemic control in newly diagnosed type 2 diabetic patients by transient intensive insulin treatment. *Diabetes Care* 20:1353-1356, 1997.

[133] Ohkubo Y, Kishikawa H, Araki E, et al.: Intensive insulin therapy prevents the progression of diabetic microvascular complications in Japanese patients with non-insulin-dependent diabetes mellitus: a randomized prospective 6-year study. *Diabetes Res Clin Pract* 28:103-117, 1995.

[134] Georgopoulos A, Margolis S, Bachorik P, and Kwiterovich PO: Effect of improved glycemic control on the response of plasma triglycerides to ingestion of a saturated fat load in normotriglyceridemic and hypertriglyceridemic diabetic subjects. *Metabolism* 37:866-871, 1988.

[135] Bolli GB, Gerich JE: The "dawn phenomenon"--a common occurrence in both non-insulin-dependent and insulin-dependent diabetes mellitus. *N Engl J Med* 310(12):746-750, 1984.

[136] Reutrakul S, Wroblewski K, Brown RL. Clinical Use of U-500 Regular Insulin: Review and Meta-Analysis. *J Diabetes Sci Technol* 6(2):412-420, 2012.

[137] White P: Pregnancy complicating diabetes. *Am J Med* 7:609-616, 1949.

[138] Pedersen J, Molsted-Pedersen L and Andersen B: Assessors of fetal perinatal mortality in diabetic pregnancy. *Diabetes* 23:302-305, 1974.

[139] Pedersen J: Fetal mortality in diabetics in relation to management during the latter part of pregnancy. *Acta Endocrinol* 15:282-294, 1954

[140] Pedersen J and Brandstrup E: Fetal mortality in pregnant diabetics: strict control of diabetes with conservative obstetric management. *Lancet* I:607a-612, 1956.

[141] Fuhrmann K, Reiher H, Semmler K, Fischer F, Fisher M and Glockner E: Prevention of congenital malformations in infants of insulin-dependent diabetic mothers. *Diabetes Care* 6:219-223, 1983.

[142] Kitzmiller JL, Gavin LA, Gin GD, Jovanovic-Peterson L, Main EK and Zigrang WD: Preconception care of diabetes: Glycemic control prevents congenital anomalies. *JAMA* 265:731-736, 1991.

[143] Rosenn B, Miodovnik M, Combs CA, Khoury J and Siddiqi TA: Preconception management of insulin-dependent diabetes: Improvement of pregnancy outcome. *Obstet Gynecol* 77:846-849, 1991.

[144] Steel JM, Johnstone FD, Hepburn DA and Smith A: Can prepregnancy care of diabetic women reduce the risk of abnormal babies? *Br Med J* 301:1070-1074, 1990.

[145] Miodovnik M, Skillman C, Holroyde JC, Butler JB, Wendel JS and Siddiqi TA: Elevated maternal glycohemoglobin in early pregnancy and spontaneous abortion among insulin-dependent diabetic women. *Am J Obstet Gynecol* 153:439-442.

[146] Mills JL, Simpson JL, Driscoll SG, Jovanovic-Peterson L, Van Allen M, Aarons JH, Metzger B, et.al.: The National Institute of Child Health and Human Development: Diabetes in Early Pregnancy Study: Incidence of spontaneous abortion among normal women and insulin-dependent diabetic women whose pregnancies were identified within 21 days of conception. *NEJM* 319:1617-1623, 1988.

[147] Jovanovic-Peterson L, Druzin M and Peterson CM: Effect of euglycemia on the outcome of pregnancy in insulin-dependent diabetic women as compared with normal control subjects. *Am J Med* 71:921-927, 1981.

[148] Combs CA, Wheeler B, Gunderson E, Gavin L, and Kitsmiller JL: Significance of microproteinuria in the first trimester of pregnancies complicated by diabetes. *Diabetes* 39:36A, 1990.

[149] Bo S, et al: Clinical characteristics and outcome of pregnancy in women with gestational hyperglycaemia with or without antibodies to beta-cell antigens. *Diab Med* 20 (1):64-68, 2003.

[150] Ostlund I and Hanson U: Occurrence of gestational diabetes mellitus and the value of different screening indicators for the oral glucose tolerance test. *Acta Obstet Gynecol Scand* 82 (2):103-108, 2003.

[151] Sheffield JS, Butler-Koster EL, Casey BM, McIntire DD, Leveno KJ: Maternal diabetes and infant malformations. *Obstet Gynecol* 100 (5 Pt 1):925-930, 2002.

[152] International Association of Diabetes and Pregnancy Study Groups Consensus Panel. International association of diabetes and pregnancy study groups recommendations on the diagnosis and classification of hyperglycemia in pregnancy. *Diabetes Care* 33(3):676-82, 2010.

[153] Jovanovic-Peterson L and Peterson CM: Dietary manipulation as a primary treatment strategy for pregnancies complicated by diabetes. *J Am Coll Nutr* 9:320-325, 1990.

[154] Rosenn B, Miodovnik M, Combs CA, Khoury J and Siddiqi TA: Preconception management of insulin-dependent diabetes: Improvement of pregnancy outcome. *Obstet Gynecol* 77:846-849, 1991.

[155] Jovanovic L, Knopp RH, Brown Z, Conley MR, Park E, Mills JL, Metzger BE, Aarons JH, Holmes LB, Simpson JL: Declining insulin requirement in the late first trimester of diabetic pregnancy. *Diabetes Care* 24(7):1130-1136, 2001.

[156] Langer O, Conway DL, Berkus MD, Xenakis EM, Gonzales ON: A comparison of glyburide and insulin in women with gestational diabetes mellitus. *N Engl J Med* 343(16):1134-1138, 2000.

[157] Yajnik CS: Fetal Programming of Diabetes: Still So Much to Learn! *Diabetes Care* May 2010 vol. 33 no. 5 1146-1148

[158] American College of Obstetricians and Gynaecologists. Diabetes and pregnancy. ACOG technical bulletin 200. Washington, DC: ACOG, 1995.

[159] Davidson PC, Hebblewhite HR, Bode BW, et al. An empirical basis for modifying the "1500 rule" [abstract]. *Diabetes* 51(suppl 2):A128, 2002.

[160] Davidson PC, Hebblewhite HR, Steed RD, and Bode BW. Analysis of guidelines for basal-bolus insulin dosing: basal insulin, correction factor, and carbohydrate-to-insulin ratio. *Endocr Pract.* 14:1095-1101, 2008.

School Care Plan for an Insulin Pump

Re: _____   Date: _____/_____/_____

To Whom It May Concern:

_____ is a patient in our Center with Type 1 Diabetes Mellitus (Insulin Dependent Diabetes Mellitus). To better control his/her diabetes, he/she is using insulin pump therapy.

An insulin pump is simply another way to deliver insulin. Through the pump, _____ receives insulin around the clock via a small needle or plastic tube which is inserted in the abdomen. He/she has been taught how to program the pump to deliver insulin, as needed. This means he/she will program the pump before each meal to give insulin in a dose determined by his/her fingerstick blood glucose test.

To care for his/her diabetes at school, _____ will need to have the following items with him/her:

— The insulin infusion pump, which is worn
— Backup pump supplies (syringes, tubing, infusion sets, insulin), and regular syringe
— Glucagon injection kit for severe low blood sugar
— Blood glucose testing supplies (meter, strips, lancet device, and lancets)
— Snack foods and water (to handle extremes of blood glucose)
— Ketostix (to test urine ketones as needed)
— _____

There may be times when he/she will need to be excused to test a blood sugar or for ketones, or to use the bathroom.

In case of a low blood sugar emergency, the pump can be stopped for 30 to no more than 60 minutes, although it is usually more important to raise the blood sugar with a drink or food that contains sugar. _____ can show you how to detach the line ahead of time. If a severe low blood sugar occurs, the catheter can be temporarily detached from the infusion set near the skin site, but it is important to reattach within 30 to 60 minutes.

Pump therapy is a safe and effective way to manage diabetes. We are confident that this individual can handle this tool properly.

If you need further information, please contact his/her family or our office.

Sincerely,

_____   ( ) _____-_____

Glossary

A1c

Glycosylated hemoglobin (A1c) levels reflect the average glucose level over the previous two to three months. Normal A1c levels are generally 4% to 6%.

Albuminuria

A condition in which high levels of a protein called albumin are found in the urine. Excess albumin in the urine is often a sign of early kidney disease.

Autoimmune antibodies

Antibodies in the blood stream of a person with an autoimmune disease. Type 1 and Type 1.5 are characterized by these.

Autoimmune disease

A disease caused by a defect in which the body's internal defense system attacks a part of the body itself. Type 1 diabetes is an autoimmune disease.

Basal/Bolus balance

Created by having the basal and bolus a balanced percentage of the Total Daily Dose (TDD), such as 50% basal/50% bolus. Assessing the basal/bolus balance is one way to troubleshoot poor control.

Basal insulin or rate

A continuous 24-hour delivery of insulin that matches background insulin need. When the basal rate is correctly set, the blood sugar does not rise or fall during periods in which the pump user is not eating. Basal rates are given as units/hour, with typical rates between 0.4 u/hr and 1.6 u/hr for many pumpers.

Bolus See Carb Bolus or High Blood Sugar Bolus.

Beta cells (b-cells) Cells that make insulin and are found in the Islets of Langerhans within the pancreas.

Blood glucose level

The concentration of glucose in the blood (blood sugar). It is measured in milligrams per deciliter (mg/dl) in the U.S. or in millimoles (mmol/l) in other countries.

Body mass index (BMI)

A unit of measurement (kg/m^2) that describes weight in relation to height for people 20 to 65 years old.

C-peptide

Plasma C-peptide is a by-product of insulin production with a longer half-life than insulin. It measures how much insulin a person is able to make. A level below 0.3 is defined as type 1 diabetes.

Carbohydrate

One of the three main constituents (carbohydrates, fats, and proteins) in foods and the most important for glucose control. Carbohydrates (four calories per gram) are composed mainly of sugars and starches.

Carb bolus

A spurt of insulin delivered quickly to match carbohydrates in an upcoming meal or snack. Most pumpers use between 1 unit of rapid insulin for each 5 grams of carbohydrate and 1 unit for each 25 grams.

Carb counting

Counting the grams of carbohydrate in any food eaten. This is an effective way to determine the amount of insulin needed to maintain a normal blood sugar.

Carb factor (CarbF)

The number of grams of carbohydrate one unit of insulin covers for a person. This varies from person to person.

Catheter

The plastic tube through which insulin is delivered between the pump and the insertion set.

Continuous glucose monitor (CGM)

A device often consisting of a sensor implanted under the skin sending glucose readings via radio waves to a transmitter. Often displays individual readings taken every 5 minutes, graphs of the readings over time and trend arrows. Often provides high and low blood sugar alarms.

Correction bolus

A spurt of insulin delivered quickly to bring a high blood sugar back within a person's target range before a meal, after a meal, or a bedtime.

Correction factor (CorrF)

The distance a high blood sugar will drop for one unit of insulin for a person. Measured in mg/dl in the U.S. and mmol/L in other countries. Varies from person to person; determined from 1960 Rule.

CSII Continuous subcutaneous insulin infusion, another name for an insulin pump.

DCCT

The Diabetes Control and Complications Trial. The DCCT was a 9-year study of more than 1,400 people with Type 1 diabetes. Sponsored by the National Institute of Health, it showed that tight blood sugar control significantly reduced the risk of diabetic retinopathy, neuropathy, and nephropathy.

Dawn Phenomenon

An early morning rise in blood glucose levels, caused largely by the normal release of growth hormone that blocks insulin's effect during the early morning hours.

Diabetic coma

Loss of consciousness due to very high glucose levels. (See ketoacidosis)

Diabetic nephropathy

Kidney disease resulting from diabetes that usually has been poorly controlled for several years. There rarely are symptoms until very late in the disease.

Diabetic neuropathy

Damage to the nervous system most often resulting from poor control. Three different forms of neuropathy can be distinguished: peripheral neuropathy, sensory neuropathy, and autonomic neuropathy. *Peripheral neuropathy* affects the motor nerves, which can lead to problems with muscle movement and size. *Sensory neuropathy* impairs the nerves that control touch, sight, and pain perception. *Autonomic neuropathy* affects the nerves involved in such involuntary functions as digestion. Symptoms such as pain, loss of sensation, loss of reflexes, and/or weakness may occur.

Diabetic retinopathy

Damaged small blood vessels in the eye that can cause vision problems, including blindness.

Fasting plasma glucose (FPG) test

A lab test is taken after fasting for 8 to 10 hours, typically overnight. FPG level less than 100 mg/dl is normal; one between 100 and 125 mg/dl indicates impaired glucose tolerance, one of 126 mg/dl or greater supports a provisional diagnosis of diabetes.

Fat

One of the three main constituents (carbohydrate, fats, and protein) of foods. Fats occur alone as liquids or solids, such as oils and margarines, or they may be a component of other foods. Fats may be of animal or vegetable origin. They have a higher energy content than any other food (9 calories per gram).

Gestational diabetes

Elevated blood sugars usually diagnosed during the last half of pregnancy and triggered by insulin resistance. Gestational diabetes increases the risk of perinatal mortality and development of diabetes in the mother years after the pregnancy.

Glucagon

A hormone made by the pancreas that raises blood sugar levels. It is injected during severe low blood sugars to raise the blood sugar quickly by releasing glucose stored in the liver.

Glucose

A simple sugar, also known as dextrose, that is found in the blood and is used by the body for energy.

Glycemic Index (GI)

A method to classify foods, especially carbohydrates, according to how they affect the blood glucose level.

Glycogen

Glycogen is the form in which the liver and muscles store glucose. It may be broken down to active blood glucose during a low blood sugar, fasting, or exercise.

Glycosylated hemoglobin See A1c.

Gram

A small unit of weight in the metric system. Used in weighing food. One ounce equals 28 grams.

Hormone

A chemical substance produced by a gland or tissue and carried by the blood to other tissues or organs, where it stimulates action and causes a specific effect. Insulin and glucagon are hormones.

Hyperglycemia

A higher than normal level of glucose in the blood (high blood sugar).

Hypertension

High blood pressure (excess blood pressure in the blood vessels). Found to aggravate diabetes and diabetic complications.

Hypoglycemia

A lower than normal glucose level in the blood (low blood sugar), usually less than 70 mg/dl (3.9 mmol/l). Symptoms vary from confusion, nervousness, sweating, shakiness, headaches, and drowsiness to moodiness, or numbness in the arms and hands. Untreated, severe hypoglycemia can cause loss of consciousness, convulsions, or even death.

Infusion set

The hub, tubing, insertion set, and cannula used to transfer insulin from the pump through an infusion line to below the skin.

Insertion set

The part of the infusion set inserted through the skin. It may be a fine metal needle or a larger metal needle, which is removed to leave a small Teflon catheter/cannula under the skin.

Insulin

A hormone secreted by the beta cells of the Islets of Langerhans in the pancreas. Needed by many cells to use glucose for energy.

Insulin pump

A small, computerized, programmable device about the size of a beeper that can be programmed to deliver basal insulin and give a bolus of insulin for a meal or high blood sugar. It replaces insulin injections. A pump delivers fast-acting insulin via a plastic catheter to either a teflon infusion set or a small metal needle inserted through the skin for gradual absorption into the bloodstream.

Insulin resistance syndrome (IRS, metabolic syndrome, syndrome X)

A basic metabolic abnormality underlying Type 2 diabetes. Insulin resistance describes reduced insulin sensitivity of cells to the action of insulin.

Interstitial fluid

A relatively clear fluid between cells in which glucose measurements can be made with a CGM.

Islets of Langerhans

Special groups of pancreatic cells that produce insulin and glucagon.

Ketoacidosis

A very serious condition in which the body does not have enough insulin. An excess release of free fatty acids causes high levels of ketones in the blood and urine. This acidic state takes hours or days to develop, with symptoms of abdominal pain, nausea, and vomiting. It also causes dehydration, electrolyte imbalance, rapid breathing, coma, and possibly death.

Ketones Acidic byproducts of fat metabolism.

Nephropathy See Diabetic nephropathy

Neuropathy See Diabetic neuropathy

Oral glucose tolerance test (OGTT)

A 2 or 3-hour test of plasma glucose with values over 200 mg/dl (> 11.1 mmol/L) used to confirm a suspected diagnosis of diabetes.

Pancreas

A gland positioned near the stomach that secretes insulin, glucagon, and many digestive enzymes.

Protein

One of the three main constituents (carbohydrate, fat, and protein) of foods. Proteins are made up of amino acids and are found in foods such as milk, meat, fish, and eggs. Proteins are essential constituents of all living cells and form important structures and enzymes. Proteins (four calories per gram) are burned at a slower rate than fats or carbohydrates.

Proteinuria

Protein in the urine. This may be a sign of kidney damage.

Reservoir/Syringe/Cartridge A container which holds the fast-acting insulin inside a pump.

Retina

A very thin light-sensitive layer of nerves and blood vessels at the back of the inner surface of the eyeball.

Smart insulin pump

An insulin pump with smart features. Became available in late 2002.

Total Daily Dose (TDD)

The amount of insulin a person uses in a day. Calculations are made using the TDD to determine the basal rate, carb factor and correction factor.

Type 1 diabetes

In Type 1 diabetes the pancreas makes little or no insulin because the insulin-producing beta cells have been destroyed. It is an autoimmune disease caused by a defect in which the body's internal defense system attacks a part of the body itself. This type of diabetes usually appears suddenly, is more common in people younger than 30, but can be seen at any age. Treatment consists of daily insulin injections or use of an insulin pump, a planned diet, regular exercise, and daily self-monitoring of blood glucose through finger sticks or continuous monitoring.

Type 1.5 diabetes

Also called LADA. A slower form of Type 1 diabetes in adults in which only one or two types of autoimmune antibodies is present.

Type 2 diabetes

Type 2 diabetes is associated with insulin resistance and impaired beta cell function. It sometimes is controlled by diet, exercise, and daily monitoring of glucose levels, but at other times oral antihyperglycemic agents or insulin injections are needed. Type 2 diabetes accounts for 90% to 95% of diabetes cases.

Index

lows, see *hypoglycemia*
    fear of, 204
    frequent lows, 234
    high to low, 183
    low to high, 183

M

macular edema, 11
macrosomia, 287-290
Mastisol, 85
MDI (multiple daily injections), 8
medical ID, 34
Medicare, 70
medication
    Bydureon, 215
    Byetta, 215
    Glycet, 213
    metformin, 267, 287, 294
    Precose, 213
    Symlin, 213-215
Medtronic pump, 102, 103
    sensor 37, 39, 41, 43
menses
    complicates control, 204
    teens, 268
metabolic syndrome, 277, 279
meter download sheet, 186
metformin, 267, 287, 294
metric conversion table, 24
Micropore tape, 85
microalbumin test, 289
microalbuminuria, see *kidney disease*

N

nausea,
    symptom of DKA, 197
    pregnancy, 286, 295
nephropathy, see *kidney disease*
neuropathy, 8
nighttime lows, see *lows,* and
    hypoglycemia
NIH, 277
nutrition, 27-31

O

O-rings
    care, 82
    leaks, 82
Omnipod, 102, 103

opensourcediabetes.org, 94
oral medications
    and pregnancy, 293-294
other issues impact control, 203-209
over-the-counter products effect on
    control, 207

P

pancreas as model, 6
parents, questions for, 17-18
patterns, glucose
    definition, 173
    common ones, 177-184
    find unwanted, 173-175
    fix unwanted, 175-176, 181, 182
    frequent highs, 179-185
    no pattern, 176, 177
    review records for, 173
    stop lows first, 177-178
    use meter, 174-175, 186
    use CGM, 173-174
PCOS, 288. 294
peritoneal insulin delivery, 52
plasma vs whole blood,
post-meal glucose goals, 149-150
post-meal spiking,
    causes, 212
    how to reduce, 212-213
    medications to control, 213-215
    tips to prevent, 212-213
Precision Xtra, ketones, 89, 90
Precose, 213
pregnancy
    bad signs, 285
    birth defects, 284, 285, 286
    blood glucose targets, 284
    blood glucose monitoring, 289
    blood pressure, 290
    breast feeding, 296
    C-section, 288
    carb adjustments, 292-293
    care following delivery, 296
    CGM, 286, 289, 290
    complications by trimester, 284
    conception, 286
    diagnosis, 289
    exercise, 293
    fasting plasma glucose, 288, 289

gestational diabetes (GDM), 287-288
    glucagon, 295
    glucose control, 283-285
    high glucose levels, 283
    insulin adjustments, 290
    insulin choices, 292
    ketoacidosis, 285, 295
    labor & delivery, 296
    macrosomia, 287, 288, 290
    management program, 289
    miscarriage, 285
    nausea and vomiting, 286, 295
    nutrition therapy, 292-293
    OGTT oral glucose tolerance test
        288, 289
    oral medication, 293-294
    other pregnancy tests, 290
    polyhydrammios, 290
    preeclampsia, 285, 290
    prediabetes, 287
    preparation, 286-287
    random plasma glucose, 288
    risk factors for GDM, 288
    Rule of 18ths, 289, 292-293
    screening for GDM, 289
    start insulin, 294
    TDD rise, 289, 290-292
    tight glucose, 285-286
    toxemia, 285, 290
    Type 2, 283-296
    use of injection overnight, 295
    when to start insulin, 294-295
protein, effect on blood sugar, 28
pump alarms, 75
pump bumps, 237
Pump Tune-Up Checklist, 14
pump, see *insulin pump*

Q

quick carbs, 222

R

rapid breathing, and DKA, 197
rapid heartbeat
    symptom of hypoglycemia, 221
records, 53, 55
reminders and alerts, pump, 75
retinopathy, 8, 11, 289-290

Order Pumping Insulin and Other Helpful Diabetes Books

Send me _____ copy(ies) of **Pumping Insulin** 5th edition at $27.95 each, plus shipping. (California residents add 7.75% sales tax.) This and many other diabetes books and products are available at www.diabetesnet.com/dmall/ with a 30% discount. Please call for discounts on quantity orders.

Name _____

Address _____

City _____ State _____ Zip _____

Phone   (____) _____ – _____   Email _____@_____

_____ **Pumping Insulin** 5th edition at $27.95 each ($30.12 in Calif.) $ _____

_____ **Using Insulin** at $23.95 each ($25.81 in Calif.) $ _____

_____ *Smart Charts* (refill for 4 mos.) at $8.95 ($9.64 in Calif.) $ _____

_____ *Smart Charts* (refill for 12 mos.) at $21.45 ($23.11 in Calif.) $ _____

Shipping: ❑ Priority Mail $5.50   ❑ Bookrate $3.50 $ _____
(+ $1.25 for each add.)   (+ $0.50 for each add. item)

Total $ _____

Payment: ❑ Check   ❑ Visa   ❑ Master Card   ❑ Amer Express   ❑ Discover

Card #: _____ Expires: _____ / _____

Signature: _____

Mail to:

Torrey Pines Press /   *Call:*   (800) 988-4772
Diabetes Mall   *Fax:*   (619) 497-0900
1030 West Upas St.   *Online:*   www.diabetesnet.com/dmall/
San Diego, CA 92103